Lesley V. D'Anglada, Elizabeth D. Hilborn and
Lorraine C. Backer (Eds.)

Harmful Algal Blooms (HABs) and Public Health: Progress and Current Challenges

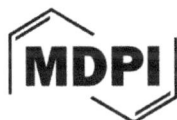

MDPI

This book is a reprint of the Special Issue that appeared in the online, open access journal, *Toxins* (ISSN 2072-6651) from 2014–2015 (available at: http://www.mdpi.com/journal/toxins/special_issues/HABs?sort=asc).

Guest Editors
Lesley V. D'Anglada
U.S. Environmental Protection Agency
USA

Elizabeth D. Hilborn
United States Environmental Protection Agency
USA

Lorraine C. Backer
National Center for Environmental Health
USA

Editorial Office
MDPI AG
Klybeckstrasse 64
Basel, Switzerland

Publisher
Shu-Kun Lin

Managing Editor
Chao Xiao

1. Edition 2016

MDPI • Basel • Beijing • Wuhan • Barcelona

ISBN 978-3-03842-155-9 (Hbk)
ISBN 978-3-03842-156-6 (PDF)

Table of Contents

Chapter 1: Environmental Fate of Toxins in Water Systems

Chapter 2: Human Health Risk Assessment

Chapter 3: Guideline Development

Chapter 4: Monitoring Efforts in Freshwater and Marine Water Systems

Chapter 5: Treatment Techniques for Toxin Removal and Control in Reservoirs and Drinking Water

List of Contributors

Anabella Aguilera: INBIOTEC-CONICET y CIB-FIBA, Vieytes 3103, Mar del Plata 7600, Argentina.

Farah S. Ahmed: Kansas Department of Health and Environment, 1000 SW Jackson Street, Suite 075, Topeka, KS 66612, USA.

Darío Andrinolo: Toxicología, Facultad de Ciencias Exactas, Universidad Nacional de La Plata, 48 y 115, La Plata 1900, Argentina.

Ali Atoui: Laboratory of Microorganisms and Food Irradiation, Lebanese Atomic Energy Commission-CNRS, P.O. Box 11-8281, Riad El Solh, Beirut 1107 2260, Lebanon.

Lorraine C. Backer: National Center for Environmental Health, Centers for Disease Control and Prevention, 4770 Buford Highway NE, Chamblee, GA 30341, USA.

Letizia Bauzá: Toxicología, Facultad de Ciencias Exactas, Universidad Nacional de La Plata, 48 y 115, La Plata 1900, Argentina.

Val R. Beasley: Department of Veterinary and Biomedical Sciences, College of Agricultural Sciences, the Pennsylvania State University, University Park, PA 16802, USA.

Birgit Bolton: International Trachoma Initiative, the Task Force for Global Health, 325 Swanton Way, Decatur, GA 30030, USA.

Gregory L. Boyer: Department of Chemistry, College of Environmental Science and Forestry, State University of New York, Syracuse, NY 13210, USA.

Edward Carney: Kansas Department of Health and Environment, 1000 SW Jackson Street, Suite 075, Topeka, KS 66612, USA.

Liah X. Coggins: Aquatic Ecology and Ecosystem Studies, School of Civil, Environmental and Mining Engineering, the University of Western Australia, 35 Stirling Highway, M015, Crawley, WA 6009, Australia.

Marina Counter: Public Health Division, Oregon Health Authority, 800 NE Oregon Street, Suite 640, Portland, OR 97232, USA.

Curtis Cud: Public Health Division, Oregon Health Authority, 800 NE Oregon Street, Suite 640, Portland, OR 97232, USA.

Lesley V. D'Anglada: Environmental Protection Agency, Office of Science and Technology, Office of Water, 1200 Pennsylvania Ave., N.W., Washington, DC 20460, USA.

Jamie DeMent: Florida Department of Health, 4052 Bald Cypress Way, Tallahassee, FL 32399, USA.

Dariusz Dziga: Department of Plant Physiology and Development, Faculty of Biochemistry, Biophysics and Biotechnology, Jagiellonian University, Gronostajowa 7, 30387 Kraków, Poland.

Ricardo Echenique: División Ficología, Facultad de Ciencias Naturales y Museo, Universidad Nacional de La Plata, Paseo del Bosque s/n°, La Plata 1900, Argentina.

Elisabeth J. Faassen: Aquatic Ecology and Water Quality Management Group, Department of Environmental Sciences, Wageningen University, P.O. Box 47, 6700 AA Wageningen, The Netherlands.

Ali Fadel: Laboratory of Microorganisms and Food Irradiation, Lebanese Atomic Energy Commission-CNRS, P.O. Box 11-8281, Riad El Solh, Beirut 1107 2260, Lebanon; LEESU (UMR MA-102) Université Paris-Est, Ecole des Ponts ParisTech, AgroParisTech, Marne-la-Vallée F-77455, France.

David Farrer: Public Health Division, Oregon Health Authority, 800 NE Oregon Street, Suite 640, Portland, OR 97232, USA.

Anas Ghadouani: Aquatic Ecology and Ecosystem Studies, School of Civil, Environmental and Mining Engineering, the University of Western Australia, 35 Stirling Highway, M015, Crawley, WA 6009, Australia.

Leda Giannuzzi: Toxicología, Facultad de Ciencias Exactas, Universidad Nacional de La Plata, 48 y 115, La Plata 1900, Argentina.

Patricia Haines-Lieber: Kansas Department of Health and Environment, 1000 SW Jackson Street, Suite 075, Topeka, KS 66612, USA.

F. Joan Hardy: Washington State Department of Health, Olympia, WA 98504, USA.

Elizabeth D. Hilborn: National Health and Environmental Effects Research Laboratory, Office of Research and Development, United States Environmental Protection Agency, Research Triangle Park, NC 27711, USA.

Rebecca Hillwig: Public Health Division, Oregon Health Authority, 800 NE Oregon Street, Suite 640, Portland, OR 97232, USA.

Thomas Langer: Kansas Department of Health and Environment, 1000 SW Jackson Street, Suite 075, Topeka, KS 66612, USA.

Bruno J. Lemaire: LEESU (UMR MA-102) Université Paris-Est, Ecole des Ponts ParisTech, AgroParisTech, Marne-la-Vallée F-77455, France; Department of Forest, Water and Environmental Sciences and Engineering, AgroParisTech, Paris F-75005, France.

Rebecca LePrell: Virginia Department of Health, 109 Governor Street, Richmond, VA 23219, USA.

Magdalena Lisznianska: Department of Plant Physiology and Development, Faculty of Biochemistry, Biophysics and Biotechnology, Jagiellonian University, Gronostajowa 7, 30387 Kraków, Poland.

Miquel Lürling: Aquatic Ecology and Water Quality Management Group, Department of Environmental Sciences, Wageningen University, P.O. Box 47, 6700 AA Wageningen, The Netherlands; Department of Aquatic Ecology, Netherlands Institute of Ecology (NIOO-KNAW), P.O. Box 50, 6700 AB Wageningen, The Netherlands.

Deana Manassaram-Baptiste: American Cancer Society, 250 Williams Street, Quad 6C, Atlanta, GA 30303, USA.

Henri Ménager: Kansas Department of Health and Environment, 1000 SW Jackson Street, Suite 075, Topeka, KS 66612, USA.

Debin Meng: Aquatic Ecology and Water Quality Management Group, Department of Environmental Sciences, Wageningen University, P.O. Box 47, 6700 AA Wageningen, The Netherlands.

Janet Neff: Kansas Department of Health and Environment, 1000 SW Jackson Street, Suite 075, Topeka, KS 66612, USA.

Kevin P. Price: Department of Agronomy, College of Agriculture, Kansas State University, 2004 Throckmorton Plant Science Center, Manhattan, KS 66506, USA; Current Address: EVP Research and Technology Development, AgPixel LLC, 5530 West Parkway, Suite 300, Johnston, IA 50131, USA.

Elke S. Reichwaldt: Aquatic Ecology and Ecosystem Studies, School of Civil, Environmental and Mining Engineering, the University of Western Australia, 35 Stirling Highway, M015, Crawley, WA 6009, Australia.

Justine R. Schmidt: Department of Chemistry, College of Environmental Science and Forestry, State University of New York, Syracuse, NY 13210, USA.

James L. Sinclair: Office of Groundwater and Drinking Water, Technical Support Center, USEPA, Cincinnati, OH 45268, USA.

Kamal Slim: Laboratory of Microorganisms and Food Irradiation, Lebanese Atomic Energy Commission-CNRS, P.O. Box 11-8281, Riad El Solh, Beirut 1107 2260, Lebanon.

Haihong Song: Aquatic Ecology and Ecosystem Studies, School of Civil, Environmental and Mining Engineering, the University of Western Australia, 35 Stirling Highway, M015, Crawley, WA 6009, Australia.

Benjamin Southwell: Environmental Analysis Laboratory, Lake Superior State University, Sault Ste. Marie, MI 49783, USA.

Richard P. Stumpf: National Centers for Coastal Ocean Science, National Oceanic and Atmospheric Administration, 1305 East-West Highway, Silver Spring, MD 20910, USA.

David C. Szlag: Chemistry Department, Oakland University, Rochester, MI 48309, USA.

Vera L. Trainer: NOAA, Northwest Fisheries Science Center, Marine Biotoxins Program, Seattle, WA 98112, USA.

Ingrid Trevino-Garrison: Kansas Department of Health and Environment, 1000 SW Jackson Street, Suite 075, Topeka, KS 66612, USA.

Deon van der Merwe: Department of Diagnostic Medicine/Pathobiology, College of Veterinary Medicine, Kansas State University, 1800 Denison Avenue, Manhattan, KS 66506, USA.

Brigitte Vinçon-Leite: LEESU (UMR MA-102) Université Paris-Est, Ecole des Ponts ParisTech, AgroParisTech, Marne-la-Vallée F-77455, France.

Judy A. Westrick: Lumigen Instrument Center, Department of Chemistry, Wayne State University, Detroit, MI 48202, USA.

Steven W. Wilhelm: Department of Microbiology, University of Tennessee, Knoxville, TN 37996-0845, USA.

Benedykt Wladyka: Department of Analytical Biochemistry, Jagiellonian University, Gronostajowa 7, 30387 Kraków, Poland; Malopolska Centre of Biotechnology, Jagiellonian University, Gronostajowa 7, 30387 Kraków, Poland.

Timothy T. Wynne: National Centers for Coastal Ocean Science, National Oceanic and Atmospheric Administration, 1305 East-West Highway, Silver Spring, MD 20910, USA.

About the Guest Editors

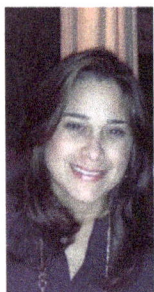

Lesley V. D'Anglada is a senior microbiologist with the United States Environmental Protection Agency (EPA). She currently leads the Harmful Algal Blooms related efforts for the Office of Science and Technology, Office of Water. Lesley is the manager of the EPA Drinking Water Health Advisories for Cyanotoxins and is the Office of Water representative on the Interagency Working Group for HABHRCA (Harmful Algal Blooms, Hypoxia, Research and Control Act). She has been a member of the WHO's Water Quality and Health Technical Advisory Group (WQTAG) since 2010 and an ex-officio member of the National HABs Committee since 2013. She received her Doctorate in Public Health and her Masters on Environmental Health from the University of Puerto Rico, Medical Science Campus, and her Bachelor Degree in Industrial Microbiology from the University of Puerto Rico, Mayaguez Campus.

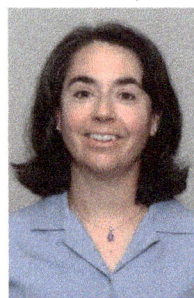

Elizabeth D. Hilborn is a senior health scientist (epidemiologist) in the Environmental Public Health Division, Office of Research and Development, United States Environmental Protection Agency (EPA). Dr. Hilborn's expertise is in the human health effects of waterborne contaminants including toxic cyanobacteria. She currently serves on the Interagency Working Group for the Harmful Algal Blooms, Hypoxia, Research and Control Act, on the Scientific Committee for the 10th International Conference on Toxic Cyanobacteria, and on multiple cyanobacteria-focused EPA committees and workgroups. Dr. Hilborn earned a Bachelor of Science in Biology from the University of North Carolina (UNC) at Chapel Hill, a Doctor of Veterinary Medicine at North Carolina State University College of Veterinary Medicine, and a Master of Public Health at the UNC at Chapel Hill. Dr. Hilborn served in the Centers for Disease Control and Prevention's Epidemic Intelligence Service, and is board-certified with the American College of Veterinary Preventive Medicine.

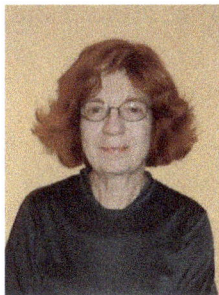

Lorraine Backer is a senior scientist and environmental epidemiologist at the Centers for Disease Control and Prevention (CDC), National Center for Environmental Health (NCEH) in Atlanta, Georgia. She received her PhD in genetic toxicology from the University of Kansas in Lawrence, Kansas, and her MPH in epidemiology from the University of North Carolina, Chapel Hill, North Carolina. She has been with the CDC since 1994. Dr. Backer created and led the Clean Water for Health Program for NCEH, which focused on the public health effects associated with drinking water from private wells, from 2007 to 2015. She oversaw numerous projects, including a cooperative agreement with 10 states to conduct data discovery for private wells and private well water quality. Dr. Backer has led CDC's HAB-related efforts since 1998, when *Pfiesteria piscicida* was found in the Chesapeake Bay, Maryland, USA. The topics of her research included the public health effects from exposure to Florida red tides and recreational exposure to cyanobacteria and related toxins.

Preface

Reprinted from *Toxins*. Cite as: Lesley V. D'Anglada. Editorial on the Special Issue "Harmful Algal Blooms (HABs) and Public Health: Progress and Current Challenges". *Toxins* **2015**, *7*, 4437-4441.

Harmful Algal Blooms (HABs) affect the quality of fresh and marine waters and adversely affect both animals and humans. Public health risks include exposure to toxins through consumption of contaminated drinking water and fish and shellfish, and by recreating on or in contaminated waters. Federal and State professionals and researchers contributed to this Special Issue on HABs and Public Health with research papers and reviews on various aspects of public health including the occurrence and fate of toxins in the environment, monitoring efforts in freshwater and marine water systems, human health risk assessment, effectiveness of treatment techniques, and guideline development.

Understanding the processes cyanobacteria and their toxins undergo in the environment is considered in the papers by Schmidt *et al.* [pp. 21–55], Fadel *et al.* [pp. 3–20], and Song *et al.* [pp. 56–74]. Schmidt *et al.* [pp. 21–55] discussed the environmental fate of microcystins, cyanobacterial toxins, and their toxicokinetics (absorption, metabolism, distribution, and excretion) in the body. Regarding environmental fate, the authors not only discussed the process of photodegradation of microcystins, but also the contribution of bacterial degradation that transforms the parent compounds into a series of conjugated products. This detoxification process, which according to the authors, is not well understood, could form toxic conjugates. Toxin degradation is also considered in the paper by Fadel *et al.* [pp. 3–20]. The authors recorded the degradation of cylindrospermopsin, another cyanobacterial toxin, due by sedimentation in lakes or by degradation, even in the presence of cylindrospermopsin-forming cyanobacterium blooms. This research emphasized that although it was not possible to definitely determine the relationship of cylindrospermopsin with other environmental factors, such as nutrients, water levels and temperature, the toxin was not correlated with cyanobacterium biovolume since it was observed at high concentrations even long after the cyanobacterium bloom had senesced. Sedimentation of microcystin in lakes, and their relationship with biological and physicochemical variables was explored by Song *et al.* [pp. 56–74]. Microcystin was detected in all sediment samples, and spatial variability was observed among microcystins and cyanobacterial biomass in different water levels and in sediments, highlighting the importance of the interaction between water and sediments in the distribution of microcystins in aquatic systems.

HABs have an adverse impact in recreational waters by fouling beaches and shoreline, affecting the quality of the water, and limiting recreational activities such as fishing, swimming, and boating. The adverse effect of the occurrence of both marine and freshwater toxic algal blooms in recreational waters in Washington State was discussed by Trainer and Hardy [pp. 171–200], with a focus on monitoring efforts and the role of these efforts in the protection of public health. In addition to regular monitoring practices for cyanotoxins, the authors described the effectiveness of partnering state regulatory programs with citizen and user-fee sponsored monitoring efforts in the surveillance and reporting of HABs and how the combination of technologies provides a comprehensive system for the protection of public health from exposure to HABs in fresh and marine waters. Trainer and Hardy also discussed the role of forecasting systems for marine and freshwater HABs, the basis for Wynne and Stumpf's paper [pp. 201–215]. Wynne and Stumpf discussed in their paper the usefulness of satellite data to examine spatial patterns of blooms and help local communities and managers in planning. Satellites may help managers identify patterns of bloom development and the areas most commonly impacted, some of them being public water supplies or recreational areas. Spatial and temporal distribution of blooms is also the topic of the paper by Van der Merwe and Price [pp. 157–170], though here the emphasis is on the use of data from unmanned aircraft systems, then to correlate it with cyanobacterial biomass densities at the water surface. The authors demonstrate how these methods can provide valuable information that could help improve risk assessments and risk management derived from traditional risk assessment methods.

HABs also could be present in drinking water and could potentially affect drinking water treatment. Taste-and-odor problems have led some utilities to change processes during the drinking-water treatment to decrease tastes and odors in finished drinking water caused by algal blooms in the supply reservoir. Another problem is the presence of cyanobacterial cells and toxins in finished drinking water. In the paper by Szlag et al. [pp. 252–274], the authors concluded that conventional treatment effectively removed cyanobacterial cells and toxins. The authors conducted monitoring of three toxins (microcystins, anatoxin-a, and cylindrospermopsin), and toxin-producing cyanobacteria on raw and finished water samples from five conventional drinking water treatment plants experiencing cyanobacterial blooms in their raw water. One of the toxins, anatoxin-a, was not detected in any of the utilities, and all finished water samples showed toxins levels below the analytical methods detection limits.

Human health risks from exposure to HABs is another topic discussed in this special issue. The paper by Hilborn and Beasley [pp. 108–129] used harmful cyanobacteria-associated animal illnesses and deaths as sentinel events to warn of potential human health risks. The paper primarily focuses on the One Health concept to integrate and collaborate among disciplines as a way to effectively monitor environmental and animal health as a way to assess human health risks. The authors concluded that illnesses or deaths among livestock, dogs, and fish are all potentially useful as predictors for the presence of cyanobacteria-associated human health risks. Human health risks surveillance is also the topic of the paper by Backer et al. [pp. 77–93], with a focus on the reports from States describing bloom events and associated adverse human and animal health events collected in the Harmful Algal Bloom-related Illness Surveillance System (HABISS) from 2007 to 2010. States used monitoring data to develop a wide range of public health prevention and response activities including issuing public health advisories or beach closures, and the development of public outreach activities. This work is indicative of the need of attention to public health risks associated with human and animal exposures to cyanobacteria and algae blooms. As mentioned before, HABs can cause adverse health effects in both humans and animals as recorded in Kansas by Trevino-Garrison *et al.* [pp. 94–107]. In this paper, the authors described the human and animal HAB-associated health events in 2011, including reports of dog illnesses and several deaths, and human illnesses, some of them requiring hospitalization. As part of its surveillance activities, the Kansas Department of Health and Environment, in conjunction with their local and national partners, developed a Harmful Algal Bloom Policy and Response Plan. This plan included the investigation of reports of HAB-related cases, the evaluation of water sample data, and education to the public of the public health risks. The authors highlighted the importance of the development of policies and guidelines to prevent morbidity and mortality among humans and animals.

Numerous techniques already exist for managing blooms in reservoirs. However, the effectiveness of these techniques is relative. For example, Bauzá *et al.* [pp. 219–237] exposed water samples from a recreational lake with cyanobacteria to different concentrations of hydrogen peroxide. Densities of cyanobacterial cells collapsed after exposure to the highest concentration over a 48 hour period in the presence of light. The authors concluded that the use of hydrogen peroxide could be used in hypertrophic systems. As in Bauzá *et al.* [pp. 219–237], the paper by Lürling *et al.* [pp. 275–296] also evaluates the effectiveness of hydrogen peroxide to reduce cyanobacterial cells and their toxins in freshwater systems, albeit this time also evaluating the effectiveness of ultrasound. Peroxide effectively reduced toxin-producing cyanobacteria biomass at similar levels to those found by Bauzá *et al.*, and proved to be ineffective at low levels. However, although a reduction of toxins was observed, still a significant release of the toxins into the water was detected. Ultrasound treatment only caused minimal growth inhibition and some release of toxins into the water, showing the treatment to be ineffective at controlling cyanobacteria. In these proposals, toxin reducing bacterial strains are used in water reservoirs as another option that may help in the reduction of microcystins occurrence. The use of bioreactors to eliminate microcystins is suggested by Dziga *et al.* [pp. 238–251] as an alternative to chemical methods of cyanotoxins elimination. This paper describes the effectiveness of using genetically engineered bacteria to degrade microcystins, based on further research on the optimization of the technique and to follow-up the long-term stability of the designed systems in natural conditions.

This special issue also includes a paper describing the development of guideline values for cyanotoxins in the state of Oregon. In the United States, drinking water contaminants are regulated under the Safe Drinking Water Act (SDWA). Currently, there are no regulations for cyanotoxins in drinking water under the SDWA, but EPA developed in June 2015, Health Advisories (HAs) for the cyanotoxins microcystins and cylindrospermopsin, to assist federal, state and local officials in protecting public health from exposure to these two toxins in drinking water systems. Regulations or guidelines have not been developed either for aquatic life, aesthetics, or recreation in any body of water under the Clean Water Act (CWA). In the absence of these guidelines, many US States, including Oregon (Farrer *et al.* [pp. 133–153]) have developed guidelines for cyanotoxins. The Oregon Health Authority (OHA) developed guideline values for drinking water, human recreational exposure, and dog recreational exposures for the four most common cyanotoxins in Oregon's fresh waters. This study shows that having cyanotoxin guidelines can give rise to the development of toxin-based monitoring programs, which reduce the number of health advisories, an important step in the protection of public health.

Public health professionals have taken measures to protect public health by assessing and monitoring HABs occurrence and health effects, developing guidelines and HAB-related public health programs, and implementing remediation and treatment technologies. Despite these efforts, it is reasonable to say that the factors that promote HABs and their toxin production, the health impacts, and the fate of these blooms and their toxins in the environment is not totally understood. The different studies published in this special issue recognized these knowledge gaps including the spatial variability among cyanobacteria and their toxins in water and sediments, the complexity of monitoring and inconsistency in treatment techniques, and the importance of the development of guidelines for the protection of public health.

Lesley V. D'Anglada
Guest Editor

Chapter 1:
Environmental Fate of Toxins in Water Systems

Dynamics of the Toxin Cylindrospermopsin and the Cyanobacterium *Chrysosporum* (*Aphanizomenon*) *ovalisporum* in a Mediterranean Eutrophic Reservoir

Ali Fadel, Ali Atoui, Bruno J. Lemaire, Brigitte Vinçon-Leite and Kamal Slim

Abstract: *Chrysosporum ovalisporum* is a cylindrospermopsin toxin producing cyanobacterium that was reported in several lakes and reservoirs. Its growth dynamics and toxin distribution in field remain largely undocumented. *Chrysosporum ovalisporum* was reported in 2009 in Karaoun Reservoir, Lebanon. We investigated the factors controlling the occurrence of this cyanobacterium and vertical distribution of cylindrospermopsin in Karaoun Reservoir. We conducted bi-weekly sampling campaigns between May 2012 and August 2013. Results showed that *Chrysosporum ovalisporum* is an ecologically plastic species that was observed in all seasons. Unlike the high temperatures, above 26 °C, which is associated with blooms of *Chrysosporum ovalisporum* in Lakes Kinneret (Israel), Lisimachia and Trichonis (Greece) and Arcos Reservoir (Spain), *Chrysosporum ovalisporum* in Karaoun Reservoir bloomed in October 2012 at a water temperature of 22 °C during weak stratification. Cylindrospermopsin was detected in almost all water samples even when *Chrysosporum ovalisporum* was not detected. *Chrysosporum ovalisporum* biovolumes and cylindrospermopsin concentrations were not correlated ($n = 31$, $r^2 = -0.05$). Cylindrospermopsin reached a maximum concentration of 1.7 µg L^{-1}. The vertical profiles of toxin concentrations suggested its possible degradation or sedimentation resulting in its disappearance from the water column. The field growth conditions of *Chrysosporum ovalisporum* in this study revealed that it can bloom at the subsurface water temperature of 22 °C increasing the risk of its development and expansion in lakes located in temperate climate regions.

Reprinted from *Toxins*. Cite as: Fadel, A.; Atoui, A.; Lemaire, B.J.; Vinçon-Leite, B.; Slim, K. Dynamics of the Toxin Cylindrospermopsin and the Cyanobacterium *Chrysosporum* (*Aphanizomenon*) *ovalisporum* in a Mediterranean Eutrophic Reservoir. *Toxins* **2014**, *6*, 3041-3057.

1. Introduction

Many lakes and reservoirs throughout the world suffer from toxic cyanobacterial blooms e.g., [1–5]. *Chrysosporum ovalisporum*, previously known as *Aphanizomenon ovalisporum* [6] is a toxic bloom-forming cyanobacterium that was reported in several freshwater bodies mainly in Australia and around the Mediterranean Sea [7–10]. *Chrysosporum ovalisporum* is a planktonic nostocalean that can colonize freshwater bodies due to different competitive strategies. Its eco-physiological characteristics are presented in Table 1. In a stratified water column, its gas vacuoles enable it to migrate between surface layers with high light availability and deeper layers with high nutrient availability [11]. Its colonies are characterized by thick wall cells called heterocysts, dedicated to atmospheric nitrogen fixation during nitrogen limitation periods [12]. Moreover, its filamentous morphology and colony size offer protection against grazing [13].

Table 1. Eco-physiological characteristics of *Chrysosporum ovalisporum*.

Parameter	*Chrysosporum ovalisporum*
Laboratory optimal growth temperature (°C)	28 ± 2 [a]
	33 ± 2 [b]
	32.8 ± 0.9 [c]
	26 ± 1 [d]
Maximum growth rate at optimal temperature (day^{-1})	0.3 [a]
	0.36 [c]
Filament flotation rate (m h^{-1})	<0.04 [e]
Optimal solar irradiation (W m^{-2})	80 [a]

Source: [a] [14]; [b] [15]; [c] [16]; [d] [9]; [e] [17].

Chrysosporum ovalisporum produces cylindrospermopsin (CYN), a toxin that poses serious threats to human and environmental health. CYN is produced by some cyanobacterial species other than *Chrysosporum ovalisporum* including *Chrysosporum* (*Anabaena*) *bergii*, *Cylindrospermopsis raciborskii*, *Raphidiopsis curvata*, and *Umezakia natans* [18,19]. This toxin, produced by *Cylindrospermopsis raciborskii* is believed to be responsible for the severe hepatoenteritis that affected 148 people in 1979 on Palm Island, Queensland, Australia [20]. CYN is a water soluble alkaloid hepatotoxin that was found to cause damage to kidneys, lungs and heart. It was also reported as protein synthesis inhibitor, genotoxic [21] and carcinogenic [22].

A large fraction of CYN can be found in extracellular water because it is released from cells under physiological stress by temperature and light [23]. CYN persists in many water bodies because of its chemical stability and slow degradation; after 10 weeks at 50 °C, cylindrospermopsin had degraded to 57% of the original concentration [24]. Recently, it was found in high extracellular concentrations in many freshwater bodies throughout the world: 18.4 µg L^{-1} in Lake Albano, Italy [25], 9.4 µg L^{-1} by *Chrysosporum ovalisporum* in Arcos Reservoir, Spain [9] and 12.1 µg L^{-1} in German lakes [26].

Understanding the mechanisms and processes that control the growth and succession of cyanobacterial species is of great concern. Karaoun Reservoir is the largest freshwater body in Lebanon, with a maximum capacity of 224×10^6 m^3. Before 1996, the reservoir was dominated by diatoms that constituted 80% of the total population [27]. After the year 2000, the dinoflagellate *Ceratium hirundinella* and filamentous green algae were the main phytoplankton species documented in the reservoir [28]. *Chrysosporum ovalisporum* blooms were first reported in Karaoun Reservoir in May 2009 [29,30]. *Chrysosporum ovalisporum* is not as widely spread as other cyanobacteria species like *Microcystis aeruginosa*. It was documented in some water bodies around the Mediterranean Sea but its growth dynamics were not sufficiently studied. As well, cylindrospermopsin toxin profiles were poorly studied at field. In this paper, we describe the dynamics and controlling factors of this blooming cyanobacterium as well as CYN distribution in the water column of Karaoun Reservoir.

2. Results

2.1. Physical-Chemical Conditions

During 2012 and 2013, subsurface water temperature in Karaoun Reservoir ranged from 13 to 26 °C (Figure 1). Comparison between water temperatures at 1 and 10 m in 2012 and 2013 showed that the reservoir was stratified from May to August. The water was weakly stratified (less than 1 °C between the surface and the lake bottom) or fully mixed in September, October and November 2012. The water level ranged from 837 to 859 m above sea level. The reservoir was full at the beginning of May in 2012 and 2013. Then, the water level decreased by 20 m due to small inflows and regular withdrawals in the dry season, between May and October. Subsurface orthophosphate concentration was close to detection limit (0.01 mg P L^{-1}) in 2012. In 2013, it decreased from 0.95 mg L^{-1} in March down to under the detection limit in summer. Total phosphorus varied greatly between campaigns and some of its peaks were correlated with total phytoplankton biovolume peaks. Nitrate nitrogen did not exceed 0.2 mg L^{-1} except on October 16, 2012 (0.47 mg L^{-1}) (Figure 2). TN:TP ratio did not exceed 22:1 during the study period.

2.2. Dynamics of Chrysosporum ovalisporum in Karaoun Reservoir

Chrysosporum ovalisporum in Karaoun Reservoir was already blooming at the beginning of the survey on May 15, 2012 with a biovolume of 8.2 mm^3 L^{-1} in a sample taken at the edge of the reservoir (S$_B$, see section 4.1.). At that time, the reservoir was full. This bloom had declined a week after the water level had begun to decrease on May 24, 2012. *Chrysosporum ovalisporum* bloomed again in June but disappeared in July. Subsurface nitrate nitrogen concentration was 0.16 mg N L^{-1} and water temperature was 25 °C at that time. *Chrysosporum ovalisporum* was not detected from August to September 2012 when the reservoir was dominated by *Microcystis aeruginosa* that had a maximum biovolume of 6.7 mm^3 L^{-1} on September 12, 2012. In mid-October 2012, *Microcystis aeruginosa* was not detected and was replaced by *Chrysosporum ovalisporum* colonies with trichomes of 150 ± 75 μm without heterocysts (Figure 3a). It was a mixing period, orthophosphate concentration was close to detection limit (0.01 mg P L^{-1}), nitrate concentration was 0.47 mg N L^{-1}, water level was low (10 m depth at S$_M$, 841 m above sea level), daily average irradiance was 120 W m^{-2} and water temperature was 22 °C. After 2 weeks, *Chrysosporum ovalisporum* was not detected anymore and was replaced by dinoflagellate *Ceratium hirundinella* which bloomed in November.

In 2013, *Chrysosporum ovalisporum* was observed in March and July but its biovolumes did not exceed 1.3 mm^3 L^{-1}. In March, *Chrysosporum ovalisporum* trichomes of 130 ± 50 μm showed visible heterocysts (Figure 3b), while nitrate nitrogen concentration was 0.15 mg N L^{-1}.

In summary, during both years, *Chrysosporum ovalisporum* was seen both at high and low water levels, during stratified and unstratified conditions, in a wide range of daily average irradiance (100–260 W m^{-2}).

Figure 1. Daily mean values of physical variables at the sampling dates: water level, solar irradiance, water temperature at 1 and 10 m, and biovolumes of total phytoplankton and *Chrysosporum ovalisporum* in 2012 and 2013 at S_M in Karaoun Reservoir, except on May 15, 2012 where samples were taken at S_B.

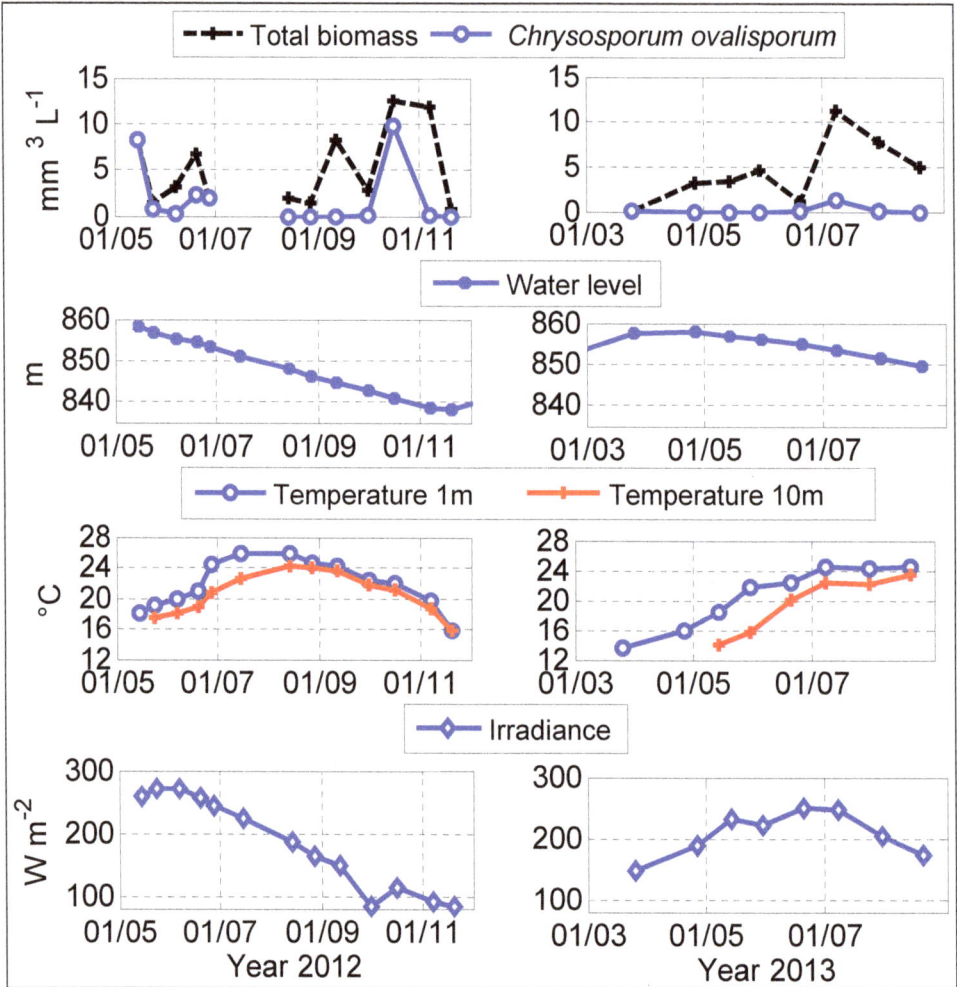

Figure 2. Concentrations of nitrate nitrogen, total nitrogen, total phosphorus, orthophosphate phosphorus and *TN/TP* ratio in 2012 and 2013 at S$_M$ in Karaoun Reservoir.

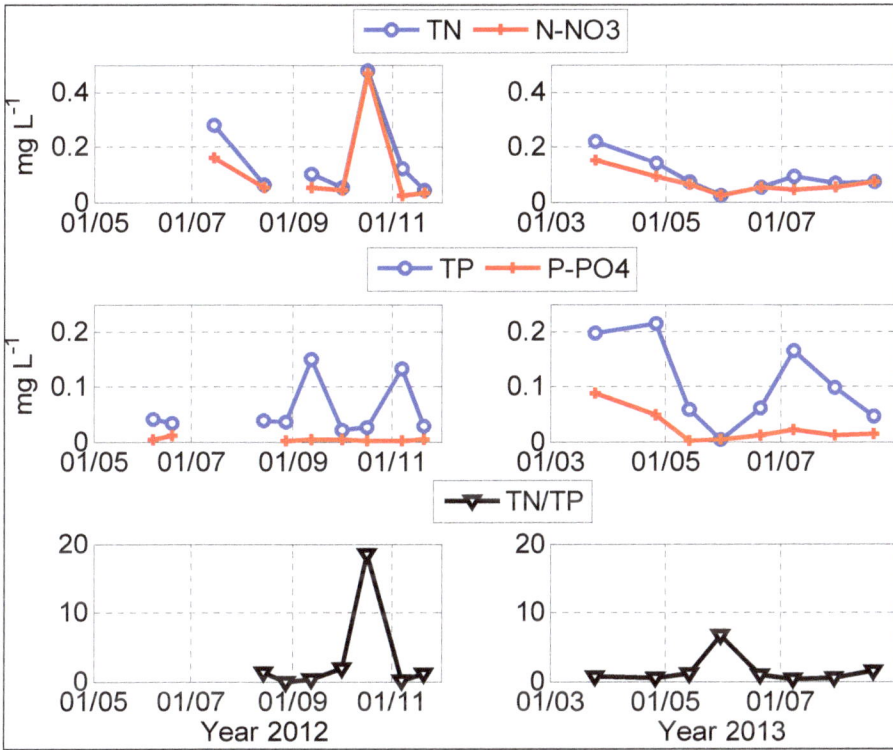

Figure 4 presents the phycocyanin profiles of *Chrysosporum ovalisporum* measured in 2012 and 2013. The relative proportion of each cyanobacterial species with respect to the total biovolume of cyanobacteria group was calculated using microscopic counting. This proportion was then used to calculate their corresponding phycocyanin values measured by Trios fluoremeter. Phycocyanin profiles showed the seasonal variation of *Chrysosporum ovalisporum* profiles. In late spring, May and June 2012, when daily irradiance ranged between 230 and 270 W m^{-2}, *Chrysosporum ovalisporum* was present in the top 5 m, in the euphotic zone of Karaoun Reservoir, and was concentrated between 1 and 3 m. In autumn, in October 2012, when irradiance was 100 ± 20 W m^{-2}, *Chrysosporum ovalisporum* exhibited a surface bloom.

Figure 3. *Chrysosporum ovalisporum* at Karaoun Reservoir (**a**) colony on October 16, 2012; (**b**) visible heterocyst on March 25, 2013.

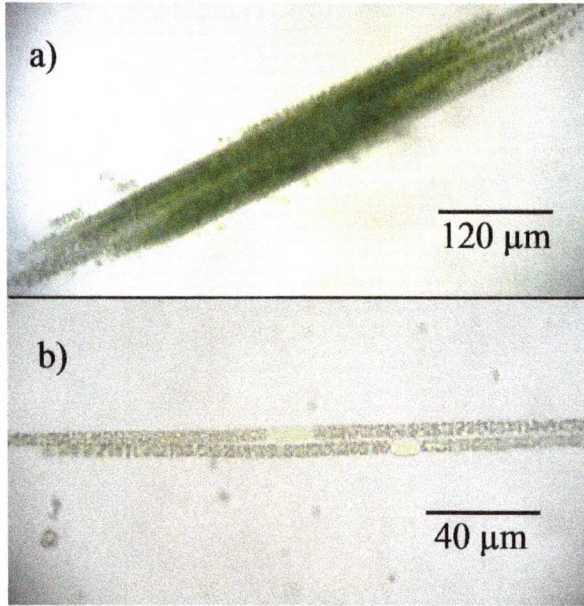

Figure 4. Phycocyanin fluorescence profiles, proxies of *Chrysosporum ovalisporum* concentration in the water column at S_M in Karaoun Reservoir in 2012 and 2013.

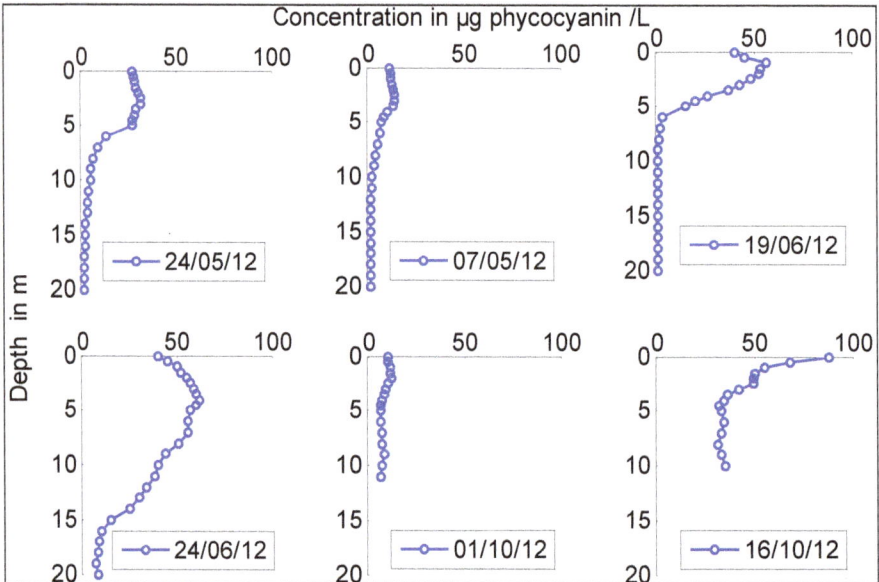

2.3. Cylindrospermopsin Quantification

Subsurface concentrations of CYN in Karaoun Reservoir ranged from 0.38 to 1.72 µg L^{-1} in 2012 and 2013 (Figure 5). The lowest concentration (0.38 µg L^{-1}) was recorded at the beginning of a *Chrysosporum ovalisporum* bloom on May 15, 2012. This concentration showed an increasing trend in the first four campaigns (May 15, May 24, June 7 and June 19, 2012). The highest concentration (1.7 µg L^{-1}) was recorded both on August 28, 2012 and April 26, 2013, in the absence of *Chrysosporum ovalisporum* in the water column.

Figure 5. Subsurface cylindrospermopsin (CYN) concentration and biovolumes of *Chrysosporum ovalisporum* in 2012 and 2013 at S$_M$ in Karaoun Reservoir, except on May 15, 2012 where sample were taken at S$_B$.

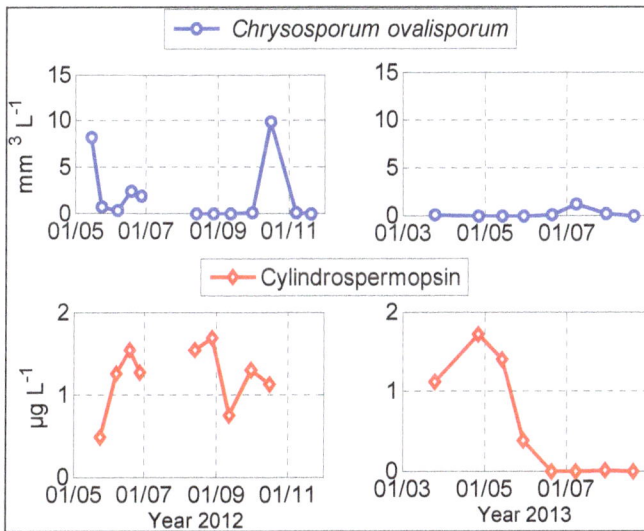

2.4. Comparison Between Chrysosporum ovalisporum and CYN Distribution in the Water Column

Chrysosporum ovalisporum was the only CYN producing cyanobacteria species recorded in the reservoir in both 2012 and 2013. We therefore tried to compare the distribution of the cyanobacterium and of the toxin in the water column. In 2013, *Chrysosporum ovalisporum* was first observed on March 25. It was not detected in April, May and June 2013 but it was detected again in July 2013 at a low biovolume (Figure 6). On March 25, 2013, CYN concentrations were higher than 1 µg L^{-1} at the surface and at 5 m and 10 m depths. In April 2013, the CYN concentration increased from 1.1 to 1.7 µg L^{-1} at the surface and remained constant at 5 m and 10 m depth. On May 14, 2013, it decreased from 1.7–1.4 µg L^{-1} at the surface and from 1.3 to 0.9 µg L^{-1} at 10 m and increased from 1.29 to 1.7 µg L^{-1} at 5 m. On May 30, 2013, it decreased from 1.4 to 0.38 µg L^{-1} at the surface and from 1.7 to 1.1 µg L^{-1} at 5 m depth. This decrease at 1 and 5 m was accompanied by an increase from 0.9 to 1.5 µg L^{-1} at 10 m depth. CYN was not detected down to 5 m depth on June 20, 2013 and was at a low concentration of 0.2 µg L^{-1} at 10 m depth. On July 8, 2013, CYN was not detected at the surface and 10 m and was 0.09 µg L^{-1} at 5 m depth. On July 30, 2013 following *Chrysosporum ovalisporum* detection on July 8, 2013, CYN increased only at 5 m, from 0.09 to 0.25 µg L^{-1}.

Figure 6. Vertical profiles of *Chrysosporum ovalisporum* biovolumes (10^{-3} mm^3 L^{-1}) and CYN concentrations (µg L^{-1}) in Karaoun Reservoir during the year 2013. Error-bars are the standard deviations on the runned triplicates.

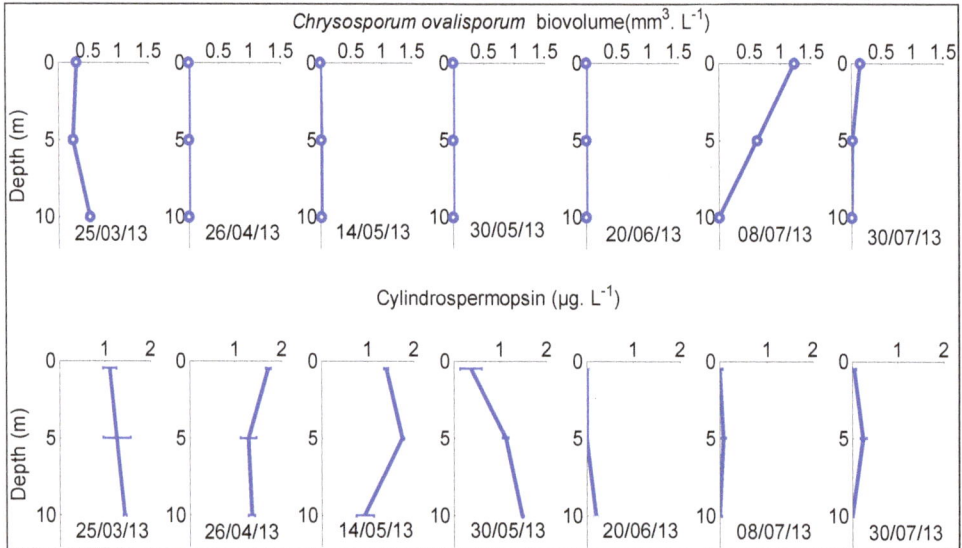

2.5. Absence of Correlation between Cylindrospermopsin Concentration and Chrysosporum ovalisporum Biovolumes

To measure the strength of the linear relationship between *Chrysosporum ovalisporum* biovolumes and cylindrospermopsin concentrations, Pearson's correlation coefficients were computed on 31 samples taken at 0, 5 and 10 m depths in 2012 and 2013. A negative low value of $r^2 = -0.05$ showed the absence of any correlation between CYN concentrations and *Chrysosporum ovalisporum* biovolumes. Although *Chrysosporum ovalisporum* biovolumes in 2013 was eight times lower than in 2012, cylindrospermopsin was 1.72 µg L^{-1}, as high as in 2012.

3. Discussion

3.1. Chrysosporum ovalisporum Blooms in Karaoun Reservoir

Cyanobacterial blooms are a new phenomenon in Karaoun Reservoir compared to the near Lake Kinneret (Israel), located 80 km to the south of Karaoun Reservoir. In Lake Kinneret, winter and spring blooms of *Microcystis* sp. were reported since the 1960s [31]. Also, an intense bloom of *Chrysosporum ovalisporum* occurred for the first time in the summer of 1994 [10]. Although there is no direct evidence for this, viable cells of *Chrysosporum ovalisporum* could have been transported from Lake Kinneret to Karaoun Reservoir by migratory birds and they could have bloomed when environmental conditions became favorable.

Horizontal displacement, nitrogen availability and water temperature could be the factors controlling the growth and succession of *Chrysosporum ovalisporum* in Karaoun Reservoir. In mid May 2012, *Chrysosporum ovalisporum* dominated in samples taken at the edge of the reservoir. Its concentration greatly decreased within 10 days. Profiles of *Chrysosporum ovalisporum* on May 24, 2012 showed that it was concentrated in the top 5 m. Between May 14 and 24, 2012, the reservoir was full and overflowed. Horizontal transport of buoyant *Chrysosporum* by wind and current may have caused their loss after they exit the reservoir through the spillway. Horizontal displacement is considered as the limiting factor that causes the loss of floating colonial cyanobacteria through outflow. It was reported to be the main reason affecting the horizontal distribution of phytoplankton, especially buoyant cyanobacteria, in Lake Taihu [32] and in four Andalusian reservoirs in Spain [33].

Nitrogen limitation is a factor that can promote *Chrysosporum ovalisporum* growth [34]. The bloom of *Chrysosporum* ovalisporum in October 2012 was preceded by a period of very low nitrogen levels and N:P ratios that did not exceed 22:1 during the study period. According to Smith *et al.* (1995), lake water TN:TP ratios below 22:1 favour the dominance of N_2-fixing cyanobacteria [35]. Similar effects of low N:P ratios have been seen in Lake Kinneret where the invasion of the nitrogen-fixing cyanobacterium *Chrysosporum ovalisporum* was consistent with the trend towards increasing *N*-deficiency in the water column [36].

Chrysosporum ovalisporum occurred at different water temperatures in other freshwater bodies. In July 1999, *Chrysosporum* ovalisporum dominated at subsurface water temperatures between 29 and 31 °C, in the warm monomictic Lakes Lisimachia and Trichonis in Greece [7]. Laboratory experiments showed that *Chrysosporum ovalisporum* of Lake Kinneret has an optimal temperature of 26–30 °C [14]. In Arcos Reservoir, *Chrysosporum ovalisporum* dominated in October and September at a subsurface temperature of 26 °C [9]. Unlike the temperature conditions that were associated with blooms of *Chrysosporum ovalisporum* in Lakes Kinneret, Lisimachia, Trichonis and Arcos Reservoir, *Chrysosporum ovalisporum* in Karaoun Reservoir peaked in October 2012, with a maximum biovolume of 9.8 mm^3 L^{-1}, when water temperature was 22 °C. Although there is a difference in the water temperature at which *Chrysosporum ovalisporum* blooms in Lake Kinneret and Karaoun Reservoir, climate change is thought to be one of the drivers of *Chrysosporum ovalisporum* blooms. Slim *et al.* [29] revealed that changes in climate regime, increase in air temperature and decrease in precipitation between 2000 and 2010 have altered Karaoun Reservoir biodiversity and resulted in low diversity dominated by *Chrysosporum ovalisporum* and *Microcystis aeruginosa* blooms. In Lake Kinneret, Hadas *et al.* [37] proposed that the appearance and establishment of *Chrysosporum ovalisporum* since 1994 was linked to increased water temperature and limited nitrogen availability. Using a temperature based model, Mehnert *et al.* [16] hypothesized a future northward expansion of *Chrysosporum ovalisporum* in Europe under the global warming scenario. In Karaoun Reservoir, *Chrysosporum ovalisporum* bloomed at a water temperature of 22 °C. This supports the possibility of *Chrysosporum ovalisporum* blooms in European lakes in which subsurface water temperature can exceed 22 °C like Lake Bourget in France [38], Lake Mondsee in Austria [39], and Lake Zurich in Switzerland [40].

As in Cobaki Village Lake in Australia [41], *Chrysosporum ovalisporum* in Karaoun Reservoir was present in the epilimnion with the highest cell concentrations occurring at a depth of 1 to 3 m in spring 2012 when irradiance was 250 ± 20 W m^{-2}. Its highest filament concentrations then occurred at top 1 m when irradiance was 100 ± 20 W m^{-2}. *Chrysosporum ovalisporum* in Karaoun Reservoir is probably also sensitive to photoinhibition as in Lake Kinneret where the rate of photosynthesis of *Chrysosporum ovalisporum* reaches maximum at about 80 W m^{-2} and declines at higher irradiance, due to photoinhibition [14].

3.2. Relation between Cylindrospermopsin Concentrations and Chrysosporum ovalisporum

CYN can be present in water body as extracellular and intracellular. The extracellular fraction can exceed the intracellular fraction [20]. The low correlation between CYN concentrations and *Chrysosporum ovalisporum* biovolumes can be explained by the ability of this cyanobacterium to liberate high levels of CYN that remains stable even after the decline of the cyanobacterium. CYN is relatively stable under a variety of conditions; it decomposes slowly in temperatures ranging from 4 to 50 °C at pH 7. After 10 weeks at 50 °C, cylindrospermopsin degraded to 57% of the original concentration [24]. According to Preußel *et al.* [23] several temperature–light combinations which constitute physiological stresses seem to trigger CYN production and particularly CYN release from cells. Shaw *et al.* [42] found that the extracellular cylindrospermopsin fraction was at least 85% in Ocean Park ponds and Palm Lakes in Australia, indicating that *Chrysosporum ovalisporum* releases cylindrospermopsin to water. For that, analyses based on *Chrysosporum ovalisporum* cell counts cannot decipher cylindrospermopsin concentration because they do not take into account extracellular CYN.

3.3. Disappearance of CYN from Water Column by Degradation or Sedimentation

Vertical profiles of CYN in Karaoun Reservoir showed that its concentration decreased at the surface and increased at deeper depths during summer. Information about the vertical distribution of CYN and its disappearance from the water column in other freshwater bodies are scarce. Settling after adsorption to particulate material or degradation may have resulted in the disappearance of CYN from the surface.

In situ photodegradation of CYN was observed, but rate is affected by both the turbidity of the water and the depth of the photic zone [24]. Little information is available regarding the effect of temperature on the biodegradation of cyanobacterial toxins [43]. There are conflicting reports regarding the efficiency of the biodegradation of these metabolites in water bodies [43]. For example, Smith *et al.* [44] documented biodegradation in water supplies that had a history of toxic *Cylindrospermopsis raciborskii* blooms in North Pine Dam in Queensland, Australia, while Wormer *et al.* [45] did not observe any biodegradation of cylindrospermopsin produced by *Chrysosporum ovalisporum* in Santillana Reservoir in Spain. The profiles presented on Figure 6 represent both intracellular and extracellular CYN. A large fraction of CYN was in extracellular form when it started to decrease at 1 m depth because *Chrysosporum ovalisporum* was not detected. Extracellular toxins may adsorb to clays and organic material in the water column [46]. The settling velocity of CYN was about 1 m per week which means that it might have been adsorbed on organic material rather than clay that needs months to settle. In Cobaki Village Lake, Australia, the maximum toxin concentration was present in the hypolimnion during a *Chrysosporum ovalisporum* bloom [41]. This suggests that the decrease of CYN concentration at surface in Karaoun Reservoir might de due to CYN settling or degradation.

4. Experimental Section

4.1. Study Site

Karaoun Reservoir (33°34'N, 35°41'E), located in the southern part of the Bekaa valley, between the two Lebanese mountain chains, is the largest freshwater body in Lebanon (Figure 7, Table 2). The reservoir was constructed between 1958 and 1965 on the Litani River for power production and irrigation. Most of the river inflow (90% of the mean annual inflow) occurs mainly in the wet season, from October to May, while the withdrawals are regular throughout the year, which causes a large level variation, by about 20 m [47].

Figure 7. Karaoun Reservoir and sampling sites: S_M (33°34'05"N, 35°41'44"E) and S_B (33°34'37"N, 35°41'20"E).

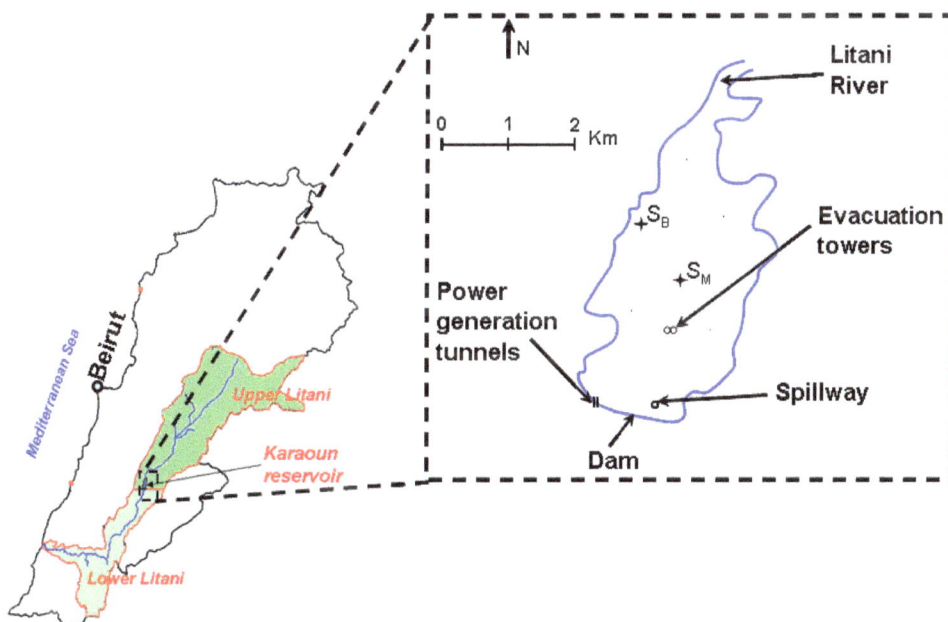

Table 2. Karaoun Reservoir morphometric and hydrologic characteristics.

Morphometry and hydrology	Values
Surface area at full capacity	12 km^2
Maximum storage capacity	224×10^6 m^3
Maximum depth	60 m
Mean depth at full capacity	19 m
Altitude at maximum level (m)	860 m
Catchment area	1600 km^2
Mean residence time of water	9 months

4.2. Sampling Procedure

Measurements and samples were taken at the most representative point (S$_M$), located in the middle of the lake (33°34'05"N, 35°41'44"E). However, for safety reasons during high water level, the sample of May 15, 2012 was taken at the reservoir side, S$_B$ (Figure 7). Campaigns were performed bi-weekly between 11:00 and 13:00. Water samples were collected at 0.5 m depth from May to November 2012 and at 0.5, 5 and 10 m depths from March to August 2013 with a vertical Niskin bottle of 2.2 L capacity (Wildco 1120-D42, Florida, United States). Samples were stored at 4 °C until further processing in the laboratory. Different volumes and bottles were used for phytoplankton identification and counting, nutrient analysis and cylindrospermopsin quantification.

4.3. Water Temperature and Phycocyanin Measurements

Water temperature was measured with temperature sensors (Starmon mini, Star-Oddi, Gardabaer, Iceland) at 1 and 10 m depths to monitor thermal stratification. The sensor measuring temperature range is −2 to 40 °C with an accuracy of ±0.05 °C. A submersible fluorometer (TriOS microFlu-blue, Rastede, Germany) was used to measure fluorescence profiles of phycocyanin, a pigment specific to cyanobacteria. It is equipped with ultra-bright red LEDs, of an excitation wavelength 620 nm, detection wavelength 655 nm and band-width 10 nm. It gives a linear response to phycocyanin concentration up to 200 µg L^{-1} with an accuracy of 0.02 µg L^{-1}. Measurements were performed every half meter between the surface and the bottom of the reservoir by descending the cable manually at a speed of 5 cm s^{-1} and waiting for 30 s for values to become stable.

4.4. Microscopic Identification and Counting

The subsamples used for phytoplankton counting were fixed by formaldehyde and preserved at 4 °C (4% of sample volume). The phytoplankton species were determined on the sampling day according to taxonomic keys based on cell structure and dimensions, colony morphology, and mucilage characteristics [48,49]. Microscopic identification and enumeration were carried out under a phase contrast microscope (Nikon TE200, Nikon, Melville, NY, USA), under a ×40 objective and using Nageotte chamber that accepts 100 µL on 40 bands. The number of bands counted depended on sample concentration. Each subsample was counted on triplicate.

4.5. Nutrient Analysis

Subsamples used for the analysis of nutrients (total phosphorus, orthophosphate, nitrate, and ammonium) were preserved at 4 °C after addition of 2 mL of 18 M H_2SO_4 Soluble phosphorus (orthophosphate), nitrate, and ammonium subsamples were then filtrated through a 0.45 μm cellulose acetate filter (MF-Millipore, HAWP04700, American Fork, UT, USA).

Nitrate and ammonium concentrations were estimated by colorimetry with a photometer (Palintest Photometer 7000se, Gateshead, UK). Total phosphorus and orthophosphate concentrations were determined at 880 nm by UV/VIS spectrophotometer (Thermospectronic, LaboTech, Beirut, Lebanon) using colorimetric ascorbic acid method (EPA Standard Method 365.3, Washington, DC, USA). The quantification range for nitrate nitrogen is 0.1–30 mg N L^{-1}, ammonium nitrogen 0.1–12 mg N L^{-1}, and phosphorus 0.01–1.2 mg P L^{-1}.

4.6. Cylindrospermopsin Analysis

Samples for cylindrospermopsin analysis were collected in borosilicate bottles, transported in the dark and preserved at 4 °C until analysis date. To measure the concentration of both intracellular and extracellular toxin forms, samples were vortexed before analysis but not filtered. According to Humpage *et al.* [50], high amounts of cyanobacterial cell material or a relatively high organic load, even in wastewater, do not have a significant effect on the analysis result. ELISA kit (Abraxis, product number: 522011, Warminster, UK) was used to evaluate extracellular cylindrospermopsin concentration. Each sample was run in triplicate. The absorbance of the coloured product of antibody-conjugated enzymes was read at 450 nm using a microplate ELISA photometer (Stat Fax 303 Plus, Palm City, FL, USA). The subsequent quantification was based on calibration curves of the semi-logarithmic relationship between relative absorbance and toxin concentration using the six standards provided with the kit. The quantification range for cylindrospermopsin by ELISA is 0.04–2 μg L^{-1}.

4.7. Meteorological and Hydrological Data

Solar radiation, precipitation and wind speed measurements were obtained from Tal-Amara meteorological station of the Lebanese Agriculture Research Institute located in the Bekaa valley (33°51'50"N, 35°59'06"E), 40 km North of Karaoun Reservoir. Daily water level measurements were provided by the Litani River Authority (LRA), responsible for the management of the reservoir.

5. Conclusions

Chrysosporum ovalisporum in Karaoun Reservoir was detected in all seasons. It is difficult to decide conclusively its relationship with all the environmental factors and nutrient availability in particular. *Chrysosporum ovalisporum* dominated both during periods of high and low water level, stratification and mixing in a wide range of light irradiances and water temperatures. Light irradiation higher than 250 W m^{-2} photoinhibited *Chrysosporum ovalisporum* and resulted in its concentration between 1 at 3 m depths. Among the main hypotheses for explaining its decline in Karaoun Reservoir is water temperature higher than 25 °C and horizontal transport and withdrawal.

Unlike high temperature conditions which were associated with blooms of *Chrysosporum ovalisporum* in lakes located in the Middle-East or in Southern Europe, *Chrysosporum ovalisporum* in Karaoun Reservoir bloomed at water temperature of 22 °C. Lakes in which water temperature exceeds 22 °C are susceptible to blooms of *Chrysosporum ovalisporum*. Our results suggest that within a period of a month, CYN produced by *Chrysosporum ovalisporum* disappeared from the water column either by sedimentation or degradation. It also shows that CYN concentrations were not correlated with *Chrysosporum ovalisporum* biovolumes and it can be observed at high concentrations even long after the end of *Chrysosporum ovalisporum* blooms.

On the local level, it shows that Karaoun Reservoir contains cylindrospermopsin. Presence of cylindrospermopsin long after blooms of *Chrysosporum ovalisporum* requires regular monitoring of cylindrospermopsin in the Reservoir, to avoid health problems when using Karaoun water for irrigation or for drinking water supply.

Acknowledgments

This work was funded by the Lebanese National Council for Scientific Research, Ecole des Ponts ParisTech, the French Ministry for Higher Education and Research and the French Ministry for Foreign Affairs through the CEDRE program (project 10 EF 38/L9).

Author Contributions

All authors conceived and designed the experiments. Ali Fadel, Kamal Slim and Ali Atoui conducted the experiments. All authors participated in data analysis. Ali Fadel wrote the paper. All co-authors participated in revising the article critically for important intellectual content. All authors approved the final paper.

Conflicts of Interest

The authors declare no conflict of interest.

References

1. Li, D.; Kong, F.; Shi, X.; Ye, L.; Yu, Y.; Yang, Z. Quantification of microcystin-producing and non-microcystin producing *Microcystis* populations during the 2009 and 2010 blooms in Lake Taihu using quantitative real-time PCR. *J. Environ. Sci.* **2012**, *24*, 284–290.
2. Liu, Y.; Tan, W.; Wu, X.; Wu, Z.; Yu, G.; Li, R. First report of microcystin production in *Microcystis smithii* Komárek and Anagnostidis (Cyanobacteria) from a water bloom in Eastern China. *J. Environ. Sci.* **2012**, *23*, 102–107.
3. Messineo, V.; Bogialli, S.; Melchiorre, S.; Sechi, N.; Luglia, A.; Casiddu, P.; Mariani, M.A.; Padedda, B.M.; Corcia, A.D.; Mazza, R.; *et al.* Cyanobacterial toxins in Italian freshwaters. *Limnologica* **2009**, *39*, 95–106.

4. Ballot, A.; Pflugmacher, S.; Wiegand, C.; Kotut, K.; Krienitz, L. Cyanobacterial toxins in Lake Baringo, Kenya. *Limnologica* **2003**, *33*, 2–9.

5. Rejmánková, E.; Komárek, J.; Dix, M.; Rejmánková, J.; Girón, N. Cyanobacterial blooms in Lake Atitlan, Guatemala. *Limnologica* **2011**, *41*, 296–302.

6. Zapomělová, E.; Skácelová, O.; Pumann, P.; Kopp, R.; Janeček, E. Biogeographically interesting planktonic Nostocales (Cyanobacteria) in the Czech Republic and their polyphasic evaluation resulting in taxonomic revisions of *Anabaena bergii* Ostenfeld 1908 (*Chrysosporum* gen. nov.) and *A. tenericaulis* Nygaard 1949 (*Dolichospermum tenericaule* comb. nova). *Hydrobiologia* **2012**, *698*, 353–365.

7. Gkelis, S.; Moustaka-Gouni, M.; Sivonen, K.; Lanaras, T. First report of the cyanobacterium *Aphanizomenon ovalisporum* Forti in two Greek lakes and cyanotoxin occurrence. *J. Plankton Res.* **2005**, *27*, 1295–1300.

8. Messineo, V.; Melchiorre, S.; Di Corcia, A.; Gallo, P.; Bruno, M. Seasonal succession of *Cylindrospermopsis raciborskii* and *Aphanizomenon ovalisporum* blooms with cylindrospermopsin occurrence in the volcanic Lake Albano, Central Italy. *Environ. Toxicol.* **2010**, *25*, 18–27.

9. Quesada, A.; Moreno, E.; Carrasco, D.; Paniagua, T.; Wormer, L.; Hoyos, C.D.; Sukenik, A. Toxicity of *Aphanizomenon ovalisporum* (Cyanobacteria) in a Spanish water reservoir. *Eur. J. Phycol.* **2006**, *41*, 39–45.

10. Pollingher, U.; Hadas, O.; Yacobi, Y.Z.; Zohary, T.; Berman, T. *Aphanizomenon ovalisporum* (Forti) in Lake Kinneret, Israel. *J. Plankton Res.* **1998**, *20*, 1321–1339.

11. Reynolds, C.S.; Oliver, R.L.; Walsby, A.E. Cyanobacterial dominance: The role of buoyancy regulation in dynamic lake environments. *N. Z. J. Mar. Freshwater Res.* **1987**, *21*, 379–390.

12. Reynolds, C.S. Nutrient uptake and assimilation in phytoplankton. In *The Ecology of Phytoplankton*; Cambridge University Press: Cambridge, UK, 2006; pp. 145–175.

13. Kardinaal, W.; Visser, P. Dynamics of cyanobacterial toxins. In *Harmful cyanobacteria*; Huisman, J., Matthijs, H.C.P., Visser, P.M., Eds.; Springer Netherlands: Dordrecht, The Netherlands, 2005; pp. 41–63.

14. Hadas, O.; Pinkas, R.; Malinsky-Rushansky, N.; Shalev-Alon, G.; Delphine, E.; Berner, T.; Sukenik, A.; Kaplan, A. Physiological variables determined under laboratory conditions may explain the bloom of *Aphanizomenon ovalisporum* in Lake Kinneret. *Eur. J. Phycol.* **2002**, *37*, 259–267.

15. Cirés, S.; Wörmer, L.; Timón, J.; Wiedner, C.; Quesada, A. Cylindrospermopsin production and release by the potentially invasive cyanobacterium *Aphanizomenon ovalisporum* under temperature and light gradients. *Harmful Algae* **2011**, *10*, 668–675.

16. Mehnert, G.; Leunert, F.; Cirés, S.; Jöhnk, K.D.; Rücker, J.; Nixdorf, B.; Wiedner, C. Competitiveness of invasive and native cyanobacteria from temperate freshwaters under various light and temperature conditions. *J. Plankton Res.* **2010**, *32*, 1009–1021.

17. Porat, R.; Teltsch, B.; Perelman, A.; Dubinsky, Z. Diel Buoyancy Changes by the Cyanobacterium *Aphanizomenon ovalisporum* from a Shallow Reservoir. *J. Plankton Res.* **2001**, *23*, 753–763.

18. Boopathi, T.; Ki, J.S. Impact of Environmental Factors on the Regulation of Cyanotoxin Production. *Toxins* **2014**, *6*, 1951–1978.

19. Stucken, K.; John, U.; Cembella, A.; Soto-Liebe, K.; Vásquez, M. Impact of nitrogen sources on gene expression and toxin production in the diazotroph *Cylindrospermopsis raciborskii* CS-505 and non-diazotroph *Raphidiopsis brookii* D9. *Toxins* **2014**, *6*, 1896–1915.

20. Griffiths, D.J.; Saker, M.L. The Palm Island mystery disease 20 years on: A review of research on the cyanotoxin cylindrospermopsin. *Environ. Toxicol.* **2003**, *18*, 78–93.

21. Humpage, A.R.; Fenech, M.; Thomas, P.; Falconer, I.R. Micronucleus induction and chromosome loss in transformed human white cells indicate clastogenic and aneugenic action of the cyanobacterial toxin, cylindrospermopsin. *Mutat. Res. Genet. Toxicol. Environ. Mutagenesis* **2000**, *472*, 155–161.

22. Falconer, I.R.; Humpage, A.R. Cyanobacterial (blue-green algal) toxins in water supplies: Cylindrospermopsins. *Environ. Toxicol.* **2006**, *21*, 299–304.

23. Preußel, K.; Wessel, G.; Fastner, J.; Chorus, I. Response of cylindrospermopsin production and release in *Aphanizomenon flos-aquae* (Cyanobacteria) to varying light and temperature conditions. *Harmful Algae* **2009**, *8*, 645–650.

24. Chiswell, R.K.; Shaw, G.R.; Eaglesham, G.; Smith, M.J.; Norris, R.L.; Seawright, A.A.; Moore, M.R. Stability of cylindrospermopsin, the toxin from the cyanobacterium, *Cylindrospermopsis raciborskii*: Effect of pH, temperature, and sunlight on decomposition. *Environ. Toxicol.* **1999**, *14*, 155–161.

25. Bogialli, S.; Bruno, M.; Curini, R.; Di Corcia, A.; Fanali, C.; Laganà, A. Monitoring algal toxins in lake water by liquid chromatography tandem mass spectrometry. *Environ. Sci. Technol.* **2006**, *40*, 2917–2923.

26. Rücker, J.; Stüken, A.; Nixdorf, B.; Fastner, J.; Chorus, I.; Wiedner, C. Concentrations of particulate and dissolved cylindrospermopsin in 21 *Aphanizomenon*-dominated temperate lakes. *Toxicon* **2007**, *50*, 800–809.

27. Slim, K. Contribution to the study of the flora of the basin of the Litani basin. *Leb. Sci. Res. Rep.* **1996**, *1*, 65–73.

28. Saad, Z.; Slim, K.; Elzein, G.; Elsamad, O. Evaluation of the water quality of Karaoun reservoir (Lebanon). *Bull. Soc. Neuchatel. Sci. Nat.* **2005**, *128*, 71–80.

29. Slim, K.; Fadel, A.; Atoui, A.; Lemaire, B.J.; Vinçon-Leite, B.; Tassin, B. Global warming as a driving factor for cyanobacterial blooms in Lake Karaoun, Lebanon. *Desalination Water Treat.* **2014**, *52*, 2094–2101.

30. Atoui, A.; Hafez, H.; Slim, K. Occurrence of toxic cyanobacterial blooms for the first time in Lake Karaoun, Lebanon. *Water Environ. J.* **2013**, *27*, 42–49.

31. Pollingher, U. Phytoplankton periodicity in a subtropical lake (Lake Kinneret, Israel). *Hydrobiologia* **1986**, *138*, 127–138.

32. Chen, Y.; Qin, B.; Teubner, K.; Dokulil, M.T. Long-term dynamics of phytoplankton assemblages: *Microcystis*-domination in Lake Taihu, a large shallow lake in China. *J. Plankton Res.* **2003**, *25*, 445–453.

33. Moreno-Ostos, E.; Cruz-Pizarro, L.; Basanta-Alvés, A.; Escot, C.; George, D.G. Algae in the motion: Spatial distribution of phytoplankton in thermally stratified reservoirs. *Limnetica.* **2006**, *25*, 205–216.

34. Whitton, B.; Potts, M.; Oliver, R.; Ganf, G. Freshwater Blooms. In *The Ecology of Cyanobacteria*; Springer Netherlands: Dordrecht, The Netherlands, 2002; pp. 149–194.

35. Smith, V.H.; Bierman, V.J.; Jones, B.L.; Havens, K.E. Historical trends in the Lake Okeechobee ecosystem IV. Nitrogen:phosphorus ratios, cyanobacterial dominance, and nitrogen fixation potential. *Arch. Hydrobiol.* **1995**, *107*, 71–88.

36. Gophen, M.; Smith, V.H.; Nishri, A.; Threlkeld, S.T. Nitrogen deficiency, phosphorus sufficiency, and the invasion of Lake Kinneret, Israel, by the N2-fixing cyanobacterium *Aphanizomenon ovalisporum. Aquat. Sci.* **1999**, *61*, 293–306.

37. Hadas, O.; Pinkas, R.; Malinsky-Rushansky, N.; Nishri, A.; Kaplan, A.; Rimmer, A.; Sukenik, A. Appearance and establishment of diazotrophic cyanobacteria in Lake Kinneret, Israel. *Freshw. Biol.* **2012**, *57*, 1214–1227.

38. Vinçon-Leite, B.; Lemaire, B.J.; Khac, V.; Tassin, B. Long-term temperature evolution in a deep sub-alpine lake, Lake Bourget, France: How a one-dimensional model improves its trend assessment. *Hydrobiologia* **2014**, 1–16.

39. Wu, Q.L.; Hahn, M.W. High predictability of the seasonal dynamics of a species-like *Polynucleobacter* population in a freshwater lake. *Environ. Microbiol.* **2006**, *8*, 1660–1666.

40. Peeters, F.; Livingstone, D.M.; Goudsmit, G.H.; Kipfer, R.; Forster, R. Modeling 50 years of historical temperature profiles in a large central European lake. *Limnol. Oceanogr.* **2002**, *47*, 186–197.

41. Everson, S.; Fabbro, L.; Kinnear, S.; Eaglesham, G.; Wright, P. Distribution of the cyanobacterial toxins cylindrospermopsin and deoxycylindrospermopsin in a stratified lake in north-eastern New South Wales, Australia. *Mar. Freshw. Res.* **2009**, *60*, 25–33.

42. Shaw, G.R.; Sukenik, A.; Livne, A.; Chiswell, R.K.; Smith, M.J.; Seawright, A.A.; Norris, R.L.; Eaglesham, G.K.; Moore, M.R. Blooms of the cylindrospermopsin containing cyanobacterium, *Aphanizomenon ovalisporum* (Forti), in newly constructed lakes, Queensland, Australia. *Environ. Toxicol.* **1999**, *14*, 167–177.

43. Ho, L.; Sawade, E.; Newcombe, G. Biological treatment options for cyanobacteria metabolite removal: A review. *Water Res.* **2012**, *46*, 1536–1548.

44. Smith, M.J.; Shaw, G.R.; Eaglesham, G.K.; Ho, L.; Brookes, J.D. Elucidating the factors influencing the biodegradation of cylindrospermopsin in drinking water sources. *Environ. Toxicol.* **2008**, *23*, 413–421.

45. Wörmer, L.; Cirés, S.; Carrasco, D.; Quesada, A. Cylindrospermopsin is not degraded by co-occurring natural bacterial communities during a 40-day study. *Harmful Algae* **2008**, *7*, 206–213.

46. Cyanobacteria and Cyanotoxins: Information for Drinking Water Systems. Available online: http://water.epa.gov/scitech/swguidance/standards/criteria/nutrients/upload/cyanobacteria_factsheet.pdf (accessed on 23 October 2014).

47. Fadel, A.; Lemaire, B.J.; Atoui, A.; Vinçon-Leite, B.; Amacha, N.; Slim, K.; Tassin, B. First assessment of the ecological status of Karaoun Reservoir, Lebanon. *Lakes Res.* **2014**, *19*, 142–157.

48. Komárek, J.; Anagnostidis, K. Cyanoprokaryota, part 1: Chroococcales. In *Süßwasserflora von Mitteleuropa*; Elsevier: Heidelberg, Germany, 1998.

49. Komárek, J.; Anagnostidis, K. Cyanoprokaryota, part 2: Oscillatoriales. In *Süsswasserflora von Mitteleuropa*; Elsevier: Heidelberg, Germany, 2005.

50. Humpage, A.R.; Froscio, S.M.; Lau, H.M.; Murphy, D.; Blackbeard, J. Evaluation of the Abraxis Strip Test for Microcystins™ for use with wastewater effluent and reservoir water. *Water Res.* **2012**, *46*, 1556–1565.

The Fate of Microcystins in the Environment and Challenges for Monitoring

Justine R. Schmidt, Steven W. Wilhelm and Gregory L. Boyer

Abstract: Microcystins are secondary metabolites produced by cyanobacteria that act as hepatotoxins in higher organisms. These toxins can be altered through abiotic processes, such as photodegradation and adsorption, as well as through biological processes via metabolism and bacterial degradation. Some species of bacteria can degrade microcystins, and many other organisms metabolize microcystins into a series of conjugated products. There are toxicokinetic models used to examine microcystin uptake and elimination, which can be difficult to compare due to differences in compartmentalization and speciation. Metabolites of microcystins are formed as a detoxification mechanism, and little is known about how quickly these metabolites are formed. In summary, microcystins can undergo abiotic and biotic processes that alter the toxicity and structure of the microcystin molecule. The environmental impact and toxicity of these alterations and the metabolism of microcystins remains uncertain, making it difficult to establish guidelines for human health. Here, we present the current state of knowledge regarding the alterations microcystins can undergo in the environment.

Reprinted from *Toxins*. Cite as: Schmidt, J.R.; Wilhelm, S.W.; Boyer, G.L. The Fate of Microcystins in the Environment and Challenges for Monitoring. *Toxins* **2014**, *6*, 3354-3387.

1. Introduction

Cyanobacteria (blue-green algae) are photosynthetic organisms found in both marine and freshwater environments. These organisms can be benthic or pelagic [1]. Selected strains of cyanobacteria are capable of fixing atmospheric nitrogen, giving them a competitive edge over other algal species [1,2]. Cyanobacteria can also avoid predation by forming colonies and elongated shapes, making predatory grazing difficult [3]. Many species of cyanobacteria produce secondary metabolites, some of which are toxic to higher organisms [4]. Toxic metabolites are classified into four categories: hepatotoxins, dermatoxins, neurotoxins and cytotoxins [5–7]. The occurrence of algal blooms has increased over time [8], and anthropogenic input of phosphorus and nitrogen into natural water bodies are contributors to this increase in toxic algal blooms [9]. The risk to human health due to the increasing presence of these toxins is of concern [9–11].

Microcystins are a group of over 90 hepatotoxins produced by cyanobacteria, of which microcystin-LR (MC-LR) is the most common [7,12,13] (Figure 1). Their toxicities resulted from the inhibition of protein phosphatases and disrupted formation of the cytoskeleton [7]. They also promote oxidative stress in liver tissues [2]. Microcystins can be introduced to tissues of organisms through the diet or by ingestion of contaminated water [2,14,15]. The log of the octanol/water distribution ratio, (*i.e.*, $\log D_{ow}$ in reference [16]) of microcystin-LR is approximately -1 at pH 7 (estimated from Figure 2 in reference [16]), indicating that microcystins are readily water-soluble and not likely to passively diffuse into tissues from the surrounding water. Instead, microcystins accumulate in the liver via the bile acid transport system [7,14,17,18]. The bile acid transport system is comprised of proteins that actively transport peptides and biliary acids into hepatocytes [19]. The methyl-dehydroalanine (Mdha) and 3-amino-9-methyoxy-2,6,8-trimethyl-10-phenyl-4,6-decadienoic acid (ADDA) groups are integral to binding of microcystins to protein phosphatases in organisms (Figure 1) [20].

The toxicity of microcystins varies according to the combination of amino acids at the two variable positions on the peptide ring (Figure 1) [12,21]. The oral LD_{50} for MC-LR in rats and mice is 5 mg/kg of body weight [22,23]. For comparison, the oral LD_{50} for cyanide is 3 mg/kg of body weight [24]. The oral LD_{50} for microcystin-RR (MC-RR), a microcystin congener with two arginine groups attached to the peptide ring, is ten-fold higher than that of MC-LR [23]. The LD_{50} for MC-RR and MC-LR administered intraperitoneally in mice are 235.4 and 43 µg/kg body weight, respectively [15]. MC-RR is more polar than MC-LR and is not as easily transported via the bile acid transport system as MC-LR, hence the observed difference in toxicity [12]. Microcystin-LA (MC-LA), which has leucine and alanine at the two variable positions on the peptide ring, has an intraperitoneal LD_{50} identical to that of MC-LR [25–28]. Different microcystin congeners vary in their response to the protein phosphatase inhibition assay (PPIA). For example, the half maximal inhibitory concentrations (IC_{50}) ranged from below 0.06 µg/mL for [D-Asp3, Z-Dhb7] MC-LR to greater than 10 µg/mL for MC-RR in the PPIA [29]. MC-LR is an environmental health concern due to its widespread presence in freshwater bodies worldwide.

Figure 1. The structure of microcystin-LR. The 3-amino-9-methyoxy-2,6,8-trimethyl-10-phenyl-4,6-decadienoic (ADDA) and methyl-dehydroalanine (Mdha) groups are important in binding of microcystin-LR to the protein phosphatase enzyme. The microcystin ring system contains two variable sites (A and B), which can contain variable amino acids. This forms the basis of microcystin nomenclature. Microcystin-LR contains leucine at site A and arginine at site B, microcystin-RR contains arginine at both sites, *etc.*

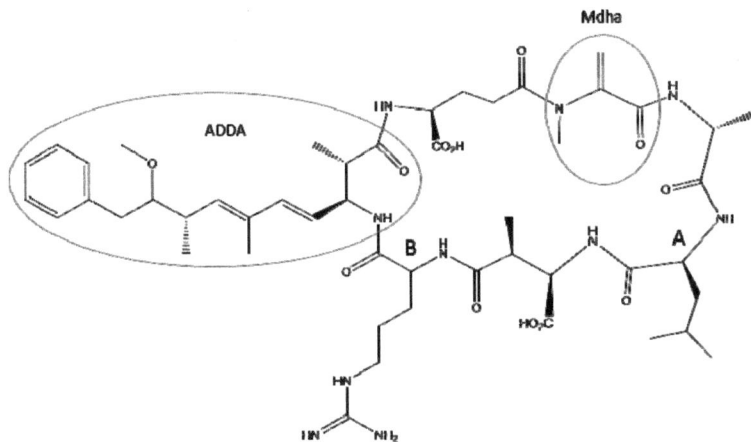

Human exposure to microcystins is recognized as a global health issue [9–11]. Incidents of human sickening [30] and death [31] due to microcystin exposure have been documented. Microcystin exposure may promote liver tumors [32] and has been linked to liver cancer in humans [33]. Chronic exposure to low levels of microcystins can promote the growth of tumors in the liver and other organs [23]. Human health guidelines have been made for the unaltered toxins in water and in tissues [23,34,35], but updating these regulations to include correction factors for environmental alterations is a challenging problem. The environmental fate of microcystins affects its impact on human health.

1.1. Abiotic Transformations

Dilution is a major process by which microcystin toxicity is reduced in natural waters [36,37]. Microcystins are released into the surrounding environment after a bloom senesces or cells are ruptured. Dilution of microcystins occurs when they are introduced to a large volume of water, such as that of a lake. However, dilution may not always reduce microcystin abundance below the critical point for organisms, as some deep oligotrophic lakes are also subject to toxic algal blooms [38]. Breakdown of microcystins due to high temperatures has also been cited as a means for detoxification [23,39]. However, thermal decomposition is usually partnered under laboratory conditions with low pH to increase the degradation rate, as microcystins are stable at high temperatures and can withstand boiling [23,36].

Microcystins are adsorbed onto suspended particulate matter (SPM) in aquatic systems [40,41]. Adsorption by SPM is an important mechanism of removal for contaminants in both freshwater and marine environments [41,42]. This process limits exposure of fish and other biota to free microcystins by binding to particles and may decrease the risk of microcystin food web transfer [41,43]. The extent to which microcystin is adsorbed by SPM is a function of the pH [16].

The microcystin molecule contains two carboxyl groups and one amino group not built into the peptide ring, which are able to be ionized (Figure 1) [44]. However, the very low pH necessary to ionize these carboxylic acid groups (approximately pH 2.1) is rarely seen in natural systems [16]. The pH of a water body increases during a productive algal bloom and can exceed pH 8 due to the consumption of dissolved carbon dioxide [45,46]. The adsorption of microcystins onto SPM is dependent on the hydrophilicity of the microcystin congeners at pH ranges found in natural waters (e.g., pH 6–9).

Despite the hydrophilic nature of microcystins in natural systems, microcystins are adsorbed onto sediments. Adsorption to sediments was stronger with more hydrophilic microcystins, such as microcystin-RR (microcystin-arginine and arginine, Figure 1), than with less hydrophilic congeners [37]. The affinity of microcystin-RR for sediments is dependent on the different mechanisms for microcystin adsorption onto particles. Adsorption can begin with hydrophilic groups on the microcystin structure interacting with sediments [37]. The most hydrophobic part of the microcystin molecule, the ADDA moiety (Figure 1), may not strongly interact with sediments. Alternatively, naturally occurring clays can be used to adsorb microcystins via interactions with the ADDA moiety, making hydrophobic binding the dominant process over hydrophilic interactions in these cases [40]. The precise mechanism for binding of microcystins to sediments is uncertain.

Microcystins are also subject to transformation from exposure to sunlight in the presence of photosensitizers [47,48]. Isomerization of the conjugated ADDA side chain from the "E" to "Z" configuration of the microcystin molecule can occur [49–51]. This process requires low concentrations of photosensitizers, such as humic acids or pigments; microcystins cannot be transformed by sunlight alone [47,48,52]. The rate of microcystin transformation by light is dependent on several factors, including pH, concentration of humic acids and wavelength of light. In natural systems, large concentrations of humic acids may shield microcystins from being altered by sunlight, which explains the persistence of microcystins in water samples exposed to lower energy ultraviolet light and sunlight [43,51,53].

Breakdown of microcystins can also occur through photodegradation [36,43,49]. MC-LR has been degraded at the conjugated diene and aromatic ring of ADDA and at the double bond at the Mdha position using titanium oxide in the presence of ultraviolet light or coupled hydrogen peroxide and an iron-yttrium complex in the presence of visible light [41,53–57]. Complete degradation of microcystins was observed within five days using 365-nm light and within only 1 h using 254-nm light [43]. The majority of MC-LR (79%) was degraded when exposed to the full spectrum of ultraviolet light for 22 days [52]. The half-life of MC-LR in a natural system is estimated at 90–120 days per meter of water depth [48]. A decrease in the pH of a water body will increase the rate of microcystin photolysis [51], but the pH of the surrounding water increases during a productive algal bloom. Thus, the transformation of microcystins is only significant in shallow water bodies due to the availability of sunlight [48]. High pH and high concentrations of humic acids may prevent exposure of organisms to critical levels of microcystins in natural systems.

1.2. Biological Processes

1.2.1. Microbial Degradation

Microbial degradation of microcystins has been confirmed as a detoxification mechanism in selected strains of fungi [58,59] and bacteria [60–62]. In selected strains of bacteria, three enzymes collectively referred to as microcystinase operate in a sequential pathway to degrade MC-LR [61]. The first enzyme linearizes MC-LR through the cleavage of the peptide ring at the ADDA-arginine bond. The second enzyme cleaves this linear intermediate at the alanine-leucine bond, yielding a peptide intermediate of ADDA-Glu-Mdha-Ala (Figure 2) [60–62]. The final enzyme degrades the products formed by the first two enzymes and liberates ADDA from the tetrapeptide intermediate (Figure 2). ADDA is non-toxic up to 10 mg/kg [63].

Degradation of MC-LR in a laboratory study began almost immediately once the bacterium *Sphingopyxis* sp. C-1 was introduced to MC-LR [64]. After 24 h, 25% of the MC-LR was degraded. The levels of MC-LR were at or below the World Health Organization "safe" level of 1 μg/L in drinking water by the eighth day of treatment with *Sphingopyxis* sp. C-1 [27]. Bacterial degradation contributes to the detoxification of microcystins in a laboratory setting at neutral pH.

Figure 2. Degradation pathway of microcystin-LR by bacteria. The first step is the cleavage of the peptide ring at the ADDA-arginine bond, followed by subsequent degradation of the linear microcystin-LR product to yield a tetrapeptide intermediate and the ADDA moiety. Sites of enzymatic cleavage are indicated with dashed lines (derived from mechanism proposed by [60]).

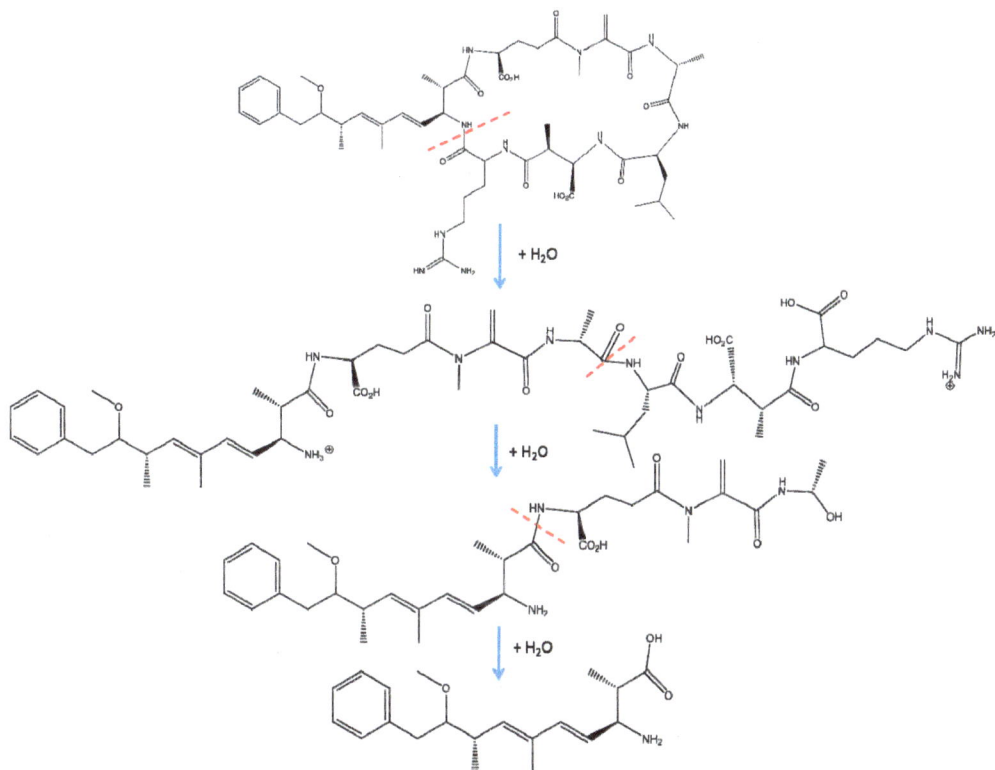

Bacteria that thrive in water with productive algal blooms need to be tolerant of alkaline conditions [46]. The maximum degradation rate of MC-LR was observed between pH 6.5 and 8.5 for *Sphingopyxis* sp. C-1, an alkaline-tolerant bacterium, even though the optimal pH for growth of the bacterium was at approximately pH 7.0 [65]. Immediately after MC-LR was added to lake water containing native microbes and a culture of the microcystin-producing cyanobacterium, *Microcystis aeruginosa*, degradation of MC-LR was initiated, and the diversity of microbes increased [66]. The microbial community surrounding a cyanobacterial bloom in natural environments may vary by location [67]. *Oscillatoriales*, *Chroococcales* and *Nostocales* were dominant in three lakes with toxic blooms over two continents, indicating that the bacterial community in a toxic bloom at a phylogenetic level is conserved across lakes [67]. The phyla of the bacterial communities in these lakes were different; genetic signatures for nitrogen uptake in Lake Erie and Grand Lake St. Marys in North America were dominated by cyanobacteria, whereas the bacterial community in Lake Tai, China, was dominated by Proteobacteria [67]. In Lake Tai, certain species of eubacteria may be closely linked to blooms and could potentially use toxins produced by the bloom event as a carbon source [68].

Although bacteria are numerous and very diverse, not all bacterial strains are able to break down microcystins. Selected strains of *Sphingomonas sp.* and *Sphingopyxis sp.* are capable of microcystin degradation [61,64,69–71]. Novel bacterial species that degrade microcystins have also been identified in water [72,73]. Lahti *et al.* (1998) characterized 17 strains of bacteria that degrade microcystins [74]. Berg (2009) identified 460 strains of bacteria present in water bodies with frequent cyanobacterial blooms, in which *Sphingomonas* was the dominant species [75]. Microcystins could accumulate and remain in the water column if the particular bacterial strains that degrade microcystins are not present during a toxic bloom [69,74]. Bacterial species capable of degrading microcystins have also been identified in soils [28].

1.2.2. Metabolism and Conjugation

The ADDA group on MC-LR is important for the binding of the toxin to its target enzyme, protein phosphatases 1 and 2A [76]. The Mdha group in microcystins can subsequently covalently bind to a cysteine in a protein phosphatase enzyme [20]. Microcystins permanently block the active site and destroy the functionality of the protein phosphatase enzyme. Organisms subject to microcystin exposure have developed detoxification mechanisms to resist microcystin intoxication. Animal metabolism utilizes two classes of enzymes to eliminate xenobiotics [77,78]. The primary phase I enzymes are usually the cytochrome P-450 enzymes, which catalyze the addition of oxygen-containing groups to toxins through oxidation-reduction reactions. Products of phase I enzymes are often reactive and could negatively affect the cell if not metabolized further by phase II enzymes. These products are then conjugated to glucuronic acid, sulfates or peptides to prevent cellular damage [78].

Glutathione (GSH) is a common peptide used in phase II biotransformations (Figure 3) [78]. Formation of the glutathione conjugate by the phase II enzyme, glutathione-*S*-transferase (GST), is one of the most common types of xenobiotic modification. This reaction occurs between a nucleophilic center on the toxin and the sulfhydryl group of the reduced glutathione (Figure 3) [79]. In microcystins (Figure 1), this nucleophilic center is provided by the Mdha group. Conjugation of GSH to a xenobiotic increases its water-solubility so that the toxin can be eliminated. Glutathione-conjugated xenobiotics can be eliminated via bile [80,81], although this is rare [78].

GSH-conjugation is often the first in a series of metabolic alterations to a xenobiotic, ultimately producing an *N*-acetyl-cysteine (mercapturic acid) conjugate that is quickly excreted by the organism (Figure 3) [78]. The γ-glutamic acid group of the GSH molecule is enzymatically cleaved by gamma glutamyl transferase, forming the γ-glutamylcysteine intermediate (Figure 3) [78,82]. The glycine of this γ-glutamylcysteine intermediate is then cleaved by a dipeptidase to yield the cysteine-conjugated product, which is subsequently oxidized to form the mercapturic acid metabolite (Figure 3) [78]. This mercapturic acid derivative is easily excreted in urine, although there is potential for the other conjugates in the metabolic pathway to be removed from cells for excretion [78]. A glutathione-*S*-pump is an active transport protein, which moves GSH-conjugated toxins out of cells and could potentially transport microcystins, although no experiments with this pump transporting MC-LR-GSH have been conducted [83–85].

The processing of MC-LR either occurs via irreversible covalent binding to proteins or biotransformation through the glutathione pathway into intermediate products (Figure 3) [86–90]. It is assumed that covalently-bound microcystins are not a major vector for microcystin exposure [91]. However, bound microcystins have the potential to be cleaved enzymatically, releasing peptide fragments, which can be liberated from tissues [92,93]. These microcystins with their attached peptide fragments still possess some degree of protein phosphatase inhibition by PPIA [92]. This represents an additional pool of potentially toxic microcystin analogs in the cell. These fragments could be released over a period of time as enzymatic cleavage occurs, creating another source of microcystins for potential exposure to organisms.

Conjugation of microcystins to GSH or other proteins is a major portion of the microcystin pool in natural systems [91]. Proteins that microcystins can bind to may be within the toxic bloom itself rather than in the cells of an exposed organism. Microcystins can bind to cysteine residues in several proteins in *Microcystis* through a Michael addition in the same manner as they conjugate to GSH [94]. This binding occurs more rapidly when *Microcystis* cells are under oxidative stress, which is similar to the intercellular environment of organisms in the presence of microcystins [94]. These conjugated microcystins may not be detected using traditional analytical methods, such as LC-MS or ELISA, due to the many possible proteins that can react with microcystins [91,95].

Studies on the zooplankton, *Daphnia magna*, the freshwater mussel, *Dreissena polymorpha*, and the macrophyte, *Ceratophyllum demersum*, suggest that the first step in the biotransformation pathway is the attachment of glutathione onto the Mdha residue of MC-LR [87,89]. This pathway is conserved between these highly diverse organisms. The glutathione conjugate is enzymatically converted into the cysteine conjugate through a cysteine-glycine intermediate. The final conjugate formed in this biochemical pathway is the mercapturic acid conjugate (Figure 3). Free (unconjugated) MC-LR can be eliminated via urine and feces in mice [96] and bivalves [97,98]. Conjugate intermediates have also been detected in feces [18] and bile [78,99–101] of rats. MC-LR-GSH was concentrated in feces in rats, and MC-LR-Cys was concentrated in kidneys, indicative of excretion [18]. Both the glutathione-conjugated MC-LR (MC-LR-GSH) and cysteine-conjugated microcystin-LR (MC-LR-Cys) conjugates have been identified in mice [85,102], rats [103], fish [104–108], shrimp [106] and snails [106]. The MC-LR-GSH conjugate has also been identified in humans [109].

These biological detoxification pathways are important in determining the toxicity of microcystins in an ecosystem. Biotransformation removes microcystins from the organism and releases them back into the environment. MC-LR-GSH is three- to ten-times less toxic to mammals than free MC-LR [18,110,111]. The effects of the glutathione and cysteine conjugates of MC-LR are the same as those noted from exposure to free toxin, such as hepatocyte damage [18,110,112]. Non-covalently bound MC-LR in zooplankton was readily taken up by the intestines of the planktivorous sunfish, *Lepomis gibbosus* [113]. More than 80% of free, non-covalently bound microcystin in the zooplankton *Bosmina* fed to *Lepomis gibbosus* was directly transferred to the sunfish. Free and conjugated microcystin-LR (MC-LR-GSH, MC-LR-Cys, *etc.*) can travel up the aquatic food web [113]. MC-LR was more efficiently transferred between organisms using zooplankton as a vector than by direct transfer of the toxin to *Lepomis gibbosus* through exposure to contaminated water. However, these results are complicated by the use of the enzyme-linked immunosorbent assay (ELISA) to determine microcystin concentrations in tissues. Matrix effects from tissue extracts complicate the use of ELISA to determine microcystin concentrations below 5.9 µg/kg dry weight [114]. MC-LR and its conjugates could transfer to organisms after excretion and be released into the environment [113]. *Daphnia* has been implicated as a potential vector for food web transfer of microcystins due to its consumption of toxic cyanobacteria as a food source [115].

The World Health Organization (WHO) has instituted a daily tolerable intake for lifetime human exposure of MC-LR of 0.04 µg/kg of body weight/day limit from food, based on studies in rats [22,23,27]. This has been expanded upon to create seasonal daily exposure tolerable intake of MC-LR in food of 300 µg/kg of food for adults and 40 µg/kg of food for children [34]. An acceptable daily limit of 39 µg/kg of fish for adults (aged 17 and above) and 24 µg/kg of fish for children (aged 2–16) was derived based on the No Observed Adverse Effect Level (NOAEL) of 40 µg/kg/day [35]. However, these regulations are based on the toxicity of the parent toxin, not the metabolic products.

It is currently uncertain if microcystins bioaccumulate in organisms or if they biomagnify in food webs. Bioaccumulation is defined as the concentration of a compound in a specimen being higher than that of its surrounding environment, including water and food, and biomagnification is defined as the concentration of a compound being increased from one trophic level to another in a food web [116,117]. Microcystins can bioaccumulate in the liver, muscle and viscera of the omnivorous fish, *Tilapia rendalli* [118]. No microcystins were detected in the phytoplankton samples collected from the lagoon field site, but microcystins were detected in fish tissues. Similarly, microcystins were detected in the tissues of the freshwater mussel, *Anodonta grandis simpsoniana*, despite microcystin levels in the surrounding water being below detection [119]. In both cases, the levels detected in tissues were above the WHO guideline for human exposure to MC-LR [118,119]. Differences in microcystin content by trophic level have been observed. MC-LR, MC-RR and microcystin-YR were detected in fish from Lake Tai, China, with the highest levels found in omnivorous fish, followed by phytoplanktivorous fish and carnivorous fish [120]. This observed accumulation of microcystins in tissue after toxin levels were reduced below detection in water could reflect a retention of toxins in the tissue after toxins had disappeared from the water column. This could also reflect bound microcystins being gradually released within the tissue in the form of microcystin-containing peptide fragments [92].

Figure 3. Glutathione metabolic pathway for microcystin-LR. Metabolic alteration using the glutathione pathway occurs at the double bond of the methyl-dehydroalanine (Mdha) position on the peptide ring. The 3-amino-9-methyoxy-2,6,8-trimethyl-10-phenyl-4,6-decadienoic acid (ADDA) group is responsible for non-covalent binding to protein phosphatase. After the first enzymatic step, microcystin-LR is represented by a rectangle for each step, with the chemical structure of the metabolically altered groups drawn out. Glutathione is attached to the Mdha group of microcystin-LR through glutathione-S-transferase, forming the microcystin-LR-glutathione conjugate. The gamma-glutamic acid group is removed by gamma-glutamyltransferase, yielding the microcystin-LR-cysteine-glycine conjugate. The glycine group of the microcystin-LR-cysteine-glycine conjugate is removed by dipeptidase, forming the microcystin-LR-cysteine conjugate. This microcystin-LR-cysteine conjugate is oxidized through acetyl transferase, forming the microcystin-LR-mercapturic acid conjugate.

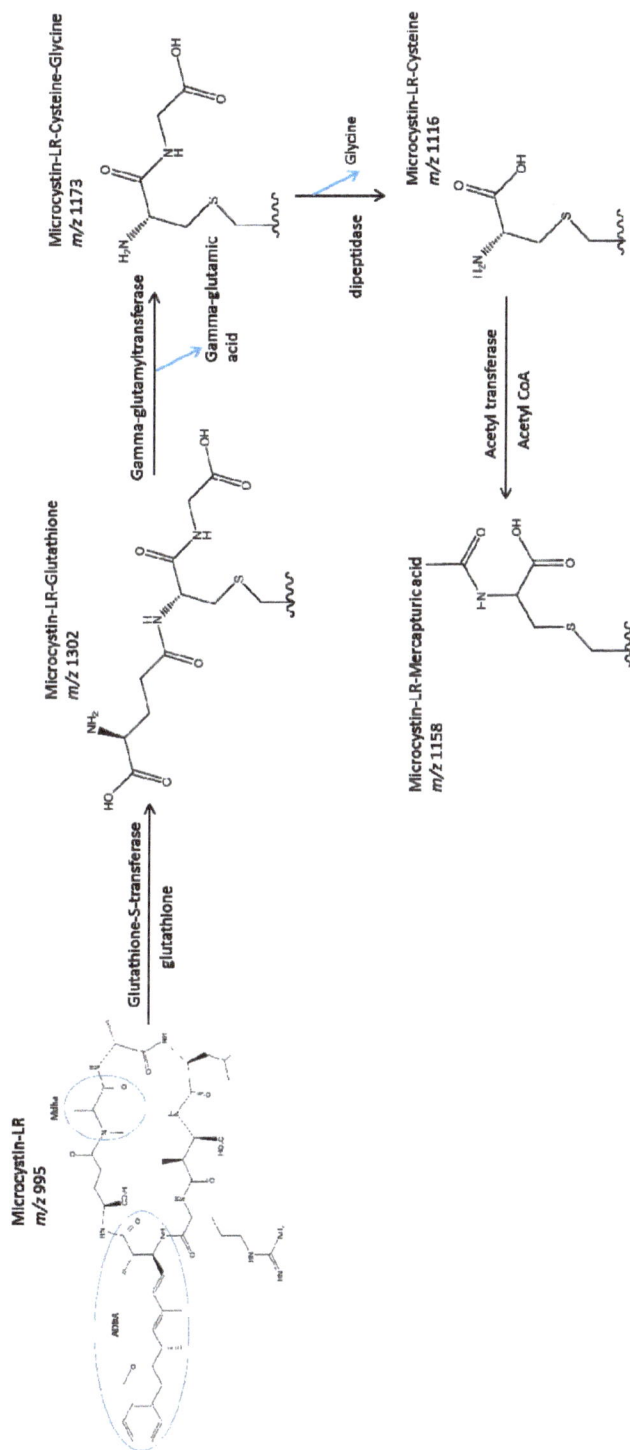

Bioaccumulation of microcystins into fish tissues is also complicated by the high variability of toxin concentration in natural systems [95,121]. Out of five species of fish taken from Grand Lake St. Marys in Ohio, USA, only two had detectable levels of MC-LR in muscle tissues [95]. This implicates a species-dependent mechanism of MC-LR uptake into fish. However, fish of the same species had a range of toxin values from non-detection to as high as 70 µg/kg, which is over three orders of magnitude above the World Health Organization guideline for tissue [95]. There is clearly variation in toxin uptake between individual fish of the same species, as well, which can be a major complicating factor when addressing human health guidelines. Even if a safe toxin threshold value is established for consumption of fish tissues of a particular species, it is impossible to determine if any given fish is below this threshold or orders of magnitude above it.

Some ecosystems have organisms with consistently high levels of microcystins in their tissues. Amrani *et al.* (2014) reported that common carp muscle was over the 0.04 µg/kg of the body weight/day guideline value from food over a one-year period of monitoring carp tissue using PPIA [122]. Both PPIA and ELISA are subject to interferences from tissue matrices [95]. Peng *et al.* (2010) reported that aquatic organisms from three lakes in China were as high as 148 times the WHO safe guideline value of 0.04 µg/kg body weight/day [123]. Over half of the fish tissues from Lake Tai in China contained levels of microcystins over the WHO guideline using tandem mass spectrometry [124]. Organisms from these Chinese lakes were considered potentially harmful to humans if consumed.

There is also evidence for biodilution, rather than biomagnification, of microcystins in aquatic food webs. Biodilution is defined as the concentration of a parent analyte (not metabolically altered) decreasing in organisms as the trophic level increases [125,126]. Accumulation of microcystins in tissues is dependent on the species [95,127]. Biodilution is dominant over biomagnification in most aquatic species, with the exceptions being zooplankton and planktivorous fish [113,127]. The entire body of the organism is generally used for toxin analysis when examining zooplankton and planktivorous fish tissues, which could account for the observed biomagnification in these species.

No evidence of bioaccumulation was found in shrimp, mussels, frogs or fish in a eutrophic lake [128]. Rather, the tissue microcystin concentration was at or below that of the phytoplankton in the lake water. The concentration of microcystins in tissues in the literature may be skewed due to comparisons between individual organs and whole organisms, such as zooplankton, giving a false impression of biomagnification [129].

2. Degree of Resistance to Microcystin Toxicity

Organisms can avoid microcystin intoxication through adaptations in their diet. Selected species of fish and zooplankton will preferentially graze on non-toxic phytoplankton when both a toxic and non-toxic strain are present [46]. By avoiding consumption of toxic algal strains, organisms reduce their risk of microcystin exposure. In environments where this selectivity is not possible, such as water bodies with very large toxic blooms, organisms can adapt by developing a tolerance to microcystin toxicity [118,130,131].

The degree to which an organism is resistant to microcystin toxicity is variable between species. Bivalves, such as *Dreissena polymorpha* and *Mytilus galloprovincialis*, can acclimate to microcystin exposure and accumulate measurable concentrations of microcystins in their tissues without mortality [86,97,132–137]. Some species of *Daphnia* also show variable sensitivity to microcystin exposure [138].

2.1. Terrestrial Organisms vs. Aquatic Organisms

There is a difference in the physiological response to microcystin toxicity between terrestrial and aquatic organisms. Oral LD_{50} measurements for microcystins are based upon rat and mouse bioassays [22,23]. Mouse mortalities from microcystin exposure resulted from hemorrhaging of hepatocytes [22]. Fish in laboratory studies dosed with microcystins can remain alive longer and at higher levels of toxin than mice [139,140]. Rainbow trout did not experience mortality when exposed to not only higher doses of microcystins than mice, but also when exposed to a longer duration of microcystin exposure [141]. There were no signs of hepatocyte hemorrhage in rainbow trout as observed in mice [141,142]. Mice that overexpressed a transcription factor associated with preventing cellular damage due to oxidative stress experienced less liver damage than mice without this overexpression when exposed to microcystin-LA [142]. Mice may thus have a mechanism for the prevention of hepatocyte damage due to microcystin exposure that is induced by oxidative stress [142].

Rats showed signs of liver hemorrhage rather than kidney damage, as seen in selected species of fish [141,143]. Hepatocyte hemorrhage was not observed in rainbow trout exposed to MC-LR, differing from studies in rats and other fish, indicating that rainbow trout may be more tolerant of microcystin exposure than other organisms [141]. Fish may have a mechanism through urinary elimination of microcystins from the liver that differs from that of rats that decreases hepatocyte damage due to microcystin exposure. Selected species of fish in environments prone to toxic blooms must have a mechanism for quick, efficient removal of microcystins to prevent mortality.

Aquatic organisms exposed to microcystins may also develop a resistance to intoxication and can adapt to toxic environments. Nymphs of the burrowing mayfly, *Hexagenia*, were able to withstand MC-LR levels up to 10 μg/L MC-LR, a concentration recorded during a very toxic bloom in a highly eutrophic lake in North America [144,145]. Only 10% of hatchlings at the WHO guideline of 1 μg/L for drinking water died during one week of exposure, and only 20% died after one week of 10 μg/L MC-LR exposure. Large nymphs experienced less mortality than smaller nymphs, though this could be due to a difference in the surface-to-volume ratio between organisms. Alternately, larger nymphs may have more developed metabolic pathways to detoxify MC-LR than younger ones. Since *Hexagenia* were taken from water bodies with histories of toxic algal blooms, these particular organisms may have developed a resistance to MC-LR due to prior exposure to the toxin, enabling them to withstand exposure to high concentrations [145].

2.2. Bivalves

Studies on freshwater bivalves have shown measureable concentrations of microcystins in the viscera [86,97,132–136]. Little to no animal mortalities were reported in these studies, indicating that these organisms may have a higher resistance to microcystins than other organisms [136]. In the freshwater mussel, *Mytilus galloprovincialis*, an increase in GST activity in the gut and a marked decrease in GST activity in the labial palps were observed when exposed to MC-LR. The labial palps may act as a control on the concentration of microcystin taken into the gut of the bivalve, as secretion of mucus by these organs would restrict intake of toxic *Microcystis* [136].

Bivalves may also resist microcystin toxicity through expulsion of *Microcystis* in the form of pseudofeces [135,136]. *Dreissena polymorpha* is indiscriminate in the uptake of cyanobacterial strains as a food resource, regardless of toxicity [134]. However, *D. polymorpha* will produce pseudofeces in the presence of toxic cyanobacteria [98]. In the laboratory, *D. polymorpha* was exposed to both toxic *Microcystis aeruginosa* and the non-toxic diatom, *Asterionella formosa* [135]. Pseudofeces produced by these zebra mussels contained mostly *Microcystis*, not the non-toxic diatom. Thus, zebra mussels were selectivity avoiding *Microcystis* [135]. A subsequent experiment that would provide more data on whether bivalves are selectively avoiding toxic *Microcystis* is to feed both toxic and non-toxic *Microcystis* to these bivalves and observe which food is eaten and excreted. This way, differences in the morphology and size of the two foods can be better controlled. Bivalves in general may have a greater resistance to toxicity than other organisms [137]. An increase in the multidrug resistance protein activity was immediately observed when *Dreissena polymorpha* was exposed to MC-LR, as well as other xenobiotics [137]. Bivalves may be better equipped than other aquatic organisms for resisting toxicity [137].

2.3. Fish

Development of microcystin tolerance has been documented in fish. The physiological response of fish to microcystins can be attributed to several factors, including the length of time of exposure and dosage [139,141]. The age and size of the fish may also be a factor, as the concentration of microcystins in muscle tissue decreased with the length of the fish [146]. Microcystin levels were over 500 µg/g dry weight from algal samples from Grand Lake St. Marys in Ohio, USA, in 2010 [95]. Fish collected in 2011 and 2012 had detectable levels of MC-LR in their muscle tissues, whereas water samples collected during 2011 and 2012 did not show microcystin concentrations above the detection limit by LC-MS(/MS) [95]. The persistence of MC-LR in fish tissues when no microcystins were detected in the lake water indicates that these fish may accumulate the toxins and may have a mechanism protecting them from experiencing mortality from microcystin exposure.

The goldfish, *Carassius auratus* L., accumulated MC-LR in the liver after intraperitoneal injection [140]. The concentration of MC-LR in liver cells increased between 0 and 48 h of microcystin exposure [140]. The ionic homeostasis of all test organisms remained unaffected by MC-LR addition, despite high levels of MC-LR. However, a rapid decrease in liver MC-LR concentration and recovery of damaged hepatocytes were observed after 48 h. A similar trend was observed in the common carp, *Cyprinus carpio* L. [139]. Damage to kidneys observed both in goldfish and in carp indicated that MC-LR was passing through kidney cells to be excreted [139,140]. MC-LR and the MC-LR-Cys conjugate were found in the kidney tissues of fish from Chinese lakes, implicating the kidney as an excretory route for MC-LR and its metabolites [106,147].

2.4. Zooplankton

Zooplankton are an important part of the food web in natural systems and exhibit species-dependent degrees of resistance to microcystin toxicity. The rate of zooplankton grazing on cyanobacteria is not dependent on microcystin concentration alone. Cyanobacteria can produce secondary metabolites, such as protease inhibitors and other anti-feedants, which reduce grazing by zooplankton [2,148]. Toxic compounds, such as microcystins, have traditionally been correlated to reduce feeding by zooplankton [149–153]. Grazing on a toxic bloom by *Daphnia sp.* was not inhibited by toxins, despite poisoning of *Daphnia* due to the ingestion of toxic cells indicated by abnormal swimming behavior [154,155]. Cyanobacteria have also been cited as a poor food source for zooplankton due to low fatty acid and overall nutritional content, which could reduce the rate of feeding [149,156–158]. It has also been suggested that *Daphnia* grazing on toxic *Microcystis* strains in an environment where non-toxic *Microcystis* is also growing helps protect the non-toxic strains, as the *Daphnia* feeding rate slows in the presence of the toxin-producing *Microcystis* [159].

MC-LR is a strong inhibitor of protein phosphatases in zooplankton [160]. The copepods, *Acartia bifilosa* and *Eurytemora affinis*, experienced a decrease in survival when exposed to MC-LR in filtered water culture medium at concentrations found in natural water bodies. These copepods were more sensitive to MC-LR than daphnids [161–163]. When toxic blooms are present, copepods have the ability to selectively feed and exclude toxic algae [164]. The copepod *Diaptomus birgei* excluded toxic cyanobacterial strains and also nontoxic cyanobacteria that had a similar morphology to toxin-producing species [151,152,164]. This selectivity provides a mechanism for copepods to prevent microcystin intoxication.

Cladocerans, such as *Daphnia*, are relatively non-selective feeders and cannot exclude toxic cyanobacterial strains from the diet [3]. *Daphnia* of different species do not have equivalent responses to microcystin exposure [138,160,165]. Of four *Daphnia* species examined, *Daphnia magna* was the least resistant to toxicity and experienced feeding inhibition in the presence of toxic *Microcystis* after 1 h of exposure [165]. *D. galeata* did not show any sign of feeding inhibition over a 1-h period under the same feeding conditions as *D. magna*, and the feeding rate of *D. pulex* was more inhibited than that of *D. pulicaria* [160,165]. Other species demonstrated varying degrees of growth inhibition. Both inhibition of feeding and growth indicate that *Daphnia* are negatively affected by the presence of toxic *Microcystis*. Varying sensitivity among species of *Daphnia* is partly due to physiological differences [161].

The age of *Daphnia* also makes a difference in response to microcystins. Younger *Daphnia* may be better adapted to survival in an environment with microcystins, as increased glutathione-S-transferase (GST) activity in response to microcystin toxicity decreased with age [131,166]. The extent of damage to organisms by microcystins varies between *Daphnia* clones, as well as by age, and it can be difficult to assess the organismal effect of microcystin exposure.

Daphnids that had prior microcystin exposure experienced less mortality when exposed to microcystins than species that did not [130,131]. *Daphnia galeata* hatched from resting eggs formed during periods of high microcystin concentration in a eutrophic lake were well-adapted to surviving microcystin exposure [167]. Resting eggs formed during periods of low microcystin concentration experienced higher inhibition of growth when exposed to microcystins [167].

2.5. Detection of Microcystins

Detection of microcystins is a challenging problem for monitoring. Historically, researchers have used antibody-based enzyme-linked immunosorbent assays (ELISAs) to study microcystin concentrations in water and in extracted bloom samples. This strategy is sufficient for relatively clean matrices, like water or algal extracts, but its use becomes limited when applied to fish. ELISAs do not differentiate between free microcystin and its conjugates nor between different congeners of microcystins [168]. In addition, ELISA often cross reacts with other non-microcystin metabolites in tissue, leading to overestimation of the actual toxin concentration in these tissues. Thus, many analyses conducted on tissue matrices using ELISA are susceptible to false positive readings for microcystins. In response, many laboratories have turned to using liquid chromatography tandem mass spectrometry for the analysis of microcystins in fish tissues. This method requires a single transition of the molecular ion to a fragment ion, which is used to identify and quantify the analyte of interest. In tissue matrices, there may be molecules with a mass to charge ratio similar or identical to that of the desired analyte. This can lead to overestimation of the true concentration of microcystins in tissues [169]. Cleanup procedures, including C-18 solid phase extraction cartridges, hexane extraction and charcoal solid phase extraction cartridges, have been used to reduce these interferences. Internal standards, such as thiol-LR, can be used to determine microcystin concentrations in fish tissues through LC-MS analysis, but this does not address the issue of interference from the tissue matrix in the single LC-MS signal of the analyte [170]. A solution to this potential overestimation is through the use of liquid chromatography tandem quadrupole mass spectrometry (LC-MS/MS), which requires fragmentation of the analyte of interest in a collision cell. This produces several fragmentation ions, which can be used to increase confidence in the correct identification of a signal as a microcystin. One ion is designated as the quantitation ion, used to determine the concentration of the microcystin in a sample. An additional ion (or more) can be used as a confirmation ion to positively identify a signal as being from a microcystin.

Liquid chromatography-mass spectrometry (LC-MS) and liquid chromatography tandem mass spectrometry (LC-MS/MS) are also much more useful in determining the speciation of microcystins. The validated procedure of the California Department of Fish and Wildlife uses LC-MS/MS to separate six microcystin variants in both tissue and water samples [171], and Schmidt et al. (2013) used LC-MS/MS to detect MC-LR in fish tissues using five LC-MS/MS fragmentation ions [95]. A summary of common procedures in the literature for the detection of MC-LR in animal tissues is given in Table 1.

The analysis of microcystins in tissues is further complicated by the large variation in recoveries of MC-LR between methods (Table 1), making it difficult to select a method for monitoring purposes. The fact that MC-LR has been emphasized over other variants also complicates these methods, as MC-LR may not be present in all microcystin-producing blooms. It is possible that other microcystin congeners would be overlooked using these methods, as the recovery of other variants of microcystins may not be identical to that of MC-LR. Other microcystin congeners and their metabolic products possess varying degrees of toxicity by PPIA [29] and by the mouse bioassay [85]. The variants of microcystins present and detected for monitoring will impact the toxicity of tissues and are an important component in monitoring.

Table 1. Extraction and cleanup protocols for microcystin-LR in tissue from the literature.

Reference	Year	Cleanup method	Analysis	Recovery of microcystin-LR
[172]	2005	C18 solid phase extraction	LC-MS	~57% (estimated from Figure 3 of reference [172])
[129]	2005	C18 solid phase extraction	LC-MS and ELISA	68%–96%
[173]	2005	C18 solid phase extraction	LC-MS and ELISA	44%–101%
[174]	2007	-	ELISA	>25%
[105]	2007	Waters Oasis solid phase extraction	LC-Photodiode array	>85%
[175]	2008	Waters Oasis solid phase extraction, Silica gel	LC-MS	>90%
[171]	2009	500 mg C18 solid phase extraction	LC-MS/MS	74%–125%
[170]	2009	-	LC-MS	80%–99%
[114]	2009	-	LC-MS	68%–73%
[95]	2013	Charcoal solid phase extraction	LC-MS/MS	54%–106%

3. Toxicokinetics

Information on the rate of microcystin metabolism in various organisms is limited, yet is essential for accurate toxicity assessments regarding microcystin exposure due to alterations in the environment, as well as via food web transfer. Potential microcystin transfer between tissues may vary by organism and impact bioaccumulation or biodilution. Speciation, prior exposure to microcystins, age of the organism and size of the organism may affect these processes. Models are useful tools for a better understanding of the toxicokinetics of microcystins in organisms and may help simplify factors for forming guidelines for human exposure.

3.1. One-Compartment Models

A one-compartment model assumes that the concentration of a toxin in the tissue is proportional to the concentration of toxin in the surrounding media. A single compartment (tissue), rather than differentiation by organ, is used to represent uptake and elimination. Uptake of a toxin is described with a first-order uptake constant (k_1) (Figure 4A) [176]. Elimination from tissue is described using an exponential term (k_2) (Figure 4A). This model only considers the parent compound and not metabolic products (GSH conjugates, *etc.*).

When metabolites of a toxin are formed, additional kinetic constants must be considered (Figure 4B). The rate constant for the uptake of the parent toxin into tissues (k_1) is considered along with the rate of the formation of metabolites (k_3) and the uptake of these metabolic products of the parent toxin by the tissue (k_4) (Figure 4B). Rate constants for the elimination of the parent toxin (k_2) and of the metabolites (k_5) are also considered, although different metabolites may not have the same rate constant in an organism (Figure 4B).

Figure 4. (**A**) One-compartment model for uptake and elimination of a toxin from an organism. Uptake rate k_1 and elimination rate k_2 are used to determine the duration of time a toxin is metabolized and eliminated from the organism during a set duration of exposure. (**B**) One-compartment model for uptake and elimination of a parent toxin and any products from the metabolism of the parent toxin. Kinetic constants k_1 and k_2 represent uptake and elimination of the parent toxin by the tissue, respectively. The rate of the formation of metabolites from the parent toxin (k_3) and uptake of these metabolites into the tissue (k_4) are modeled. The elimination of metabolites from the tissue is represented by the kinetic constant k_5. Uptake and elimination of the parent and metabolized toxin by individual organs are not considered.

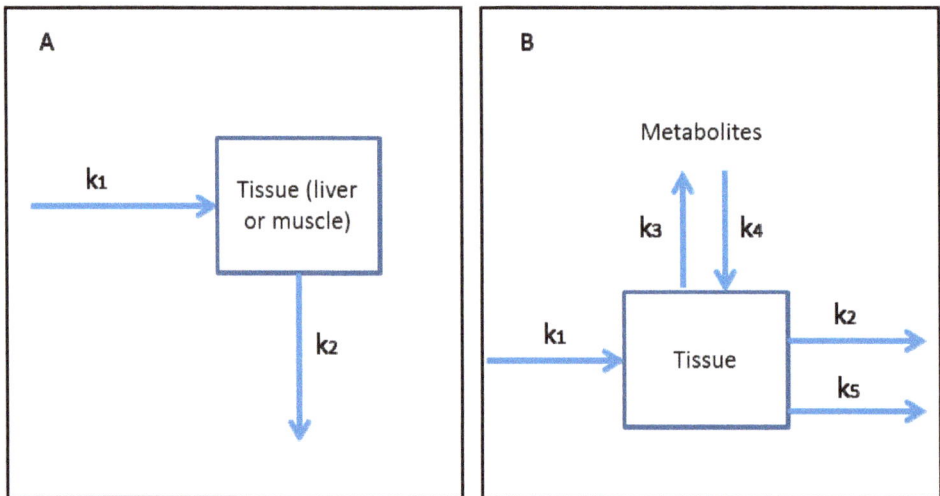

Dyble *et al.* (2011) presented a one-compartment, first order kinetic model for MC-LR elimination in yellow perch (Figure 4A) [177]. Although liver and muscle MC-LR concentrations were analyzed, the kinetic model was not differentiated by tissue type [177]. This study used only a single oral dose of MC-LR administered through a food pellet. The maximum MC-LR concentration was obtained in the liver tissue after 10 h and in muscle tissue after 12 h (estimated from Figure 2 of reference [177]). This model may not be applicable to organisms in natural systems with prolonged or variable exposure.

Concentrations in fish liver increased rapidly between 4 and 6 h of exposure and in muscle between 9 and 12 h (estimated from Figure 2 of reference [177]). MC-LR was detectable in the tank water after 4 h and increased throughout the experiment. ELISA was used to measure microcystins; thus, conjugated metabolites, such as GSH derivatives, could not be measured separately [168,177]. Intestinal uptake by fish was not analyzed, but a fish digestion model predicted that 90% of MC-LR administered by food pellet would pass through the gut within 24 h. This model suggested that consumption of contaminated fish tissues was not a major pathway for human exposure to MC-LR [177]. The accumulation and elimination of MC-LR in fish did not appear to be dose dependent. This suggests that the concentration of MC-LR in fish reached a threshold value after which the organism was unable to process the toxin or that prior exposure to the fish resulted in different rates of elimination of MC-LR [177].

The maximum MC-LR concentration in the hepatopancreas of bivalves was observed after five days of oral exposure to MC-LR in a one-compartment model [133]. MC-LR concentration rapidly increased for five days of oral exposure and reached a steady-state concentration, even when bivalves were continuously dosed for 10 days. This implies a maximum threshold MC-LR concentration may have been reached. After bivalves were introduced to non-toxic food for 15 days, rapid elimination of MC-LR was observed [133]. The test organisms used in this study were taken from a lake with prior toxic *Microcystis* blooms and depurated in non-toxic water before the experiment began. This prior exposure of these bivalves to microcystins may have impacted the threshold concentration accumulated in tissues, so as to prevent mortality. The toxicokinetic model here also varied according to time of year in which the bivalves were harvested. Higher concentrations of MC-LR were observed in tissues during colder seasons, as an increase in temperature increased the rate of elimination [133].

3.2. Multi-Compartmental Models

A multi-compartmental model produces multiple kinetic constants. It can also include multiple elimination constants that may be organ-specific. For example, the kidney and small intestine have two possible elimination routes: excretion through the urinary or gastrointestinal tracts or release of non-excreted toxin back into the blood (Figure 5). All organs have the potential to release non-metabolized toxin back into the blood for subsequent uptake by other organs. The liver has the potential to form and release metabolites into the blood or to the bile [178]. Phase II metabolites in bile may be hydrolyzed and reabsorbed by the small intestine in the enterohepatic cycle, reintroducing the toxin to the blood [178]. There are also unique uptake constants for uptake of the parent toxin into each organ (Figure 5). Unique kinetic constants for the elimination of a parent toxin from each specific organ are also assigned to account for differences between organs (Figure 5). Several studies have been conducted on microcystin uptake and elimination using multi-compartmental models.

Beasley and Stotts prepared a multi-compartment model for MC-LR metabolism in pigs. MC-LR concentration in blood peaked after 90 min following intravenous injection [179]. No conjugated metabolites were identified. After 4 h, the highest distribution of the radiolabeled MC-LR was in the liver, followed by kidneys, heart, small intestine and spleen (Figure 5) [179]. The presence of MC-LR in the kidney, small intestine and spleen are indicative of elimination. However, it is not clear at what point within the 4-h window this elimination began. MC-LR concentration was detectable in the intestines of pigs after 4 h of exposure, but the majority of MC-LR was concentrated in the liver [179]. MC-LR was detected in the bile of pigs after only 12 min of exposure, indicating that biliary elimination of MC-LR may be a major elimination pathway in pigs. Smaller doses of MC-LR resulted in higher concentrations in tissues after exposure than larger doses of MC-LR [179]. The metabolism of MC-LR is faster with lower doses than with higher doses in pigs. Higher concentrations of MC-LR could be overwhelming the elimination mechanisms of organisms, as binding of microcystins to protein phosphatases in cells is dose dependent [180]. At higher concentrations, elimination pathways may be unable to keep up with binding of microcystins to protein phosphatases.

Figure 5. Multi-compartment model for uptake and elimination of a toxin from an organism. Multiple kinetic constants for both uptake (k_1) and elimination (k_2) are possible due to the circulation of metabolite products through the organism and multiple pathways for the toxin to move through. Excretion by different organs also adds additional elimination constants to the model, such as in the kidney ($k_{kidney\ 2,1}$) and small intestine ($k_{intestine\ 2,1}$).

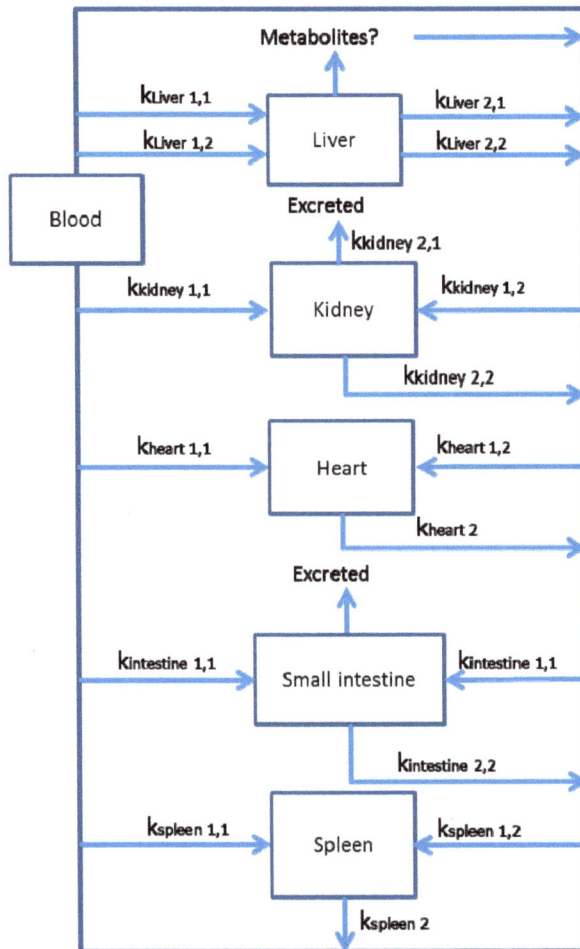

The compartmentalization of MC-LR in organs of mice after intraperitoneal injection has also been the subject of several studies. Lin (1994) observed MC-LR in serum and liver after 15 min of exposure, reaching a maximum concentration in serum after 2 h and in liver after 12 h [181]. No additional organs were analyzed. Robinson *et al.* (1990) reported maximum MC-LR concentration in liver, followed by intestine and kidney after 6 h of exposure [182]. Only small concentrations were detected in heart, spleen, lung and muscle. Like the Beasley and Stotts' (1994) study, intestine and kidney concentrations of MC-LR indicated that these were elimination routes [179]. Brooks *et al.* (1987) observed uptake of 70% of microcystin by the liver after 1 min of exposure, which increased to 90% after 3 h [183]. Uptake into other organs was less than 10%, indicating that the liver is taking up microcystin at a faster rate or containing it more efficiently than other organs in mice.

The concentration of microcystins was higher in the liver than in the muscle of common carp and silver carp after exposure to a bloom of toxic *Microcystis* for two months [174]. Rapid elimination of microcystins from both muscle and liver tissue was observed, with a higher rate of elimination in muscle than in liver. Elimination of microcystins was species-specific, as the half-life of microcystins in silver carp was shorter than that in common carp [174]. Under identical experimental conditions, the half-life of microcystins was only 0.7 days in muscle and 3.5 days in liver of silver carp, as compared to 2.8 days in muscle and 8.4 days in liver of common carp. This evidence suggests that selected species of fish have more efficient mechanisms of microcystin elimination than others.

Interestingly, Lei (2008) reported the highest microcystin concentrations in the blood, heart and kidney in crucian carp administered a mixture of MC-RR and MC-LR intraperitoneally [184]. The distribution of microcystins in this organism via the blood was an important process. The comparatively low concentration of MC-LR in the liver (0.07% of total microcystins) was different from findings in most other studies. The application of a combination of microcystin congeners may result in different distribution of microcystins between organs than observed using MC-LR alone.

Microcystin uptake and distribution within organisms is highly variable. Factors that influence this distribution include the test species, the method in which microcystins were administered to test animals, if the organisms were aquatic or terrestrial, the congener of the microcystin, the temperature of the surrounding water and any prior exposure of organisms to microcystins. The possible re-introduction of microcystins into the blood after absorption in the small intestine could also impact metabolism. The possibility that multiple pathways for the metabolism of microcystins exist in various organisms must also be considered.

3.3. Microcystin Conjugate Toxicokinetics

Little is known on how rapidly the different microcystin metabolites are formed. GSH-MC-LR was detected in the macrophyte, *Ceratophyllum demersum*, 24 h after exposure to MC-LR [87,90]. However, the study only analyzed the single conjugate species without further investigation into the rate of metabolism or metabolic pathway. An unidentified product was found by MALDI-TOF-MS with a retention time less than that of free MC-LR, but after MC-LR-GSH in *Daphnia magna*, *C. demersum* and the fish *Danio rerio* [87]. This product could be the MC-LR-Cys conjugate, but the characterization by mass spectrometry was not reported. A similar unidentified product was found in the hepatic cytosol of mice after intravenous injection after 1 and 6 h of exposure [96]. After six days of exposure, two additional products were observed by ultraviolet visible spectroscopy [96]. These three peaks could be conjugated microcystins, but were not further identified.

The MC-LR-Cys conjugate was more prevalent in fish (*Hypophthalmichthys molitrix*) tissue than the MC-LR-GSH species [106]. It was unclear if this represented direct formation of the MC-LR-Cys conjugate from free microcystin or if the conversion from MC-LR-GSH into MC-LR-Cys was a very rapid process. The GSH and Cys conjugates of both microcystin-RR and MC-LR were identified in mouse and rat liver, respectively, after 24 h of exposure [102]. Metabolism of MC-LR followed the same metabolic pathway as MC-RR, through GSH and Cys intermediates [102]. Unfortunately, there was little information on how quickly the metabolism of both the MC-LR and MC-RR species occurred.

The rate of microcystin metabolism differs between species, as does the degree of resistance to microcystin toxicity. Current information on the rate of MC-LR metabolism in different species of test organisms is limited. Toxin concentration in the hepatopancreas of *Unio douglasiae* increased for five days after being fed the MC-LR-producing cyanobacteria, *Microcystis spp.* [133]. After five days, hepatopancreatic MC-LR concentrations leveled off in a steady-state fashion. An increase in GST activity was observed for different organs of *Mytilus galloprovincialis* when exposed to microcystins [136]. GST activity increased when exposed to MC-LR for a 24-h period in *Daphnia magna*, *Ceratophyllum demersum* and *Danio rerio* [87]. The observed increase in GST activity suggests that MC-LR was being transformed to the glutathione conjugate. In contrast, a marked decrease in GST activity in the goldfish, *Carassius auratus* L., occurred after 24 h of MC-LR exposure [140].

Zooplankton also showed differentiation in response to microcystins. The estimated 48-h LD_{50} is between 10.2 and 18.3 ng of MC-LR per 1 mg of *Daphnia* (fresh weight) for *D. galeata* over the course of two days [185]. This information does not tell how prolonged exposure to MC-LR affects *D. galeata*, nor can it be used to determine how quickly the metabolism of MC-LR occurs. The LD_{50} for *E. affinis* is two orders of magnitude smaller than that of *D. magna* [162]. Unknown factors include how the toxin is accumulated within the organism or if there is a depuration period following exposure.

Below this estimated LD_{50} for MC-LR, it is possible that test organisms would metabolize MC-LR rather than suffer mortality. Sadler and von Elert (2014) did not observe any conjugation of MC-LR to GSH during a 24-h exposure of *D. magna* to microcystin [186]. MC-LR was administered to the *Daphnia* using toxic *Microcystis* as a food source for 24 h, followed by transfer to clean media and their feeding on *Cryptomonas spp.* The MC-LR concentration did not change throughout the experiment, and no transformation of the parent toxin was observed. MC-LR was not assimilated by *Daphnia*, as no MC-LR was detected after feeding with *Cryptomonas spp.* [186]. Absorption of microcystin may not have occurred or a detoxification mechanism other than the GSH metabolic pathway may be active in *Daphnia*. The elimination of MC-LR directly into the surrounding media without any biological alteration using a P-glycoprotein was suggested as a possible mechanism.

It has been suggested that glutathione conjugation to microcystins is a reversible process *in vivo* [187]. MC-RR was detected in tissues of fish injected interperitoneally with MC-RR-GSH and MC-RR-cysteine. Reversal of Michael addition reactions require low pH, suggesting that there may be an enzymatic process liberating MC-RR from its conjugated form *in vivo*. This could have major implications for monitoring, since the conjugates could comprise a large portion of the toxin pool in a natural system [91]. The metabolism of the conjugates by fish could transform microcystins into their original and most toxic form for possible excretion and uptake by other organisms in the environment. Moreover, the presence of MC-RR was dominant in the blood, not in the liver tissues [187]. This suggests another potential compartment for microcystins to occupy in fish and the importance of transport processes between organs. This could also potentially explain the presence of microcystins found in fish muscle tissues rather than liver tissues. More studies on this reversible conjugation are essential for a more complete understanding of the toxicity, transport and transformation of microcystins in living cells.

4. Conclusions and Future Direction

Microcystins are prone to physical, biological and chemical alterations in the environment. Detection of microcystins in tissues has been well-documented, yet the species of the organism and high variability between organisms of the same species with regard to uptake of microcystins complicate calculations for safety guidelines. Abiotic and microbial breakdown of microcystins, as well as the potential toxicity of the conjugated MC-LR metabolites produced by organisms in their tissues also makes the determination of human health guidelines difficult. Limited knowledge on the rate of metabolism and rate of formation of the conjugated MC-LR products is available. The potential human health risk of microcystin intoxication due to food web transfer of microcystins also remains uncertain, although microcystins and their metabolite products have been detected in some organisms of different trophic levels. The human health impact of these metabolized products being excreted and released into the environment is also uncertain.

Additional information on the rate of formation of these conjugates, as well as the rate of degradation of microcystins by microbes is needed to provide a more complete understanding of the role metabolism plays in the toxicity of MC-LR in natural systems. More data on the fate of microcystin conjugates *in vivo* are also needed to better understand the potential risk of human intoxication from tissues. The lack of the GSH-conjugated products in *Daphnia* indicates that other detoxification mechanisms may be dominant over the GSH conjugation pathway and that the use of the GSH pathway for MC-LR metabolism and elimination may not be conserved across the majority of species.

The number of microcystins and bioactive metabolites produced by cyanobacteria and impacted species is continually increasing as new and more advanced chemical techniques are applied to the identification of these compounds [188]. Microcystin congeners other than MC-LR, as well as any possible metabolites are integral to making accurate toxicity assessments and should be incorporated into the implementation of human health guidelines. One approach is to use cell-based effect assays, such as enzyme-based assays, such as the protein phosphatase inhibition assay. These assays may be effective alternatives to current monitoring techniques, especially for water samples where the concentration of matrix interferences is low. However, care must be taken to ensure that the response in these *in vitro* assays is representative of the *in vivo* toxicity, as properties, such as uptake and transport, are rarely captured by these *in vitro* tests. Structure-based assays, such as ELISA, may also give an integrated microcystin value in a sample, but it is often difficult to convert this value into a toxic effect without the knowledge of the individual congeners present. A better understanding of the occurrence of different congeners, their metabolic products and the toxicity of the between different microcystin congeners would help in this regard.

The analysis of tissue samples require different approaches, as interferences from the tissue matrix can result in false positives in both effect-based assays, such as PPIA, or structure-based assays, such as ELISA [114]. Improved cleanup methods may be able to remove these interfering compounds from the tissue matrix. Alternatively, new effect-based assays based on the mode of action of microcystins in cells may be identified that may be less sensitive to these matrix affects. Such assays would be beneficial as a screening tool for the presence of microcystins in tissues.

A second approach is to use an analysis for individual microcystin compounds. MALDI-TOF, LC-MS and LC-MS/MS are examples of such an approach, which has been applied to water and tissue samples. Analyses focus on individual compounds. The advantage of an analysis is that it is able to distinguish between different congeners of microcystins in the sample. The disadvantage is that the analytical method only considers those toxins that the operator asks it to consider, such as with LC-MS/MS, where a quantitation and confirmation ion are obtained for a particular compound of interest. With an ever-increasing number of microcystins and their metabolites being identified, these analytical methods would need to be updated constantly to incorporate new toxins. In addition, there are many compounds in complex matrices whose mass to charge ratios are similar to that of the desired analyte. Thus, both a quantitation and, possibly, multiple confirmation ions for each congener, metabolite or compound of interest would be needed. Improvements in sample cleanup techniques, as well as a better understanding of the distribution of the different congeners and metabolites in nature are essential to guide the operator in the selection of the correct method.

In practice, the ideal approach to monitoring of microcystins in tissues is likely to include a combination of assays and analyses. An effect-based assay could be used first as a screening tool to rapidly eliminate those samples that do not contain any toxins. This initial screening could then be followed up by more specific analysis using LC-MS(/MS) to confirm that the toxin(s) in question are indeed present, to eliminate potential false positives and to identify the presence of new or unknown toxins in the sample.

Acknowledgments

Funding was provided by the Ohio Environmental Protection Agency and through the National Oceanic and Atmospheric Administration Center for Sponsored Coastal Ocean Research's Prevention, Control and Mitigation of Harmful Algal Blooms Program Award Number NA11NOS4780021 to Steven W. Wilhelm and Gregory L. Boyer. This is National Oceanic and Atmospheric Administration Prevention, Control, and Mitigation (PCM) Harmful Algal Bloom program contribution PCM17.

Author Contributions

Steven W. Wilhelm and Gregory L. Boyer provided funding and laboratory materials, Justine R. Schmidt wrote the paper and designed all of the figures. Justine R. Schmidt, Gregory L. Boyer, and Steven W. Wilhelm edited and thoroughly discussed the topics in this paper.

Conflicts of Interest

The authors declare no conflict of interest.

References

1. Wehr, J.D.; Sheath, R.G. Freshwater habitats of algae. In *Freshwater Algae of North America*; Wehr, J.D., Sheath, R.G., Eds.; Academic Press: San Diego, CA, USA, 2003; pp. 11–57.
2. Smith, J.L.; Boyer, G.L.; Zimba, P.V. A Review of Cyanobacterial Odorous and Bioactive Metabolites: Impacts and Management Alternatives in Aquaculture. *Aquaculture* **2008**, *280*, 5–20.
3. Lampert, W. Laboratory Studies on Zooplankton-Cyanobacteria Interactions. *N. Z. J. Mar. Fresh.* **1987**, *21*, 483–490.
4. Carmichael, W. Cyanobacteria Secondary Metabolites—The Cyanotoxins. *J. Appl. Bacteriol.* **1992**, *72*, 445–459.
5. Carmichael, W. Health Effects of Toxin-Producing Cyanobacteria: "The CyanoHABs". *Hum. Ecol. Risk Assess.* **2001**, *7*, 1393–1407.
6. Dittman, E.; Wiegand, C. Cyanobacterial Toxins—Occurrence, Biosynthesis and Impact on Human Affairs. *Mol. Nutr. Food Res.* **2006**, *50*, 7–17.
7. Pearson, L.; Mihali, T.; Moffitt, M.; Kellmann, R.; Neilan, B. On the Chemistry, Toxicology and Genetics of the Cyanobacterial Toxins, Microcystin, Nodularin, Saxitoxin and Cylindrospermopsin. *Mar. Drugs* **2010**, *10*, 1650–1680.
8. Newcombe, G.; Chorus, I.; Falconer, I.; Lin, T. Cyanobacteria: Impacts of Climate Change on Occurrence, Toxicity and Water Quality Management. *Water Res.* **2012**, *46*, 1347–1348.
9. Paerl, H.W.; Hall, N.S.; Calandrino, E.S. Controlling Harmful Cyanobacterial Blooms in a World Experiencing Anthropogenic and Climate-induced Change. *Sci. Total Environ.* **2011**, *409*, 1739–1745.
10. De Figueiredo, D.R.; Azeiteiro, U.M.; Esteves, S.M.; Gonçalves, F.J.M.; Pereira, M.J. Microcystin-producing blooms—A serious global public health issue. *Ecotox. Environ. Saf.* **2004**, *59*, 151–163.
11. Svrcek, C.; Smith, D.W. An Overview of the Cyanobacteria Toxins and the Current State of Knowledge on Water Treatment Options. *J. Environ. Eng.* **2004**, *3*, 155–185.
12. Zurawell, R.W.; Chen, H.; Burke, J.M.; Prepas, E.E. Hepatotoxic Cyanobacteria: A Review of the Biological Importance of Microcystins in Freshwater Environments. *J. Toxicol. Environ. Health* **2005**, *8*, 1–37.
13. Niedermeyer, T.H.J.; Daily, A.; Swiatecka-Hagenbruch, M.; Moscow, J.A. Selectivity and Potency of Microcystin Congeners against OATP1B1 and OATP1B3 Expressing Cancer Cells. *PLoS One* **2014**, *9*, e91476.
14. Runnegar, M.T.C.; Berndt, N.; Kaplowitz, N. Microcystin Uptake and Inhibition of Protein Phosphatases: Effects of Chemoprotectants and Self-inhibition in Relation to Known Hepatic Transporters. *Toxicol. Appl. Pharmacol.* **1995**, *134*, 264–272.

15. Gupta, N.; Pant, S.C.; Vilayaraghavan, R.; Rao, P.V. Comparative Toxicity Evaluation of Cyanobacterial Cyclic Peptide Toxin Microcystin Variants (LR, RR, YR) in Mice. *Toxicology* **2003**, *188*, 285–296.

16. De Maagd, P.G.; Hendriks, A.J.; Seinen, W.; Sijm, D. pH-dependent Hydrophobicity of the Cyanobacteria Toxin Microcystin-LR. *Water Res.* **1999**, *33*, 677–680.

17. Eriksson, J.E.; Grönberg, L.; Nygård, S.; Slotte, P.; Meriluoto, J.A.O. Hepatocellular Uptake of ³H-dihydromicrocystin-LR, a Cyclic Peptide Toxin. *Biochim. Biophys. Acta* **1990**, *1025*, 60–66.

18. Falconer, I.R. *Cyanobacterial Toxins of Drinking Water Supplies*; CRC Press: Boca Raton, FL, USA, 2005; pp. 1–9.

19. Wolkoff, A.W.; Cohen, D.E. Hepatic Transport of Bile Acids. *Am. J. Physiol. Gastrointest. Liver Physiol.* **2003**, *284*, 175–179.

20. MacKintosh, R.W.; Dalby, K.N.; Campbell, D.G.; Cohen, P.T.W.; Cohen, P.; MacKintosh, C. The Cyanobacterial Toxin Microcystin Binds Covalently to Cysteine-273 on Protein Phosphatase 1. *FEBS Lett.* **1995**, *371*, 236–240.

21. Puerto, M.; Pichardo, S.; Jos, Á.; Cameán, A.M. Comparison of the Toxicity Induced by Microcystin-RR and Microcystin-YR in Differentiated and Undifferentiated Caco-2 Cells. *Toxicon* **2009**, *54*, 161–169.

22. Fawell, J.K.; James, C.P.; James, H.A. Toxins from Blue-Green Algae: Toxicological Assessment of micRocystin-LR and a Method for Its Determination in Water; Foundation for Water Research: Medmenham, Marlow, Bucks, UK, 1994; pp. 1–46.

23. World Health Organization. *Toxic Cyanobacteria in Water. A Guide to Public Health Consequence, Monitoring and Management*; E and FN Spon: London, UK, 1999.

24. Ballantyne, B. Toxicology and Hazard Eevaluation of Cyanide Fumigation Powders. *Fund. Appl. Toxicol.* **1988**, *26*, 325–335.

25. Kotak, B.G.; Kenefick, S.L.; Fritz, D.L.; Rousseaux, C.G.; Prepas, E.E.; Hrudey, S.E. Occurrence and Toxicological Evaluation of Cyanobacterial Toxins in Alberta Lakes and Farm Dugouts. *Water Res.* **1993**, *27*, 495–506.

26. Rinehart, K.L.; Namikoshi, M.; Choi, B.W. Structure and Biosynthesis of Toxins from Blue-green Algae (cyanobacteria). *J. Appl. Phycol.* **1994**, *6*, 159–176.

27. World Health Organization (WHO). Cyanobacterial Toxins: Microcystin-LR in Drinking Water. In *Guidelines for Drinking Water Quality*; WHO: Geneva, Switzerland, 1998.

28. Corbel, S.; Mougin, C.; Bouaïcha, N. Cyanobacterial toxins: Modes of Actions, Fate in Aquatic and Soil Ecosystems, Phytotoxicity and Bioaccumulation in Agricultural crops. *Chemosphere* **2014**, *96*, 1–15.

29. Shimizu, K.; Sano, T.; Kubota, R.; Kobayashi, N.; Tahara, M.; Obama, T.; Sugimoto, N.; Nishimura, T.; Ikarashi, Y. Effects of the Amino Acid Constituents of Microcystin Variants on Cytotoxicity to Primary Cultured Rat Hepatocytes. *Toxins* **2013**, *6*, 168–179.

30. Bláha, L.; Babica, P.; Maršálek, B. Toxins Produced in Cyanobacterial Water Blooms-toxicity and Risks. *Interdiscip. Toxicol.* **2009**, *2*, 36–41.

31. Pouria, S.; de Andrade, A.; Barbosa, J.; Cavalcanti, R.L.; Barreto, V.T.; Ward, C.J.; Preiser, W.; Poon, G.K.; Neild, G.H.; Codd, G.A. Fatal Microcystin Intoxication in Haemodialysis Unit in Caruaru, Brazil. *Lancet* **1998**, *352*, 21–26.

32. Nishiwaki-Matsushima, R.; Ohta, T.; Nishiwaki, S.; Suganuma, M.; Kohyama, K.; Ishikawa, T.; Carmichael, W.W.; Fujiki, H. Liver Tumor Promotion by the Cyanobacterial Cyclic Peptide Toxin Microcystin-LR. *J. Cancer Res. Clin. Oncol.* **1992**, *118*, 420–424.

33. Yu, S.Z. Primary Prevention of Hepatocellular Carcinoma. *J. Gastroen. Hepatol.* **1995**, *10*, 674–682.

34. Ibelings, B.W.; Chorus, I. Accumulation of Cyanobacterial Toxins in Freshwater "Seafood" and its Consequence for Public Health: A review. *Environ. Pollut.* **2007**, *150*, 177–192.

35. Mulvenna, V.; Dale, K.; Priestly, B.; Mueller, U.; Humpage, A.; Shaw, G.; Allinson, G.; Falconer, I. Health Risk Assessment for Cyanobacterial Toxins in Seafood. *Int. J. Environ. Res. Public Health* **2012**, *9*, 807–820.

36. Harada, K. Chemistry and detection of microcystins. In *Toxic Microcystis*, 1st ed.; Watanabe, M.F., Harada, K., Carmichael, W.W., Fujiki H., Eds.; CRC Press: Boca Raton, FL, USA, 1995; pp. 110–114.

37. Tsuji, K.; Masui, H.; Uemura, H.; Mori, Y.; Harada, K. Analysis of Microcystins in Sediments Using MMPB Method. *Toxicon* **2001**, *39*, 687–692.

38. Carey, C.C.; Haney, J.F.; Cottingham, K.L. First Report of Microcystin-LR in the Cyanobacterium *Gloeotrichia echinulata*. *Environ. Toxicol.* **2007**, *22*, 337–339.

39. Harada, K.I.; Tsuji, K.; Watanabe, M.F.; Kondo, F. Stability of Microcystins from Cyanobacteria—III. Effect of pH and Temperature. *Phycol.* **1996**, *35*, 83–88.

40. Morris, R.J.; Williams, D.E.; Luu, H.A.; Holmes, C.F.B.; Andersen, R.J.; Calvert, S.E. The adsorption of microcystin-LR by natural clay particles. *Toxicon* **2000**, *38*, 303–308.

41. Liu, G.; Qian, Y.; Dai, S.; Feng, N. Adsorption of microcystin-LR and -LW on suspended particular matter (SPM) at different pH. *Water Air Soil Pollut.* **2008**, *192*, 67–76.

42. Hakanson, L. *Suspended Particulate Matter in Lakes, Rivers, and Marine Systems*; Blackburn Press: West Caldwell, NJ, USA; 2006.

43. Munusamy, T.; Hu, Y.; Lee, J. Adsorption and Photodegradation of Microcystin-LR onto Sediments Collected from Reservoirs and Rivers in Taiwan: A Laboratory Study to Investigate the Fate, Transfer, and Degradation of Microcystin-LR. *Environ. Sci. Pollut. Res.* **2012**, *19*, 2390–2399.

44. Rudolph-BohÈhner, S.; Mierke, D.F.; Moroder, L. Molecular Structure of the Cyanobacterial Tumor-Producing Microcystins. *FEBS Lett.* **1994**, *349*, 319–323.

45. Seitzinger, S.P. The Effect of pH on the Release of Phosphorus from Potomac Estuary Sediments: Implications for Blue-green Algal Blooms. *Estuar. Shelf Coast. Sci.* **1991**, *33*, 409–418.

46. Codd, G.A. Cyanobacterial Toxins: Occurrence, Properties, and Biological Significance. *Water Sci. Technol.* **1995**, *32*, 149–156.

47. Tsuji, K.; Naito, S.; Kondo, F.; Ishikawa, N.; Watanabe, M.F.; Suzuki, M.; Harada, K. Stability of Microcystins from Cyanobacteria—I. Effect of Light on Decomposition and Isomerization. *Environ. Sci. Technol.* **1994**, *28*, 173–177.

48. Welker, M.; Steinberg, C. Rates of Humic Substance Photosensitized Degradation of Microcystin-LR in Natural Waters. *Environ. Sci. Technol.* **2000**, *34*, 3415–3419.

49. Tsuji, K.; Watanuki, T.; Kondo, F.; Watanabe, M.F.; Suzuki, S.; Nakazawa, H.; Suzuki, M.; Uchida, H.; Harada, K. Stability of Microcystins from Cyanobacteria—II. Effect of UV Light on Decomposition and Isomerization. *Toxicon* **1995**, *33*, 1619–1631.

50. Li, L.; Huang, W.L.; Peng, P.G.; Sheng, G.Y.; Fu, J.M. Chemical and Molecular Heterogeneity of Humic Acids Repetitively Extracted from a Peat. *Soil Sci. Soc. Am. J.* **2003**, *67*, 740–746.

51. Song, W.; Bardowell, A.; O'Shea, K. Mechanistic Study of the Influence of Oxygen on the Photosensitized Transformations of Microcystins (Cyanotoxins). *Environ. Sci. Technol.* **2007**, *41*, 5336–5341.

52. Wörmer, L.; Huerta-Fontela, M.; Cirés, S.; Carrasco, D.; Quesada, A. Natural Photodegradation of the Cyanobacterial Toxins Microcystins and Cylindrospermopsin. *Environ. Sci. Technol.* **2010**, *44*, 3002–3007.

53. Antoniou, M.G.; Shoemaker, J.A.; De La Cruz, A.A.; Dionysiou, D. Unveiling New Degradation Intermediates/Pathways from the Photocatalytic Degradation of Microcystin-LR. *Environ. Sci. Technol.* **2008**, *42*, 8877–8883.

54. Fang, Y.; Chen, D.; Huang, Y.; Yang, J.; Chen, G. Heterogeneous Fenton Photodegradation of Microcystin-LR with Visible Light Irradiation. *Chinese J. Anal. Chem.* **2011**, *39*, 540–543.

55. Antoniou, M.G.; Shoemaker, J.A.; De La Cruz, A.A.; Dionysiou, D.D. LC/MS/MS Structure Elucidation of Reaction Intermediates Formed during the TiO_2 Photocatalysis of Microcystin-LR. *Toxicon* **2008**, *51*, 1103–1118.

56. Liu, I.; Lawton, L.A.; Cornish, B.; Robertson, P.K.J. Mechanistic and Toxicity Studies of the Photocatalytic Oxidation of Microcystin-LR. *J. Photochem. Photobiol. A* **2002**, *148*, 349–354.

57. Choi, H.; Antoniou, M.G.; Pelaez, M.; De La Cruz, A.A.; Shoemaker, J.A.; Dionysiou, D.D. Mesoporous Nitrogen-doped TiO_2 for the Photocatalytic Destruction of the Cyanobacterial Toxin Microcystin-LR under Visible Light Irradiation. *Environ. Sci. Technol.* **2007**, *41*, 7530–7535.

58. Wang, Q.; Su, M.F.; Zhu, W.Q.; Li, X.N.; Jia, Y.; Guo, P.; Chen, Z.H.; Jiang, W.X. Growth Inhibition of *Microcystis Aeruginosa* by White-rot Fungus *Lopharia Spadicea*. *Water Sci. Technol.* **2010**, *62*, 317–323.

59. Jia, Y.; Du, J.; Song, F.; Zhao, G.; Tian, X. A Fungus Capable of Degrading Microcystin-LR in the Algal Culture of *Microcystis Aeruginosa* PCC7806. *Appl. Biochem. Biotechnol.* **2012**, *166*, 987–996.

60. Bourne, D.G.; Jones, G.J.; Blakeley, R.L.; Jones, A.; Negri, A.P.; Riddles, P. Enzymatic Pathway for the Bacterial Degradation of the Cyanobacterial Cyclic Peptide Toxin Microcystin-LR. *Appl. Environ. Microbiol.* **1996**, *62*, 4086–4094.

61. Bourne, D.G.; Riddles, P.; Jones, G.J.; Smith, W.; Blakeley, R.L. Characterisation of a Gene Cluster Involved in Bacterial Degradation of the Cyanobacterial Degradation of the Cyanobacterial Toxin Microcystin-LR. *Environ. Toxicol.* **2001**, *16*, 523–534.

62. Imanishi, S.; Kato, H.; Mizuno, M.; Tsuji, K.; Harada, K. Bacterial Degradation of Microcystins and Nodularin. *Chem. Res. Toxicol.* **2005**, *18*, 591–598.

63. Harada, K.; Imanishi, S.; Kato, H.; Mizuno, M.; Ito, E.; Tsuji, K. Isolation of ADDA from Microcystin-LR by Microbial Degradation. *Toxicon.* **2004**, *44*, 107–109.

64. Ho, L.; Gaudieux, A.L.; Fanok, S.; Newcombe, G.; Humpage, A.R. Bacterial Degradation of Microcystin Toxins in Drinking Water Eliminates their Toxicity. *Toxicon* **2007**, *50*, 438–441.

65. Okano, K.; Shimizu, K.; Kawauchi, Y.; Maseda, H.; Utsumi, M.; Zhang, Z.; Neilan, B.A.; Sugiura, N. Characteristics of a Microcystin-degrading Bacterium under Alkaline Environmental Conditions. *J. Toxicol.* **2009**, doi:10.1155/2009/954291.

66. Christoffersen, K.; Lyck, S.; Winding, A. Microbial Activity and Bacterial Community Structure during Degradation of Microcystins. *Aquat. Microb. Ecol.* **2002**, *27*, 125–136.

67. Steffen, M.M.; Li, Z.; Effler, C.; Hauser, L.J.; Boyer, G.L.; Wilhelm, S.W. Comparative Metagenomics of Toxic Freshwater Cyanobacteria Bloom Communities on Two Continents. *PLoS One* **2012**, *7*, e44002.

68. Wilhelm, S.W.; Farnsley, S.E.; LeCleir, G.R.; Layton, A.C.; Satchwell, M.F.; DeBruyn, J.M.; Boyer, G.L.; Zhu, G.; Paerl, H.W. The Relationships between Nutrients, Cyanobacterial Toxins and the Microbial Community in Taihu (Lake Tai), China. *Harmful Algae* **2011**, *10*, 207–215.

69. Jones, G.J.; Orr, P.T. Release and Degradation of Microcystin Following Algicide Treatment of a *Microcystis Aeruginosa* Bloom in a Recreational Lake, as 248 Determined by HPLC and Protein Phosphatase Inhibition assay. *Water Res.* **1994**, *28*, 871–876.

70. Park, H.; Sasaki, Y.; Maruyami, T.; Yanagisawa, E.; Hiraishi, A.; Kato, K. Degradation of the Cyanobacterial Heptatotoxin Microcystin by a New Bacterium Isolated from a Hypertrophic Lake. *Environ. Toxicol.* **2001**, *6*, 337–343.

71. Saito, T.; Sugiura, N.; Itayama, T.; Inamori, Y.; Matsumura, M.J. Degradation Characteristics of Microcystins by Isolated Bacteria from Lake Kasumigaura. *J. Water Supply Res. Technol.* **2003**, *52*, 13–18.

72. Rapala, J.; Berg, K.A.; Lyra, C.; Niemi, R.M.; Manz, W.; Suomalainen, S.; Paulin, L.; Lahti, K. *Paucibacter toxinivorans* gen. nov., sp. nov., a bacterium that degrades cyclic cyanobacterial hepatotoxins microcystins and nodularins. *Int. J. Syst. Evol. Micr.* **2005**, *55*, 1563–1568.

73. Maruyama, T.; Park, H.; Ozawa, K.; Tanaka, Y.; Sumino, T.; Hamana, K.; Hirashi, A.; Kato, K. *Sphingosinicella microcystinivorans* gen. nov., sp. nov., a microcystin degrading bacterium. *Int. J. Syst. Evol. Micr.* **2006**, *56*, 85–89.

74. Lahti, K.; Niemi, M.R.; Rapala, J.; Sivonen, K. Biodegradation of Cyanobacterial Hepatotoxins-Characterisation of Toxin Degrading Bacteria. In *Harmful Algae*; Reguera, B., Blanco, J., Fernández, M.L, Wyatt, T., Eds.; United Nations Educational, Scientific, and Cultural Organization: Vigo, Spain, 1988; pp. 363–365.

75. Berg, K.A.; Lyra, C.; Sivonen, K.; Paulin, L.; Suomalainen, S.; Tuomi, P.; Rapala, J. High Diversity of Cultivable Heterotrophic Bacteria in Association with Cyanobacterial Water Blooms. *ISME J.* **2009**, *3*, 314–325.

76. Goldberg, J.; Huang, H.; Kwon, Y.; Greengard, P.; Nairn, A.C.; Kuriyan, J. Three Dimensional Structure of the Catalytic Subunit of Protein Serine/threonine Phosphatase-1. *Nature* **1995**, *376*, 745–753.

77. Vermeulen, N.P.E. Role of Metabolism in Chemical Toxicity. In *Cytochromes P450: Metabolic and Toxicological Aspects*; Ioannides, C., Eds. CRC Press: Boca Raton, FL, USA, 1996; pp. 29–49.

78. Manahan, S.E. *Toxicological Chemistry and Biochemistry*, 3rd ed.; CRC Press: Boca Raton, FL, USA, 2003; pp.142–153.

79. Townsend, D.M.; Tew, K.D. The role of glutathione-*S*-transferase in anti-cancer drug resistance. *Oncogene* **2003**, *22*, 7369–7375.

80. Sies, H.; Wahlländer, A.; Waydhas, C.; Soboll, S.; Häberle, D. Functions of Intracellular Glutathione in Hepatic Hydroperoxide and Drug Metabolism and the Role of Extracellular Glutathione. *Adv. Enzyme Regul.* **1980**, *18*, 303–320.

81. Lindwall, G.; Boyer, T.D. Excretion of Glutathione Conjugates by Primary Cultured Rat Hepatocytes. *J. Biol. Chem.* **1987**, *262*, 5151–5158.

82. Lilja, H.; Jeppsson, J.; Kristensson, H. Evaluation of Serum γ-Glutamyltransferase by Electrofocusing, and Variations in Isoform Patterns. *Clin. Chem.* **1983**, *29*, 1034–1037.

83. Ishikawa, T. The ATP-Dependent Glutathione *S*-Conjugate Export Pump. *Trends Biochem. Sci.* **1992**, *17*, 463–468.

84. Müeller, M.; Meijer, C.; Zaman, G.R.; Borst, P.; Scheper, R.J.; Mulder, N.H.; DeVries, E.E.; Jansen, P.L. Overexpression of the Gene Encoding the Multidrug Resistance-associated Protein Results in Increased ATP-dependent Glutathione *S*-conjugate Transport. *J. Med. Sci.* **1994**, *91*, 13033–13037.

85. Ito, E.; Satake, M.; Yasumoto, T. Pathological Effects of Lyngbyatoxin A upon Mice. *Toxicon* **2002**, *40*, 551–556.

86. Williams, D.E.; Dawe, S.C.; Kent, M.; Andersen, R.J.; Craig, M.; Holmes, C.F.B. Bioaccumulation and Clearance of Microcystins from Salt Water Mussels, *Mytilus edulis*, and *in vivo* Evidence for Covalently Bound Microcystins in Mussel Tissues. *Toxicon* **1997**, *35*, 1617–1625.

87. Pflugmacher, S.; Wiegand, C.; Oberemm, A.; Beattie, K.A.; Krause, E.; Codd, G.A.; Steinberg, C.E.W. Identification of an Enzymatically Formed Glutathione Conjugate of the Cyanobacterial Hepatotoxin Microcystin-LR: The First Step of Detoxication. *Biochim. Biophys. Acta Gen. Subj.* **1998**, *1425*, 527–533.

88. Pflugmacher, S.; Codd, G.A.; Steinberg, C.E.W. Effects of the Cyanobacterial Toxin Microcystin-LR on Detoxication Enzymes in Aquatic Plants. *Environ. Toxicol.* **1999**, *14*, 111–115.

89. Pflugmacher, S.; Weigand, C.; Beattie, K.A.; Krause, E.; Steinberg, C.E.W.; Codd, G.A. Uptake, Effects, and Metabolism of Cyanobacterial Toxins in the Emergent Reed Plant *Phragmites Australis* (Cav.) Trin. Ex Steud. *Environ. Toxicol. Chem.* **2001**, *20*, 846–852.

90. Pflugmacher, S. Promotion of Oxidative Stress in the Aquatic Macrophyte *Ceratophyllum Demersum* during Biotransformation of the Cyanobacterial Toxin Microcystin-LR. *Aquat. Toxicol.* **2004**, *70*, 169–178.

91. Meissner, S.; Fastner, J.; Dittmann, E. Microcystin Production Revisited: Conjugate Formation Makes a Major Contribution. *Environ. Microbiol.* **2013**, *15*, 1810–1820.

92. Smith, J.L.; Schulz, K.L.; Zimba, P.V.; Boyer, G.L. Possible Mechanism for the Foodweb Transfer of Covalently Bound Microcystins. *Ecotox. Environ. Saf.* **2010**, *73*, 757–761.

93. Lance, E.; Petit, A.; Sanchez, W.; Paty, C.; Ge´rard, C.; Bormans, M. Evidence of Trophic Transfer of Microcystins from the Gastropod *Lymnaea stagnalis* to the Fish *Gasterosteus Aculeatus*. *Harmful Algae* **2014**, *31*, 9–17.

94. Zilliges, Y.; Kehr, J.; Meissner, S.; Ishida, K.; Mikkat, S.; Hagemann, M.; Kaplan, A.; Borner, T.; Dittmann, E. The Cyanobacterial Hepatotoxin Microcystin Binds to Proteins and Increases the Fitness of *Microcystis* under Oxidative Stress Conditions. *PLoS One* **2013**, *6*, e17615.

95. Schmidt, J.R.; Shaskus, M.; Estenik, J.F.; Oesch, C.; Khidekel, R.; Boyer, G.L. Variations in the Microcystin Content of Different Fish Species Collected from a Eutrophic Lake. *Toxins* **2013**, *5*, 992–1009.

96. Robinson, N.A.; Pace, J.G.; Matson, C.F.; Miura, G.A.; Lawrence, W.B. Tissue Distribution, Excretion and Hepatic Biotransformation of Microcystin-LR in Mice. *J. Pharmacol. Exp. Ther.* **1991**, *256*, 176–182.

97. Amorim, A.; Vasconcelos, V. Dynamics of Microcystins in the Mussel. *Mytilus galloprovincialis. Toxicon* **1999**, *37*, 1041–1052.

98. Vanderploeg, H.A.; Liebig, J.R.; Carmichael, W.W.; Agy, M.A.; Johengen, T.H.; Fahnenstiel, G.L.; Nalepa, T.F. Zebra Mussel (*Dreissena polymorpha*) Selective Filtration Promoted Toxic *Microcystis* blooms in Saginaw Bay (Lake Huron) and Lake Erie. *Can. J. Fish. Aquat. Sci.* **2001**, *58*, 1208–1221.

99. Hooser, S.B.; Kuhlenschmidt, M.S.; Dahlem, A.M.; Beasley, V.R.; Carmichael, W.W.; Haschek, W.M. Uptake and Subcellular Localization of Tritiated Dihydro-microcystin-LR in Rat Liver. *Toxicon* **1991**, *29*, 589–601.

100. Runnegar, M.T.C.; Gerdes, R.G.; Falconer, I.R. The Uptake of the Cyanobacterial Hepatotoxin Microcystin by Isolated Rat Hepatocytes. *Toxicon* **1991**, *29*, 43–51.

101. Sahin, A.; Tencalla, F.G.; Dietrich, D.R.; Naegeli, H. Biliary Excretion of Biochemically Active Cyanobacteria (blue-green algae) Hepatotoxins in Fish. *Toxicology* **1996**, *106*, 123–130.

102. Kondo, F.; Matsumoto, H.; Yamada, S.; Ishikawa, N.; Ito, E.; Nagata, S.; Ueno, Y.; Suzuki, M.; Harada, K. Detection and Identification of Metabolites of Microcystins formed *in Vivo* in Mouse and Rat Livers. *Chem. Res. Toxicol.* **1996**, *9*, 1355–1359.

103. Takenaka, S. Covalent Glutathione Conjugation to Cyanobacterial Hepatotoxin Microcystin-LR by F344 Rat Cytosolic and Microsomal Glutathione *S*-transferases. *Environ. Toxicol. Phar.* **2001**, *9*, 135–139.

104. Xie, L.; Xie, P.; Guo, L.; Li, L.; Miyabara, Y.; Park, H. Organ Distribution and Bioaccumulation of Microcystins in Freshwater Fish at Different Trophic Levels from the Eutrophic Lake Chaohu, China. *Environ. Toxicol.* **2005**, *20*, 293–300.

105. Xie, L.; Yokoyama, A.; Nakamura, K.; Park, H. Accumulation of Microcystins in Various Organs of the Freshwater Snail *Sinotaia histrica* and Three Fishes in a Temperate Lake, the Eutrophic Lake Suwa, Japan. *Toxicon* **2007**, *49*, 646–652.

106. Zhang, D.; Deng, X.; Xie, P.; Yang, Q.; Chen, J.; Dai, M. Determination of Microcystin-LR and its Metabolites in Snail (*Bellamya aeruginosa*), Shrimp (*Macrobrachium nipponensis*) and Silver Carp (*Hypophthalmichthys molitrix*) from Lake Taihu, China. *Chemosphere.* **2009**, *76*, 974–981.

107. He, J.; Chen, J.; Xie, P.; Zhang, D.; Li, G.; Wu, L.; Zhang, W.; Guo, X.; Li, S. Quantitatively Evaluating Detoxification of the Hepatotoxic Microcystins through the Glutathione and Cysteine Pathway in the Cyanobacterial-eating Bighead Carp. *Aquat. Toxicol.* **2012**, *116–117*, 61–68.

108. Zhang, D.; Yang, Q.; Xie, P.; Deng, X.; Chen, J.; Dai, M. The Role of Cysteine Conjugation in the Detoxification of Microcystin-LR in Liver of Bighead Carp (*Aristichthys nobilis*): A Field and Laboratory Study. *Ecotoxicology* **2012**, *21*, 244–252.

109. Buratti, F.M.; Scardala, S.; Funari, E.; Testai, E. Human Glutathione Transferases Catalyzing the Conjugation of the Hepatatoxin Microcystin-LR. *Chem. Res. Toxicol.* **2011**, *24*, 926–933.

110. Metcalf, J.S.; Beattie, K.A.; Pflugmacher, S.; Codd, G.A. Immuno-crossreactivity and toxicity assessment of conjugation products of the cyanobacterial toxin, microcystin-LR. *FEMS Microbiol. Lett.* **2000**, *189*, 155–158.

111. Campos, A.; Vasconcelos, V. Molecular Mechanisms of Microcystin Toxicity in Animal Cells. *Int. J. Mol. Sci.* **2010**, *11*, 268–287.

112. Ito, E.; Takai, A.; Kondo, F.; Masui, H.; Imanishi, S.; Harada, K. Comparison of protein phosphatase inhibitory activity and apparent toxicity of microcystins and related compounds. *Toxicon* **2001**, *40*, 1017–1025.

113. Smith, J.L.; Haney, J.F. Foodweb Transfer, Accumulation, and Depuration of Microcystins, a Cyanobacterial Toxin, in Pumpkinseed Sunfish (*Lepomis gibbosus*). *Toxicon* **2006**, *48*, 580–589.

114. Moreno, I.M.; Molina, R.; Jos, A.; Picó, Y.; Cameán, A.M. Determination of Microcystins in Fish by Solvent Extraction and Liquid Chromatography. *J. Chromatagr. A.* **2005**, *1080*, 199–203.

115. Oberhaus, L.; Gelinas, M.; Pinel-Alloul, B.; Ghadouani, A.; Humbert, J. Grazing of Two Toxic *Planktothrix* Species by *Daphnia pulicaria*: Potential for Bloom Control and Transfer of Microcystins. *J. Plankton Res.* **2007**, *29*, 827–838.

116. Smith, J.A.; Witkowski, P.J.; Fusillo, T.V. Manmade Organic Compounds in the Surface Waters of the United States—A review of Current Understanding. *U.S. Geolo. Surv. Circ.* **1988**, *1007*, 92.

117. Nowell, L.H.; Capel, P.D.; Dileanis, P.D. *Pesticides in Stream Sediment and Aquatic Biota—Distribution, Trends, and Governing Factors*; CRC Press: Boca Raton, FL, USA, 1999.

118. Freitas de Magalhães, V.F.; Soares, R.M.; Azevedo, S.M.F.O. Microcystin Contamination in Fish from the Jacarepagua Lagoon (Rio de Janeiro, Brazil): Ecological Implication and Human Health Risk. *Toxicon* **2001**, *39*, 1077–1085.

119. Prepas, E.E.; Kotak, B.G.; Campbell, L.M.; Evans, J.C.; Hrudey, S.E.; Holmes, C.F.B. Accumulation and Elimination of Cyanobacterial Hepatotoxins by the Freshwater Clam *Anodonta grandis simpsoniana*. *Can. J. Fish. Aquat. Sci.* **1997**, *54*, 41–46.

120. Zhang, D.; Xie, P.; Liu, Y.; Qiu, T. Transfer, Ddistribution and Bioaccumulation of Microcystins in the Aquatic Food Web in Lake Taihu, China, with Potential Risks to Human Health. *Sci. Total Environ.* **2013**, *7*, 2191–2199.

121. Poste, A.; Hecky, R.E.; Guildford, S.J. Evaluating Microcystin Exposure Risk through Fish Consumption. *Environ. Sci. Technol.* **2011**, *45*, 5806–5811.

122. Amrani, A.; Nasri, H.; Azzouz, A.; Kadi, Y.; Bouaïcha, N. Variation in Cyanobacterial Hepatotoxin (microcystin) Content of Water Samples and two Species of Fishes Collected from a Shallow Lake in Algeria. *Arch. Environ. Contam. Toxicol.* **2014**, *66*, 379–389.

123. Peng, L.; Liu, Y.; Chen, W.; Liu, L.; Kent, M.; Song, L. Health Risks Associated with Consumption of Microcystin-contaminated Fish and Shellfish in three Chinese Lakes: Significance for Freshwater Aquacultures. *Ecotox. Environ. Saf.* **2010**, *73*, 1804–1811.

124. Jia, J.; Luo, W.; Lu, Y.; Giesy, J.P. Bioaccumulation of Microcystins (MCs) in Four Fish Species from Lake Taihu, China: Assessment of Risks to Humans. *Sci. Total Environ.* **2014**, *487*, 224–232.

125. Leland, H.V.; Kuwabara, J.S. Trace metals. In *Fundamentals of Aquatic Toxicology*; Rand, G.M., Petrocelli, S.R., Eds.; CRC Press: New York, NY, USA, 1985; pp. 374–415.

126. Suedel, B.C.; Boraczek, J.A.; Peddicord, R.K.; Clifford, P.A.; Dillon, T.M. Trophic Transfer and Biomagnification Potential of Contaminants in Aquatic Ecosystems. *Rev. Environ. Contam. Toxicol.* **1994**, *136*, 21–89.

127. Kozlowsky-Suzuki, B.; Wilson, A.E.; Ferrão-Filho, A. Biomagnification or Biodilution of Microcystins in Aquatic Foodwebs? Meta-analyses of Laboratory and Field Studies. *Harmful Algae* **2012**, *18*, 47–55.

128. Papadimitriou, T.; Kagalou, I.; Stalikas, C.; Pilidis, G.; Leonardos, I.D. Assessment of Microcystin Distribution and Biomagnification in Tissues of Aquatic Food Web Compartments from a Shallow Lake and Evaluation of Potential Risks to Public Health. *Ecotoxicology* **2012**, *21*, 1155–1166.

129. Ibelings, B.W.; Bruning, K.; de Jonge, J.; Wolfstein, K.; Dionisio Pires, L.M.; Postma, J.; Burger, T. Distribution of Microcystins in a Lake Foodweb: No Evidence for Biomagnification. *Microbial Ecol.* **2005**, *49*, 487–500.

130. Gustafsson, S.; Hanson, L. Development of Tolerance against Toxic Cyanobacteria in *Daphnia*. *Aquat. Ecol.* **2004**, *38*, 37–44.

131. Guo, N.; Xie, P. Development of Tolerance against Toxic *Microcystis aeruginosa* in Three Cladocerans and the Ecological Implications. *Environ. Pollut.* **2006**, *143*, 513–518.

132. Pietsch, C.; Wiegand, C.; Ame, M.V.; Nicklisch, A.; Wunderlin, D.; Pflugmacher, S. The Effects of a Cyanobacterial Crude Extract on Different Aquatic Organisms: Evidence for Cyanobacterial Toxin Modulating Factors. *Environ. Toxicol.* **2001**, *16*, 535–542.

133. Yokoyama, A.; Park, H. Depuration Kinetics and Persistence of the Cyanobacterial Toxin Microcystin-LR in the Freshwater Bivalve *Unio douglasiae*. *Environ. Toxicol.* **2003**, *18*, 61–67.

134. Pires, L.M.; Bones, B.M.; Van Donk, E.; Ibelings, B.W. Grazing on Colonial and Filamentous, Toxic and Non-toxic Cyanobacteria by the Zebra Mussel *Dreissena polymorpha*. *J. Plankton Res.* **2004**, *27*, 331–339.

135. Juhel, G.; Davenport, J.; O'Halloran, J.; Culloty, S.; Ramsay, R.; James, K.; Furey, A.; Allis, O. Pseudodiarrhoea in Zebra Mussels *Dreissena polymorpha* (Pallas) Exposed to Microcystins. *J. Exp. Biol.* **2006**, *209*, 810–816.

136. Vasconcelos, V.M.; Wiegand, C.; Pflugmacher, S. Dynamics of Glutathione-*S*-transferases in *Mytilus galloprovincialis* Exposed to Toxic *Microcystis Aeruginosa* Cells, Extracts and Pure Toxins. *Toxicon* **2007**, *50*, 740–745.

137. Contardo-Jara, V.; Pflugmacher, S.; Wiegand, C. Multi-xenobiotic Resistance a Possible Explanation for the Insensitivity of Bivalves towards Cyanobacterial Toxins. *Toxicon* **2008**, *52*, 936–943.

138. Blanchette, M.; Haney, J.F. The Effect of Toxic *Microcystis Aeruginosa* on Four Different Populations of *Daphnia*. *UNH Cent. Freshw. Biol. Res.* **2002**, *4*, 1–10.

139. Råbergh, C.M.I.; Bylund, G.; Eriksson, J.E. Histopathological Effects of Microcystin-LR, a Cyclic Peptide Toxin from the Cyanobacterium (blue-green alga) *Microcystis aeruginosa*, on Common Carp (*Cyprinus carpio L.*). *Aquat. Toxicol.* **1991**, *20*, 131–146.

140. Malbrouck, C.; Trausch, G.; Devos, P.; Kestemont, P. Hepatic Accumulation and Effects of Microcystin-LR on Juvenile Goldfish *Carassius auratus L. Comp. Biochem. Phys.* **2003**, *135*, 39–48.

141. Kotak, B.G.; Semalulu, S.; Fritz, D.L.; Prepas, E.E.; Hrudey, S.E.E.; Coppock, R.W. Hepatic and Renal Pathology of Intraperitoneally Administered Microcystin-LR in Rainbow Trout (*Oncorhynchus mykiss*). *Toxicon* **1996**, *34*, 517–525.

142. Lu, Y.; Liu, J.; Wu, K.; Qu, Q.; Fan, F.; Klaassen, C.D. Overexpression of Nrf2 Protects Against Microcystin-induced Hepatotoxicity in Mice. *PLoS One* **2014**, *9*, e93013.

143. Falconer, I.R.; Jackson, A.R.B.; Langley, J.; Runnegar, M.T. Liver Pathology in Mice in Poisoning by the Blue-green Alga *Microcystis aeruginosa*. *Aust. J. Biol. Sci.* **1981**, *34*, 179–187.

144. Sivonen, K.; Jones, G.J. Cyanobacterial toxins. In *Toxic Cyanobacteria in Water: A Guide to Their Public Health Consequences, Monitoring and Management*; Chorus, I., Bartram, J., Eds.; E and FN Spon: London, UK, 1999; pp. 41–111.

145. Smith, J.L.; Boyer, G.L.; Mills, E.; Schulz, K.L. Toxicity of Microcystin-LR, a Cyanobacterial Toxin, to Multiple Life Stages of the Burrowing Mayfly, *Hexagenia*, and Possible Implications for Recruitment. *Environ. Toxicol.* **2007**, *23*, 499–506.

146. Zhang, D.; Deng, X.; Xie, P.; Chen, J.; Guo, L. Risk Assessment of Microcystins in Silver Carp (*Hypophthalmichthys molitrix*) from Eight Eutrophic Lakes in China. *Food Chem.* **2013**, *140*, 17–21.

147. Chen, J.; Xie, P.; Zhang, D.; Lei, H. In Situ Studies on the Distribution Parameters and Dynamics of Microcystins in Biomanipulation Fish-bighead Carp (*Aristichthys nobilis*). *Environ. Pollut.* **2007**, *147*, 150–157.

148. Namikoshi, M.; Rinehart, K.I. Bioactive Compounds Produced by Cyanobacteria. *J. Ind. Microbiol.* **1996**, *17*, 373–384.

149. Lampert, W. Inhibitory and Toxic Effects on Blue-green Algae on *Daphnia*. *Int. Rev. Gestamen Hydrobiol.* **1981**, *66*, 285–298.

150. Nizan, S.; Dimentman, C.; Shilo, M. Acute Toxic Effects of Cyanobacterium *Microcystis aeruginosa* on *Daphnia magna*. *Limnol. Oceanogr.* **1986**, *31*, 497–502.

151. Fulton, R.S., III; Paerl, H.W. Effects of Colonial Morphology on Zooplankton Utilization of Algal Sources during Blue-green Algal (*Microcystis aeruginosa*) Blooms. *Limnol. Oceanogr.* **1987**, *32*, 634–644.

152. Fulton, R.S., III; Paerl, H.W. Toxic and Inhibitory Effects of the Blue-green Alga *Microcystis aeruginosa* on Herbivorous Zooplankton. *J. Plankton Res.* **1987**, *9*, 837–855.

153. Benndorf, J.; Henning, M. *Daphnia* and Toxic Blooms of *Microcystis aeruginosa* in Bautzen Reservoir (GDR). *Int. Rev. Gestamen Hydrobiol.* **1989**, *74*, 233–248.

154. Rohrlack, T.; Dittmann, E.; Henning, M.; Borner, T.; Kohl, J. Role of Microcystins in Poisoning and Food Ingestion Inhibition by *Daphnia Galeata* Caused by the Cyanobacterium *Microcystis aeruginosa*. *Appl. Environ. Microbiol.* **1999**, *65*, 737.

155. Chislock, M.F.; Sarnelle, O.; Jernigan, L.M.; Wilson, A.E. Do High Concentrations of Microcystin Prevent *Daphnia* Control of Phytoplankton? *Water Res.* **2013**, *47*, 1961–1970.

156. Porter, K.G.; Orcutt, J.D. Nutritional Adequacy, Manageability, and Toxicity as Factors that Determine Food Quality of Green and Blue-green Algae for *Daphnia*. In *Evolution and Ecology of Zooplankton Communities* Kerfoot, W.C., EdS.; University Press of New England: Hanover, New Hampshire, UK, 1980; pp. 268–281.

157. Holm, N.P.; Shapiro, J.S. An Examination of Lipid Reserves and the Nutritional Status of *Daphnia pulex* Fed *Aphanizomenon flos-aquae*. *Limnol. Oceanogr.* **1984**, *28*, 677–687.

158. Ahlgren, G.; Lundstedt, L.; Brett, M.; Forsberg, C. Lipid Composition and Food Quality of Some Freshwater Phytoplankton for Cladoceran Zooplankters. *J. Plankton Res.* **1990**, *12*, 809–818.

159. Van Gremberghe, I.V.; Vanormelingren, P., Vanelslander, B.; van der Gucht, K.; D'hondt, S., de Meester, L.; Vyverman, W. Genotype-dependent Interactions among Sympatric *Microcystis* Strains Mediated by *Daphnia* Grazing. *Oikos* **2009**, *118*, 1647–1658.

160. DeMott, W.R.; Dhawale, S. Inhibition of *in-vitro* Protein Phosphatase Activity in Three Zooplankton Species by Microcystin-LR, a Toxin from Cyanobacteria. *Arch. Hydrobiol.* **1995**, *134*, 417–424.

161. DeMott, W.R.; Zhang, Q.; Carmichael, W.W. Effects of Toxic Cyanobacteria and Purified Toxins on the Survival and Feeding of a Copepod and Three Species of *Daphnia*. *Limnol. Oceanogr.* **1991**, *36*, 1346–1357.

162. Reinikainen, M.; Lindvall, F.; Meriluoto, J.A.O.; Repka, S.; Sivonen, K.; Spoof, L.; Wahlsten, M. Effects of Dissolved Cyanobacterial Toxins on the Survival and Egg Hatching of Estuarine Calanoid Copepods. *Mar. Biol.* **2002**, *140*, 577–583.

163. Ger, K.A.; Teh, S.J.; Goldman, C.R. Microcystin-LR Toxicity on Dominant Copepods *Eurytemora affinis* and *Pseudodiaptomus forbesi* of the upper San Francisco Estuary. *Sci. Total Environ.* **2009**, *407*, 4852–4857.

164. DeMott, W.R.; Moxter, F. Foraging on Cyanobacteria by Copepods: Responses to Chemical Defenses and Resource Abundance. *Ecology* **1991**, *72*, 1820–1834.

165. DeMott, W.R. Foraging Strategies and Growth Inhibition in five Daphnids Feeding on Mixtures of a Toxic Cyanobacterium and a Green Alga. *Freshwater Biol.* **1999**, *42*, 263–274.

166. Ortiz-Rodríguez, R.; Wiegand, C. Age Related Acute Effects of Microcystin-LR on *Daphnia Magna* Biotransformation and Oxidative Stress. *Toxicon* **2010**, *56*, 1342–4349.

167. Hairston, N.G.; Lampert, W.; Cáceres, C.E.; Holtmeier, C.L.; Weider, L.J.; Gaedke, U.; Fischer, J.M.; Fox, J.A.; Post, D.M. Rapid Evolution Revealed by Dormant Eggs. *Nature* **1999**, *401*, 44.

168. Geis-Asteggiante, L.; Lehotay, S.J.; Fortis, L.L.; Paoli, G.; Wijey, C.; Heinzen, H. Development and Validation of a Rapid Method for Microcystins in Fish and Comparing LC-MS/MS Results with ELISA. *Anal. Bioanal. Chem.* **2011**, *401*, 2617–2630.

169. Kohoutek, J.; Adamovský, O.; Oravec, M.; Simek, Z.; Palíková, M.; Kopp, R.; Bláha, L. LC-MS Analyses of Microcystins in Fish Tissues Overestimate Toxin Levels-critical Comparison with LC-MS/MS. *Anal. Bioanal. Chem.* **2010**, *398*, 1231–1237.

170. Smith, J.L.; Boyer, G.L. Standardization of Microcystin Extraction from Fish Tissues: A Novel Internal Standard as a Surrogate for Polar and Non-polar Variants. *Toxicon* **2009**, *53*, 238–245.

171. Mekebri, A.; Blondina, G.J.; Crane, D.B. Method Validation of Microcystins in Water and Tissue by Enhanced Liquid Chromatography Tandem Mass Spectrometry. *J. Chromatogr. A* **2009**, *1216*, 3147–3155.

172. Karlsson, K.M.; Spoof, L.E.M.; Meriluoto, J.A.O. Quantitative LC-ESF-MS Analyses of Microcystins and Nodularin-R in Animal Tissue-matrix Effects and Method Validation. *Environ. Toxicol.* **2005**, *20*, 381–389.

173. Ernst, B.; Bietz, L.; Hoeger, S.J.; Dietrich, D.R. Recovery of MC-LR in Fish Liver Tissue. *Environ. Toxicol.* **2005**, *20*, 449–458.

174. Adamovský, O.; Kopp, R.; Hilscherová, K.; Babica, P.; Palíková, M.; Pašková, V.; Navrátil, S.; Maršálek, B.; Bláha, L. Microcystin Kinetics (bioaccumulation and elimination) and Biochemical Responses in Common Carp (*Cyprinus carpio*) and Silver Carp (*Hypophthalmichthys molitrix*) Exposed to Toxic Cyanobacterial Blooms. *Environ. Toxicol. Chem.* **2007**, *26*, 2687–2693.

175. Dai, M.; Xie, P.; Liang, G.; Chen, J.; Lei, H. Simultaneous Determination of Microcystin-LR and its Glutathione Conjugate in Fish Tissues by Liquid Chromatography-tandem Mass Spectrometry. *J. Chromatogr. B* **2008**, *862*, 43–50.

176. Barron, M.G.; Stehly, G.R.; Hayton, W.L. Pharmacokinetic Modeling in Aquatic Animals I. Models and concepts. *Aquatic Toxicol.* **1990**, *18*, 61–86.

177. Dyble, J.; Gossiaux, D.; Landrum, P.; Kashian, D.R.; Pothoven, S. A Kinetic Study of Accumulation and Elimination of Microcystin-LR in Yellow Perch (*Perca flavescens*) Tissue and Implications for Human Fish Consumption. *Mar. Drugs* **2011**, *9*, 2553–2571.

178. Roberts, M.S.; Magnusson, B.M.; Burczynski, F.J.; Weiss, M. Enterohepatic Circulation: Physiological, Pharmacokinetic and Clinical Implications. *Clin. Pharmacokinet.* **2002**, *41*, 751–790.

179. Beasley, V.R.; Stotts, R.R. Toxicokinetics of Microcystin and Dihydro-microcystin in Swine. US Army report, 1994. Available online: http://www.dtic.mil/cgibin/GetTRDoc?AD= ADA280697&Location=U2&doc=GetTRDoc.pdf (accessed on 25 June 2014).

180. Li, T.; Huang, P.; Liang, J.; Fu, W.; Guo, Z.; Xu, L. Microcystin-LR (MCLR) Induces a Compensation of PP2A Activity Mediated by α4 Protein in HEK293 Cells. *Int. J. Biol. Sci.* **2011**, *7*, 740–752.

181. Lin, J.; Chu, F.S. Kinetics of Distribution of Microcystin-LR in Serum and Liver Cytosol of Mice: An Immunochemical Analysis. *J. Agric. Food Chem.* **1994**, *42*, 1035–1040.

182. Robinson, N.A.; Miura, G.A.; Matson, C.F.; Dinterman, R.E.; Pace, J.G. Characterization of Chemically Tritiated Microcystin-LR and its Distribution in Mouse. *Toxicon* **1990**, *27*, 1035–1042.

183. Brooks, W.P.; Codd, G.A. Distribution of *Microcystis Aeruginosa* Peptide Toxin and Interactions with Hepatic Microsomes in Mice. *Pharmacol. Toxicol.* **1987**, *60*, 187–191.

184. Lei, H.; Xie, P.; Chen, J.; Liang, G.; Yu, T.; Jiang, Y. Tissue Distribution and Depuration of the Extracted Hepatotoxic Cyanotoxin Microcystins in Crucian Carp (*Carassius carassius*) Intraperitoneally Injected at a Sublethal Dose. *ScientificWorldJournal* **2008**, *8*, 713–719.

185. Rohrlack, T.; Christofferson, K.; Dittmann, E.; Nogueira, I.; Vasconcelos, V.; Borner, T. Ingestion of Microcystins by *Daphnia*: Intestinal Uptake and Toxic Effects. *Limnol. Oceanogr.* **2005**, *50*, 440–448.

186. Sadler, T.; von Elert, E. Dietary Exposure of *Daphnia* to Microcystins: No *in vivo* Relevance of Biotransformation. *Aquat. Toxicol.* **2014**, *150*, 73–82.

187. Li, W.; Chen, J.; Xie, P.; He, J.; Guo, X.; Tuo, X.; Zhang, W.; Wu, L. Rapid Conversion and Reversible Conjugation of Glutathione Detoxification of Microcystins in Bighead Carp (*Aristichthys nobilis*). *Aquat. Toxicol.* **2014**, *147*, 18–25.

188. Agha, R.; Quesada, A. Oligopeptides as Biomarkers of Cyanobacterial Subpopulations. Toward an Understanding of Their Biological Role. *Toxins* **2014**, *6*, 1929–1950.

The Importance of Lake Sediments as a Pathway for Microcystin Dynamics in Shallow Eutrophic Lakes

Haihong Song, Liah X. Coggins, Elke S. Reichwaldt and Anas Ghadouani

Abstract: Microcystins are toxins produced by cyanobacteria. They occur in aquatic systems across the world and their occurrence is expected to increase in frequency and magnitude. As microcystins are hazardous to humans and animals, it is essential to understand their fate in aquatic systems in order to control health risks. While the occurrence of microcystins in sediments has been widely reported, the factors influencing their occurrence, variability, and spatial distribution are not yet well understood. Especially in shallow lakes, which often develop large cyanobacterial blooms, the spatial variability of toxins in the sediments is a complex interplay between the spatial distribution of toxin producing cyanobacteria, local biological, physical and chemical processes, and the re-distribution of toxins in sediments through wind mixing. In this study, microcystin occurrence in lake sediment, and their relationship with biological and physicochemical variables were investigated in a shallow, eutrophic lake over five months. We found no significant difference in cyanobacterial biomass, temperature, pH, and salinity between the surface water and the water directly overlying the sediment (hereafter 'overlying water'), indicating that the water column was well mixed. Microcystins were detected in all sediment samples, with concentrations ranging from 0.06 to 0.78 µg equivalent microcystin-LR/g sediments (dry mass). Microcystin concentration and cyanobacterial biomass in the sediment was different between sites in three out of five months, indicating that the spatial distribution was a complex interaction between local and mixing processes. A combination of total microcystins in the water, depth integrated cyanobacterial biomass in the water, cyanobacterial biomass in the sediment, and pH explained only 21.1% of the spatial variability of microcystins in the sediments. A more in-depth analysis that included variables representative of processes on smaller vertical or local scales, such as cyanobacterial biomass in the different layers and the two fractions of microcystins, increased the explained variability to 51.7%. This highlights that even in a well-mixed lake, local processes are important drivers of toxin variability. The present study emphasises the role of the interaction between water and sediments in the distribution of microcystins in aquatic systems as an important pathway which deserves further consideration.

Reprinted from *Toxins*. Cite as: Song, H.; Coggins, L.X.; Reichwaldt, E.S.; Ghadouani, A. The Importance of Lake Sediments as a Pathway for Microcystin Dynamics in Shallow Eutrophic Lakes. *Toxins* **2015**, *7*, 900-918.

1. Introduction

Microcystins are produced by certain species of cyanobacteria and are hazardous to humans and animals. Considered to be the most toxic group of cyanobacterial toxins, microcystins are inhibitors of specific protein phosphatases and can cause skin irritations, allergic reactions and gastroenteritis [1]. Humans are primarily exposed to microcystins via drinking water consumption and accidental ingestion of recreational water [2,3]. Recreational exposure by skin contact or inhalation to microcystins is now a recognised cause of a wide range of acute illnesses that can be life-threatening [4]. While microcystins have been reported across the world [5], the frequency of their occurrence in aquatic systems is expected to rise as a result of climate change [6–10]. To control the associated health risks, it is therefore essential to understand the fate of microcystins in aquatic systems.

In aquatic systems, microcystins can be present not only in the water but also in sediments. They have been reported in a variety of sediments, with and without the occurrence of benthic cyanobacteria [11–13]. Microcystins in lake sediments have their origin in at least three main processes (Figure 1); including the lysis of cyanobacterial cells in sediments, transfer from the dissolved form to sediments by adsorption, and grazing by aquatic animals followed by the sinking of microcystin-containing faecal pellets [14]. Their occurrence in lake sediments is a potential hazard to aquatic animals and benthic organisms, for example, by altering the organisms' metabolism [15,16]. In addition, the release of toxins that are loosely bound to the sediment might re-dissolve into the water column long after a bloom, and in absence of any visual indication of the presence of cyanobacterial blooms [17].

Studies on the distribution of total microcystins in sediments of aquatic systems are limited, likely due to technical difficulties in extracting total toxins from sediments [11]. An earlier study indicates that sediments contain two microcystin fractions: a loosely adsorbed and therefore "readily extractable" fraction, and a bound fraction [17]. The MMPB (2-methyl-3-methoxy-4-phenylbutyric acid) method is considered to be an effective analytical procedure for the quantification of total microcystins (free and bound) in lake sediments. However, this method requires a very low reaction temperature of −78 °C [11], which might be a limiting factor. Conversely, the loosely adsorbed microcystin fraction, which is possibly the more hazardous fraction for organisms due to its potential to easily re-dissolve back into the water column, is easier to extract, and some studies have focused on this fraction [14,18,19]. With conventional solvents, the extraction efficiency of loosely adsorbed microcystins strongly depends on the solvent type, the sediment characteristics, and the chemical structure of microcystins [12].

Microcystin concentrations in sediments have been shown to be highly variable on a temporal and spatial scale. High microcystin concentrations have been found in sediments during spring, followed by a decrease in the summer, when cyanobacterial biomass in the water was at a maximum [19]. Moreover, Chen et al. [14] found that the highest microcystin concentrations in sediments occurred during summer, when cyanobacterial biomass and microcystin production were at their maximum. Microcystins have been reported at different depths of sediments [11,20], with concentrations decreasing with increased depth of sediment in Lake Taihu, China [14].

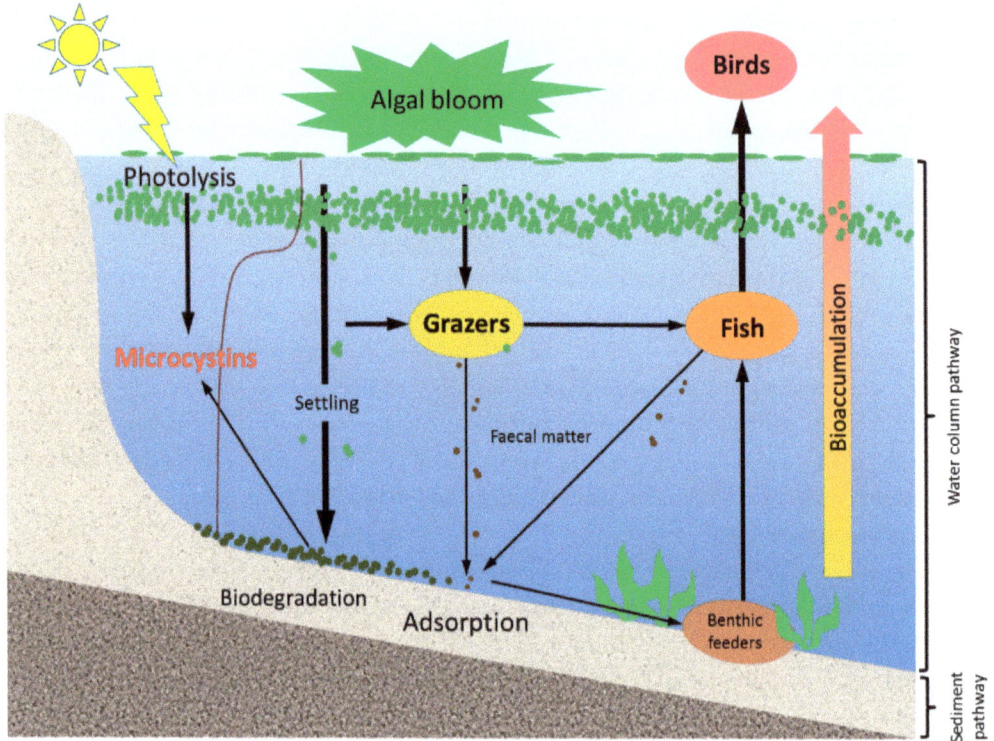

Figure 1. A schematic diagram showing the various pathways of microcystin dynamics during and following a bloom event. The sediment compartment plays a key role in release, adsorption and degradation of microcystins. Please note that stratification does not occur in all systems; especially shallow systems often have mixed water columns.

Many factors can contribute to the variability of microcystins in lake sediments. Ihle *et al.* [19] reported that microcystin concentrations in the sediments of a shallow lake correlated to *Microcystis* biomass in the sediments. Similarly, microcystin concentrations in the sediments of the Nile River and irrigation canal sediments correlated to the total count of cyanobacteria, particularly *Microcystis* spp. and intracellular microcystins in the water [18]. The concentration of microcystins in sediments can also be influenced by the sedimentation of suspended particles with absorbed microcystins [21] and the adsorption of dissolved microcystins from the water [11,12,14,18,22,23]. Furthermore, organic matter content and particle size fraction (sand, silt and clay) [14,16,22,24], as well as the physicochemical parameters of lake water, such as temperature, salinity, and pH [24–27], can influence the sediment's capacity to adsorb and degrade microcystins in aquatic systems. In shallow systems, wind-induced mixing of the water column and the associated redistribution of toxin-containing sediment potentially plays an important role in explaining the spatial distribution of toxins in the sediment.

Shallow lakes have a complex interplay between being stratified during times of high solar irradiation without wind and being completely mixed during periods of wind. Our study lake,

Lake Yangebup, which is representative of a shallow water body, is a typical example of such a system with stratification only occurring during periods of wind speed <6 m/s [28]. In such well mixed water bodies, the horizontal distribution of allochthonous contaminants in sediments can be expected to differ very little, due to the highly dynamic nature of the sediment, which is being resuspended and redeposited during mixing events [28,29]. With autochthonous substances, such as cyanotoxins, the spatial distribution of toxins in the sediment depends on the location where it is produced and on the redistribution of sediments. Thus, in the absence of wind mixing, we could expect higher concentrations of toxins in the sediment at locations that have cyanobacterial blooms (Figure 1), while these horizontal differences should be reduced during wind-induced mixing events. The spatial distribution of toxins in the sediments of shallow lakes should therefore be the result of a complex interaction of biological and physicochemical processes, including wind-driven mixing.

To date, systematic studies on the relationship between the variability of microcystins in lake sediments and the environmental factors are lacking. While a number of studies have looked at the temporal variability of microcystins in sediments, the spatial variability of microcystins within aquatic systems, especially in shallow systems has not been investigated. This study aims to identify the spatial and temporal variability of microcystins in the upper layer of sediments in a shallow, eutrophic lake, and to determine the biological and physical parameters contributing to the variability. We hypothesised that the variability of microcystin concentration in lake sediments can be predicted by a combination of biological and physical parameters such as cyanobacterial biomass in the sediments, cyanobacterial biomass and microcystins in the water, and physicochemical parameters of lake water and the sediment characteristics.

2. Results

2.1. Temporal and Spatial Variability of Microcystin Concentration in Sediments

Microcystins were detected in all sediment samples, with their concentration ranging from 0.06 (S2; September) to 0.78 µg/g dry mass (d.m.) (S2; August) (Figure 2). The average microcystin concentration in the sediments decreased from August to September and increased from September to December (Figure 3A). The lowest average concentration was observed in September (0.13 µg/g d.m.) and the maximum average concentration was observed in August (0.46 µg/g d.m.).

The temporal variability of microcystin concentrations in sediments was different for each sampling site (Figure 2). There was a significant difference in microcystin concentration in the sediments between months at sites 1–3, but not at site 4 (Table 1) which had the smallest temporal variability of microcystins in sediments (Figure 2D). Furthermore, the temporal changes in microcystin concentrations in the sediment were similar at sites 1 and 2 (Figure 2), where they decreased from August to September, followed by an increase in October, and a decrease until December. In contrast, the microcystin concentration in the sediments at site 3 decreased from August to September but then increased until December, when the maximum concentration was observed (Figure 2).

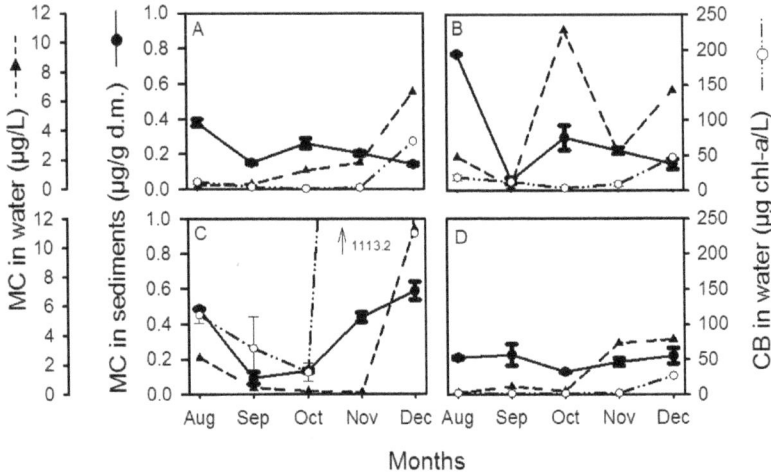

Figure 2. Microcystin concentration (MC) in sediments (●), total microcystin concentration in water (▲) and cyanobacterial biomass (CB) (○) in water as a function of time at sites 1–4 (**A–D**). CB in water is the calculated mean between CB in the surface water and the water directly overlying the sediment (overlying). Error bars represent one standard error (with $n = 3$ for MC concentration in sediments, and $n = 2$ for CB biomass in water). In November (panel C), cyanobacterial biomass was off the scale at 1113.2 µg chl-*a*/L, which is indicated by an arrow.

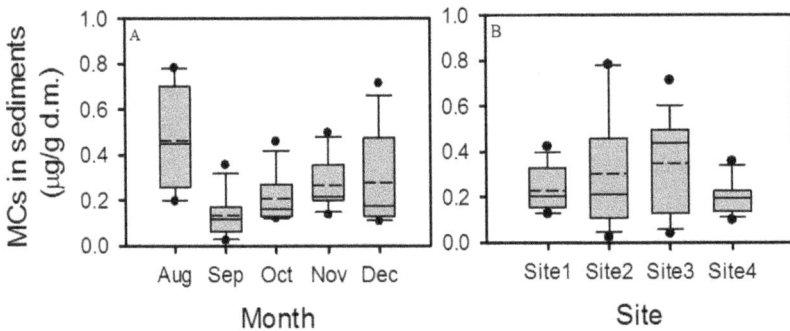

Figure 3. Spatial (**A**) and temporal variability (**B**) of microcystin concentrations in lake sediments. Boxes represent the 25th and 75th percentiles; solid lines within the boxes mark the median, dashed lines indicate the mean. Whiskers represent the largest and smallest observed values excluding the outliers. Filled circles represent outliers (>1.5 box lengths) ($n = 15$).

Table 1. Statistical results for differences between sites (one-way ANOVA or Kruskal-Wallis ANOVA on ranks) and between months (repeated-measures ANOVA or Friedman repeated-measures ANOVA on ranks) of biological and physical parameters in the sediments and water. *** indicates $p < 0.001$; ** indicates $p < 0.01$; * indicates $p < 0.05$; d.f. = degrees of freedom; n.s. = not significant; d.m. = dry mass; chl-a = chlorophyll-a.

Biological and Physical Parameters	Differences between Months	Differences between Sites
Microcystins in sediments (µg/g d.m.)	$F_{(4,8)} = 19.9$ (Site 1) *** $F_{(4,8)} = 36.2$ (Site 2) *** $F_{(4,8)} = 41.1$ (Site 3) *** n.s. (Site 4)	$H = 10.5$, d.f. = 3 (August) * n.s. (September) n.s. (October) $F_{(3,8)} = 21.5$ (November) *** $F_{(3,8)} = 21.4$ (December) ***
Cyanobacterial biomass in sediments (µg chl-a/g d.m.)	$F_{(4,8)} = 9.9$ (Site 1) ** n.s. (Site 2) n.s. (Site 3) $F_{(4,8)} = 3.9$ (Site 4) *	$H = 8.8$, d.f. = 3 (August) * $H = 9.5$, d.f. = 3 (September) * n.s. (October) n.s. (November) $H = 9.5$, d.f. = 3 (December) *
Cyanobacterial biomass in surface water (µg chl-a/L)	$\chi^2 = 12.2$, d.f. = 4 *	$H = 12.6$, d.f. = 3 **
Cyanobacterial biomass in overlying water (µg chl-a/L)	$\chi^2 = 13.6$, d.f. = 4 **	n.s.
Cyanobacterial biomass-average (µg chl-a/L)	$\chi^2 = 11.5$, d.f. = 4 *	$H = 11.3$, d.f. = 3 *
Intracellular microcystin concentration in water (µg/L)	$F_{(4,12)} = 10.9$ ***	n.s.
Dissolved microcystin concentration in water (µg/L)	$\chi^2 = 11.8$, d.f. = 4 *	n.s.
Total microcystin concentration in water (µg/L)	$F_{(4,12)} = 3.5$ *	n.s.
Organic matter (%)	$F_{(4,12)} = 31.7$ ***	n.s.

The spatial variability of microcystin concentrations in sediments was different in each month. In August, microcystin concentration in sediments at site 4 was significantly lower than at site 2, while in November and December, microcystin concentration was significantly higher at site 3 than at any other site (Table 1; Figure 2). In September and October, no significant differences in microcystin concentration between sites were observed. The largest spatial variability of microcystins in sediments occurred in August, while the smallest occurred in September (Figure 3A). On average, the microcystin concentration in sediments was highest at site 3 and lowest at site 4 (Figure 3B).

2.2. Temporal and Spatial Variability of Biological and Physical Parameters

Cyanobacterial biomass in sediments varied significantly at sites 1 and 4 over time (Table 1), and was significantly different between sites in: (i) August, when biomass at site 3 was significantly higher than at site 4; (ii) September, when biomass at site 3 was significantly higher than at sites 1 and 4; and (iii) December, when biomass at site 1 was significantly higher than at site 4 (Table 1).

Cyanobacterial biomass in the water was not significantly different between the surface water layer and the water layer directly overlying the sediment (overlying water) (*t*-test; $t = -1.23$, d.f. = 44), indicating a mixed water column. Cyanobacterial biomass, averaged over the water column (surface + overlying samples), showed a similar temporal trend at all sites and was highest at site 3 (Figure 2), with an extremely high value of 1113.2 µg chl-*a*/L in November. There was a significant difference between sites in (i) cyanobacterial biomass in surface water (Table 1), with site 3 having a higher biomass than sites 1 and 4, and (ii) cyanobacterial biomass averaged over the water column (Table 1), with site 3 having a higher biomass than site 4. There was no difference between the sites for cyanobacterial biomass in the overlying water (Table 1). Cyanobacterial biomass in surface water, overlying water, and averaged over the water column was significantly different between months (Table 1). The average cyanobacterial biomass in the water column and the cyanobacterial biomass in the surface water were higher in December than October, while the cyanobacterial biomass in the overlying water was significantly higher in December than in September.

Total microcystin concentration (intracellular + dissolved) in surface water showed a similar trend at all sites with increasing concentrations towards December (Figure 2) and was significantly different between months (Table 1). Intracellular and dissolved concentrations in the water were both significantly different between months (Table 1), with December concentrations being different to all other months. There was no difference in intracellular, dissolved, or total microcystin concentration between sites (Table 1).

Organic matter content in sediment samples was different between months, with the percentage organic matter being significantly higher in December compared to all other months (Table 1). No significant difference in organic matter between sites was detected.

2.3. Correlation between Microcystins in the Sediments and Biological and Physical Parameters

Linear correlations (Pearson's correlations) were calculated between microcystin concentration in sediments and the biological and chemical parameters studied (Table 2). Microcystin concentration in the sediments had weak but significant linear correlations with the concentration of intracellular microcystin in the water, total microcystin concentration in surface water, and cyanobacterial biomass in the water directly above the sediment (overlying).

Table 2. Pearson's correlation values (R) between microcystin concentrations (MC) in the sediments (µg/g d.m.), biological and chemical parameters. CB_{sedim}: cyanobacterial biomass in the sediments (µg chl-*a*/g d.m.); CB_{overl}, CB_{surf}, $CB_{average}$: cyanobacterial biomass in the overlying, the surface water, or averaged over the two layers (µg chl-*a*/L); MC_{intra}, MC_{diss}, tMC_{water}: intracellular, dissolved, and total microcystin concentration in the surface water (µg/L); OM: percentage (mass) of organic matter in the sediments; Sig. = p-value. All data were log transformed before analysis.

	CB_{sedim}	CB_{overl}	CB_{surf}	$CB_{average}$	MC_{intra}	MC_{diss}	tMC_{water}	OM
MC_{sedim}	−0.012	0.476	0.171	0.237	0.289	0.016	0.254	0.108
Sig.	0.929	0.000	0.193	0.068	0.025	0.906	0.050	0.418
N	60	60	60	60	60	60	60	58

2.4. Prediction of Microcystin Concentrations in Sediments from Biological and Physical Parameters

Assuming a well-mixed system, the concentration of microcystins in the sediments ($c(MC_{sedim})$) could be best predicted by:

$$\log c(MC_{sedim}) = 5.784 + 0.229 \log c(tMC_{water}) + 0.230 \log c(CB_{average}) - 0.170 \log c(CB_{sedim}) - 7.28 \log pH ,$$

with $c(tMC_{water})$ being the total microcystin concentration in the water, $\log c(CB_{average})$ being the average cyanobacterial biomass in the water column, and $c(CB_{sedim})$ being the cyanobacterial biomass in the sediment ($R^2 = 0.211$, $p < 0.05$, $F_{(4,55)} = 3.68$).

A second multiple linear regression analysis using explanatory variables expressing processes on smaller scales increased the R^2 to 0.517 ($p < 0.05$, $F_{(5,54)} = 11.055$):

$$\log c(MC_{sedim}) = 10.285 + 0.524 \log c((MC_{intra}) + 1) + 0.309 \log c(CB_{overl}) - 0.132 \log c(CB_{sedim}) -$$
$$11.402 \log pH - 0.655 \log temperature,$$ with $c(MC_{intra})$ being intracellular microcystins in the water, (CB_{overl}) being cyanobacterial biomass in the overlying water, and $c(CB_{sedim})$ being cyanobacterial biomass in the sediment.

3. Discussion

Microcystins were detected in all sediment samples in this study, including at site 4 where only a low level of cyanobacterial biomass occurred, indicating the wide presence of microcystins in the lake's sediments. Similar to previous studies [30–32], we found that cyanobacterial blooms, dominated by toxic *Microcystis* spp., and microcystins in the water occurred most of the year in Lake Yangebup. Microcystins can therefore accumulate in the sediments as a result of its long-term exposure to cyanobacterial biomass at the bottom of the lake and microcystins in the water (Figure 1).

The occurrence of microcystins in lake sediments associated with cyanobacterial blooms has been reported in earlier studies [11,12,14,18,19]. Microcystin concentrations in the sediment depend on a number of factors, including toxin production within the cyanobacterial community, and the biomass of toxic cyanobacteria in the sediment and in the water column [18,19]. Once the toxins that are produced within the water column reach the sediment, physical, chemical, and biological factors that influence the sediment's capacity to adsorb and degrade microcystins play an important role. The spatial variability of toxins in the sediment of a lake will therefore be the result of a complex interaction between the toxin producing processes in the water column, the physico-bio-chemical processes in the sediment, and a redistribution of toxin containing sediment. The latter is of extreme importance in shallow lakes, where wind is responsible for de-stratification of the water column and re-distribution of sediments [28,29]. An earlier study in Lake Yangebup showed that there is complete mixing of the water column at wind speeds >6 m/s with intermittent stratification at lower wind speeds, which can overturn within a few days [28]. Although wind speed was partially <6 m/s during our study (Figure 4B), these earlier results from Arnold and Oldham [28], in addition to the fact that we did not find a difference between the surface water layer and the water layer directly above the sediment (overlying) in cyanobacterial biomass, temperature, salinity and pH, indicates that Lake Yangebup is a typical representative of a shallow lake, that can be considered a mixed system due to wind effects and diurnal convectional cooling of the water.

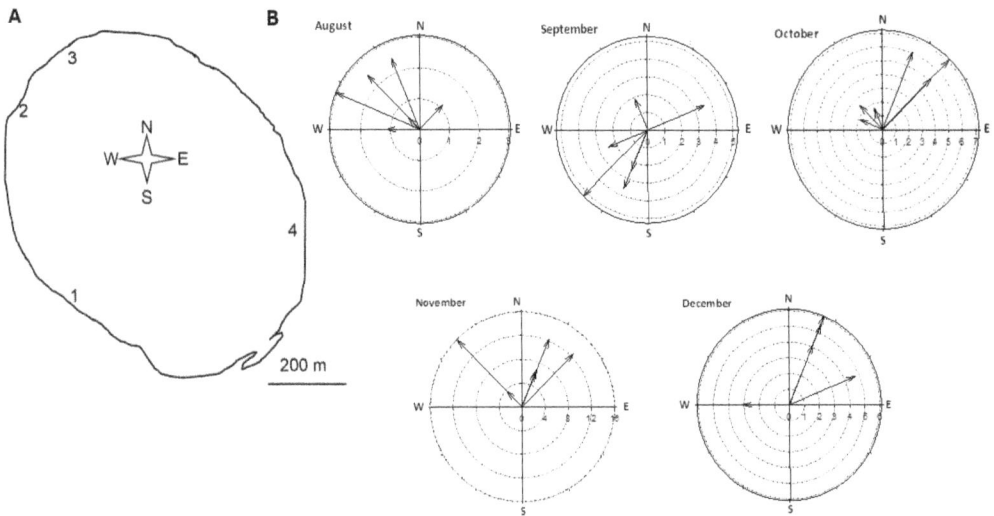

Figure 4. Study site and wind conditions. **(A)** Map of Lake Yangebup with sampling sites; **(B)** Wind speed and direction for the sampling days and the two antecedent days for each month. Wind measurements were taken at 9 am and 3 pm of each day, resulting in 6 measurements for each month. Please note different axes for wind speeds.

Interestingly, microcystin concentration and cyanobacterial biomass in the sediment was different between sites in three out of five months. This indicates that site specific processes are important for these variables, and that a re-distribution of toxin and cell containing sediment by wind-mixing might not have been complete. At the same time, we did not find a difference in the sediment toxin concentration between sites in September, when site 3 had a significantly higher cyanobacterial biomass in the water than all other sites, and differences in the sediment toxin concentration in November also did not coincide with different cyanobacterial biomass in the water column. This shows that some level of mixing is important in explaining the distribution of microcystins in the sediment. We can therefore conclude that local and wind-mixing processes are both important factors affecting the concentration of microcystin in the sediment.

We could explain the variability of microcystin concentration in the sediments by a combination of environmental variables, namely total microcystin concentration in the water, cyanobacterial biomass in the water, cyanobacterial biomass in the sediment and pH. These factors have also been shown to be of importance in previous studies, where significant and close relationships between the concentration of microcystins in sediments and intracellular microcystins or cyanobacterial biomass in the water column and the sediment have been reported [18,19]. The microcystins produced in the cyanobacteria in the water column can reach the sediment via a number of pathways, including settlement of cyanobacterial cells with subsequent cell lysis, and the adsorption of dissolved toxins to the sediment (Figure 1). The percentage of explained variability could be increased significantly by forcing variables indicative of smaller scale processes, such as cyanobacterial biomass in the overlying water, cyanobacterial biomass in the surface water, and intracellular and dissolved microcystin concentrations into the model. This clearly highlights again that, although Lake Yangebup is a mixed system, local processes are important to explain the local microcystin concentration in the sediment. Furthermore, it emphasises the importance of the link between processes in the water column in explaining the microcystin concentration in sediments [14,21].

The multiple linear regression analysis shows that microcystin concentration in sediments decreased with increasing pH and temperature. This could be due to the fact that higher temperatures increased the sediments capability to biodegrade microcystins, aiding the removal of these toxins from aquatic systems [25,33], and due to higher temperatures leading to an increased metabolic activity of the microcystin-degrading bacteria. In addition, previous studies have also shown that lower pH increases the capacity of sediments to adsorb microcystins [24,26,27], by influencing the surface charge heterogeneity of microcystins and sediment [17].

The temporal variability of microcystins in the lake's sediments was site specific, and the spatial variability in their concentration was different in each sampling month. Site 3 experienced a massive development of cyanobacterial biomass in November and December, and this possibly resulted in the increase of toxin concentration in the sediment at this site. On average, cyanobacterial biomass in the water was lowest at site 4 and highest at site 3. Wind is known to be a main driver of horizontal distribution of cyanobacterial biomass in lakes [34]. Wind speed and direction was variable in our study, however site 3 was the most downwind site in all months except September (Figure 4B). Therefore, it is likely that wind is the reason why we detected the highest biomass at this site.

The physical and chemical properties of sediments, for example, organic matter content and particle size fraction (sand, silt, and clay), will affect the sediment's capacity to adsorb and degrade microcystins [14,16,22–24]. Mohamed *et al.* [18] observed that in the Nile River, the capacity of sediments to adsorb microcystins was significantly correlated to their clay and organic matter content. Wu *et al.* [27] found that the adsorption process for microcystins to sediments mainly depended on the sediment's organic matter content. The significance of organic matter and clay in the binding and degradation of microcystins to soils and sediments has been reported in many other studies [24,35–40]. In our study, no clay was present in the sediments and no significant correlation between the concentration of microcystins and organic matter content in sediments was observed, probably due to only minor differences in the organic matter content of the samples.

4. Experimental Section

4.1. Study Site

This study was conducted at Lake Yangebup in Western Australia (32°6'40"S, 115°50'00"E). The field permit was provided by the City of Cockburn, Western Australia. The field study did not involve endangered or protected species. Lake Yangebup is a shallow, eutrophic, permanent lake with approximately 68.4 ha of open water and a mean water depth of 2.5 m [28]. Total phosphorus and total nitrogen in the water column of Lake Yangebup was previously reported to be 0.49–6.98 µM and 0.14–0.37 mM, respectively [32,41]. Toxic cyanobacterial blooms, dominated by *Microcystis* spp., frequently occur in this lake, and microcystins are present in the water for most of the year [30–32]. In a previous study in 2008–2009 [32,42], the range of concentration of microcystins in the water column was 1–80 µg equivalent microcystin-LR/L. Lake Yangebup is a groundwater through-flow lake that receives groundwater from its eastern side and discharges it towards the west. An earlier study, over 20 months using a weather station and a thermistor chain in the water column with sensors every 40 cm, showed that Lake Yangebup is mixed without stratification when wind speed is >6 m/s [28]. Sediment resuspension and redistribution during periods of wind-mixing has been hypothesised to be an important factor responsible for the horizontal distribution of sediments and contaminants in this and a neighbouring lake [28,29]. Lake Yangebup is surrounded by patches of fringing vegetation and an earlier investigation has reported the presence of a flocculate sediment layer, consisting mainly of dead and decaying organic matter covering a more consolidated sediment layer [28].

4.2. Sampling Design

Samples were taken monthly between August and December 2010, from four shore sites of Lake Yangebup with coordinates for sites 1–4 being 32°07'21"S, E115°49'45"; 32°07'07"S, 115°49'31"E; 32°6'50"S, 115°49'43"E; 32°07'11"S, 115°50'07"E, respectively (Figure 4A). Sampling sites were chosen based on their accessibility and geographic locations with the aim to distribute our sampling sites around the whole lake. All samples were taken between 7:30 am and 1:30 pm from water with a depth of 0.6–0.7 m and were stored on ice, in the dark, for transport to the laboratory. Temperature, pH, salinity were taken *in situ* from 10 cm below the water surface (referred to as "surface water") in all months, and additionally directly above the sediments (referred to as "overlying water") in October to December with probes (TPS WP-81); the average values of these parameters are given in Table 3. Dissolved oxygen was only measured at a depth of 10 cm (TPS-DO2). At each site, measurements for both surface water and overlying water were taken above the points where sediment samples were collected. There was no significant difference in temperature and salinity between the surface and the overlying water layer during the sampling period (student *t*-test; Figure 5), indicating that the water column was well mixed. Dissolved and intracellular toxins in surface water samples and cyanobacterial biomass in surface water and overlying water samples were quantified in the laboratory. For each sampling site, three sediment samples (0–4 cm) were collected using a transparent, polycarbonate sediment corer with a stainless-steel cutter (50 mm in diameter). Sediments in each sample were thoroughly mixed for homogenous quantification of cyanobacterial biomass, microcystin concentrations, and physicochemical properties. Wind direction and speed data came from the Australian Bureau of Meteorology's monitoring station at Jandakot Airport, which is 3 km from Lake Yangebup (Figure 4B).

Table 3. Physicochemical parameter means in each sampling month in Lake Yangebup. - indicates no measurement due to failure of the probe. DO = dissolved oxygen.

Month	Temperature (°C)	Salinity (mg/L)	DO (%)	DO (mg/L)	pH
August	16.4	946	44.9	4.9	8.4
September	18.9	947	54.9	5.0	8.6
October	21.4	1115	63.3	5.6	8.4
November	23.1	1202	-	-	8.6
December	22.2	1254	123.9	11.1	9.4

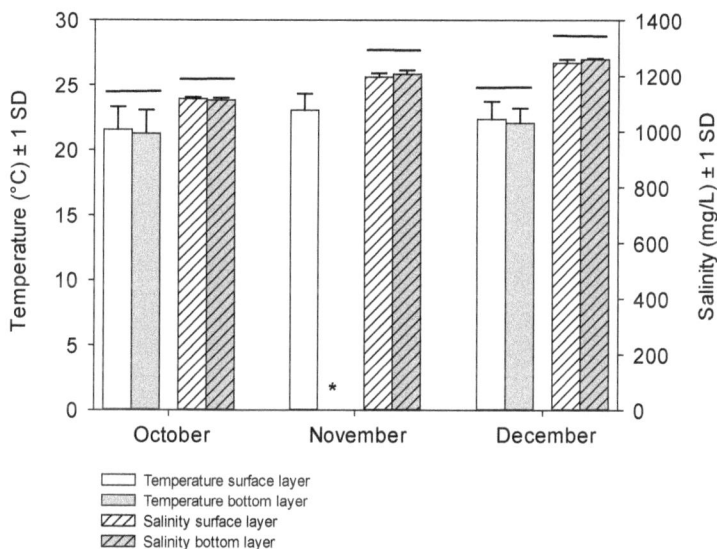

Figure 5. Mean (±1 SD) temperature (°C) and salinity (mg/L) in the surface and overlying water layers measured at the four sites in October to December in Lake Yangebup during this study. * = missing data; horizontal line indicates that no significant difference between data were detected (student *t*-test).

The mean daily air temperature, recorded at the nearest weather station to Lake Yangebup, taken over the 14 days prior to the sampling day, was used to represent surface water temperature in the data analysis. This was chosen instead of direct water temperature measurements, as water temperature strongly depends on the time of day sampling takes place. Earlier studies reported a good correlation between water temperature in shallow lakes and air temperature, and found that microcystin concentration in the water could be best predicted by mean daily air temperature of the preceding 14 days [43].

4.3. Sediment Analysis

The particle size of sediment samples was measured using a method adapted from Bowmanand Hutka [44]. The adaptations included heating the samples for a quicker digestion of the organic matter and removing the hydrogen peroxide by sequential dilution instead of evaporation. The particle size distribution analyser used was the Malvern Mastersizer 2000 with a Malvern Hydro 2000G automated wet dispersion accessory. Organic matter, measured by loss-on-ignition, was analysed according to Heiri *et al.* [45] but with samples dried in an oven at 110 °C overnight instead of freeze drying. The organic matter content of the sediment samples in Lake Yangebup ranged from 0.55% to 6.17%. With respect to particle size distribution, all sediment samples were sand, consisting of coarse and fine sand particles with a coarse sand content of 88% ± 10.12%. The particle size distribution for sediment samples at each sampling site is given in Table 4.

Table 4. Particle size fractions of sediment samples at each sampling site.

Sampling Sites	Clay % (<2 μm)	Silt % (2–20 μm)	Fine Sand % (20–200 μm)	Coarse Sand % (200–2000 μm)	Total Sand %
Site 1	0	0	13.12 ± 6.45	86.88 ± 6.45	100
Site 2	0	0	21.05 ± 2.71	78.95 ± 2.72	100
Site 3	0	0	10.66 ± 2.88	89.40 ± 2.88	100
Site 4	0	0	3.22 ± 0.87	96.78 ± 0.87	100

4.4. Analysis of Dissolved Microcystins in the Water

Surface water samples, 900–1000 mL for each water sample, were first filtered through pre-combusted GF/C filters (Whatman). Each filtrate was then applied to a solid phase extraction (SPE) cartridge (Oasis HLB 6 cc/500 mg, Waters, Rydalmere, NSW, Australia) with a flow rate <10 mL per minute for cleaning and concentration. The cartridge was then washed with 5 mL of 10% and 20% (*v/v*) methanol, in sequence, before blowing a constant air flow through the cartridge for drying. Microcystins were eluted from the cartridge with 5 mL of 100% methanol +0.1% trifluoroacetic acid (*v/v*). The elutes were dried with nitrogen gas at 45 °C before being re-dissolved in 1 mL of 30% acetonitrile (*v/v*) and analysed by high-performance liquid chromatography (HPLC) with a photodiode detector (1.2 nm resolution; Alliance 2695, Waters Corporation, Rydalmere, NSW, Australia) and an Atlantis® T3 separation column (4.6 × 150mm i.d, 3 μm, 100 Å; Waters Corporation). The HPLC gradient was identical to Lawton *et al.* [46] but with a maximum of 100% acetonitrile and, therefore, a longer run time of 37 min. Column temperature was 37.5 ± 2.5 °C and the limit of detection was 1.12 ng. Our limit of quantification was 3× the limit of detection. Peaks that showed a typical microcystin absorption spectrum with a maximum at 238.8 nm were quantified by comparing the peak area with the area of a known standard (microcystin-LR; Sapphire, Sydney, Australia).

4.5. Analysis of Intracellular Microcystins in the Water

Water samples were filtered on pre-combusted and pre-weighed GF/C filters (Whatman). The filters were dried at 60 °C, for 24 h, before being re-weighed to quantify biomass and then stored at −21 °C until microcystin extraction. Before the extraction of microcystins, the dry filters were thawed and re-frozen three times. The extraction was achieved with 6 mL of 75% methanol (*v/v*) per filter. Filters were sonicated on ice for 25 min, followed by gentle shaking for another 25 min.

The extracts were then centrifuged at 3273× g (Allegra X-12 Series; Beckman and Coulter Inc., Lane Cove, NSW, Australia) for 10 min at room temperature. Extracts were collected and filters were extracted two more times. After the three extractions, the supernatants were combined and diluted with Milli-Q water from 75% to 20% methanol (v/v) before they were applied to SPE cartridges (Oasis HLB 6 cc/500 mg, Waters, Australia). The subsequent analysis procedure was identical to that used for the dissolved microcystin analysis.

4.6. Analysis of Microcystins in the Sediments

The method used for quantification of microcystins in the sediments was adapted from Babica *et al.* [12]. In short, each freeze-dried sediment sample, 2.0–2.2 g (dry mass), was extracted twice with 20 mL of 5% acetic acid in methanol containing 0.2% v/v trifluoroacetic acid (TFA), using an ultrasonic bath for 30 min. After each extraction, the sample was centrifuged for 10 min at 3273× g (Allegra X-12, Beckman Coulter) and the supernatants from both extractions were combined, diluted with Milli-Q water from 95% to 20% methanol (v/v) and then applied to SPE cartridges (Oasis HLB 6 cc/500 mg, Waters, Australia). The subsequent analysis procedures, such as the cleaning and concentration of microcystins using SPE cartridges and the quantification of microcystins with HPLC, were identical to those used for the dissolved microcystin analysis. In a preliminary laboratory test, we determined the recovery rate for easily extractable microcystin-LR in sediment samples using this method was above 87% (data not shown).

Throughout this study, we refer to the total concentration of microcystin variants per sample as microcystin concentration. Total microcystin concentration (intracellular + dissolved) was expressed as micrograms (microcystin-LR mass equivalents) per litre water, intracellular microcystin concentration was expressed as micrograms (microcystin-LR mass equivalents) per gram cyanobacterial dry mass, and the total concentration of microcystin variants per sediment (easily extractable microcystins) was micrograms (microcystin-LR mass equivalents) per gram dry sediments.

4.7. Cyanobacterial Biomass in the Sediments and Water

The cyanobacterial biomass of each water sample was measured in the laboratory with a bench top version of the FluoroProbe (BBE Moldaenke, Schwentinental, Germany) as μg chl-a/L [47,48], for which chorophyll-a is a proxy for cyanobacterial biomass. The validation of the measurement of total chlorophyll-a with the Fluoroprobe against the values obtained from samples extracted according to standard methods [49] was described in Sinang *et al.* [32]. A strong linear correlation was found between the chlorophyll-a concentration measured with FluoroProbe and the chlorophyll-a concentration measured with the standard method (R^2 = 0.94, N = 32, p < 0.05). Sediment samples were washed with tap water until no cyanobacteria colonies in the sediments could be observed microscopically. The tap water was filtered through gauze (63 μm) to capture these colonies, which were then transferred with 30 mL of deionized water into a 100 mL glass bottle. This washing procedure was repeated twice and the cyanobacterial colonies were combined in a total of 100 mL deionized water. The concentration of cyanobacterial biomass in this bottle was quantified using the bench top version of the FluoroProbe as μg chl-a/L.

4.8. Statistical Analyses

Differences between sites were analysed using a one-way analysis of variance (ANOVA) when the data was normally distributed, and a Kruskal-Wallis ANOVA on ranks with a Bonferroni *t*-test when the data failed the normality test. Differences between months were analysed with a repeated-measures ANOVA with a Bonferroni *t*-test when the data was normally distributed, and a Friedman repeated-measures ANOVA on ranks with a Bonferroni *t*-test when the data failed the normality test. Pearson's correlations were calculated to identify the correlation between the concentration of microcystins in lake sediments and biological and physical parameters.

Two multiple linear regression analysis (backward) were carried out on the log transformed data to identify models that best explained the variability in the concentration of microcystins in the sediments. The first analysis included the following explanatory variables, which are representative for systems that are vertically well-mixed: cyanobacterial biomass in the sediment ($c(CB_{sedim})$; µg chl-a/g d.m.); total microcystin concentration in the water ($c(tMC_{water})$; µg/L); average cyanobacterial biomass in water ($c(CB_{average})$; µg/L); and pH and temperature. The second analysis included explanatory variables, which present processes on a smaller local scales: cyanobacterial biomass in the sediment ($c(CB_{sedim})$; µg chl-a/g d.m.); intracellular microcystin concentration in the water ($c(MC_{intra})$); µg/L); dissolved microcystin concentration in the water ($c(MC_{diss})$); µg/L); cyanobacterial biomass in overlying ($c(CB_{overl})$; µg/L) and surface water ($c(CB_{surf})$; µg/L); and pH and temperature. We used 0.05 as the probability of F-to-remove. Prior to the statistical analyses, the linearity of the microcystin concentration in sediments and the biological and physical parameters hypothesised to control microcystin variability were tested using scatterplots. Both dependent and independent variables were log-transformed and checked for normality using a Kologorov-Smirnov test. Statistical analyses were conducted in SigmaPlot 12.0 (Systat Software Int., San Jose, CA, USA) and IBM SPSS 21.0 (SPSS Inc., Chicago, IL, USA). Significance levels were set as $p < 0.05$ unless stated otherwise.

5. Conclusions

For the management of bloom-prone water bodies, it is important to holistically understand the fate of microcystins in the aquatic systems. Current studies and policies focusing on microcystins in aquatic systems almost exclusively concentrate on the water column, while sediments are mostly neglected. However, there is strong evidence from this and earlier studies that microcystins are widely present in sediments. In our study, the spatial variability of microcystins concentrations in sediments was different in each sampling month and their temporal variability was site specific. This highlights the fact that both local processes and lake-wide mixing contribute to the spatial distribution of microcystins in the sediment. It is interesting to note that, although we used a fairly small dataset, we could statistically identify drivers of the microcystin concentration in the sediment. We found that a significant part of the variability of the microcystin concentration in the sediments could be explained by a combination of variables in the water column, such as total microcystins in the water, cyanobacterial biomass in water, pH, and temperature. This illustrates the significance of the interaction between water and sediments in the distribution of microcystins in the sediment. In conclusion, our study highlights that cyanobacterial toxins in the sediment could pose a potential ecological hazard for the system, and that water management authorities should include sediments when assessing the potential health risks from microcystins in aquatic systems. This is especially important for shallow lakes that have an intimate link between the sediment and the water column. Further studies are required to study the role of local versus mixing processes for the microcystin distribution within sediments. In addition, long-term studies are essential to identify any seasonal patterns of sediment as a pathway for cyanotoxin dynamics.

Acknowledgments

This work was supported by the Australian Research Council Linkage Scheme (LP0776571) and the Water Corporation of Western Australia. Haihong Song was financially supported by a China Scholarship sponsored by the Chinese Scholarship Council and The University of Western Australia (UWA). The authors would like to thank the UWA Centre for Applied Statistics for statistical advice and Kristin Argall, Shian Min Liau, Randika Jayasinghe, Anna Byrne and Aninditha Dharma for comments on an earlier draft.

Author Contributions

All authors contributed to the design of this study, performed the data analysis, and jointly wrote the manuscript. All authors approved the final manuscript.

Conflicts of Interest

The authors declare no conflict of interest.

References

1. Žegura, B.; Štraser, A.; Filipič, M. Genotoxicity and potential carcinogenicity of cyanobacterial toxins—A review. *Mutat. Res.* **2011**, *727*, 16–41.
2. Chorus, I.; Falconer, I.R.; Salas, H.J.; Bartram, J. Health risks caused by freshwater cyanobacteria in recreational waters. *J. Toxicol. Env. Health B* **2000**, *3*, 323–347.
3. Funari, E.; Testai, E. Human health risk assessment related to cyanotoxins exposure. *Crit. Rev. Toxicol.* **2008**, *38*, 97–125.
4. De la Cruz, A.A.; Antoniou, M.G.; Hiskia, A.; Pelaez, M.; Song, W.H.; O'Shea, K.E.; He, X.X.; Dionysiou, D.D. Can we effectively degrade microcystins?-Implications on human health. *Anti Cancer Agent Med. Chem.* **2011**, *11*, 19–37.
5. Zurawell, R.W.; Huirong, C.; Burke, J.M.; Prepas, E.E. Hepatotoxic cyanobacteria: A review of the biological importance of microcystins in freshwater environments. *J. Toxicol. Environ. Health B* **2005**, *8*, 1–37.
6. Moore, S.; Trainer, V.; Mantua, N.; Parker, M.; Laws, E.; Backer, L.; Fleming, L. Impacts of climate variability and future climate change on harmful algal blooms and human health. *Environ. Health Glob.* **2008**, *7*, S4.

7. Paerl, H.W.; Huisman, J. Climate change: A catalyst for global expansion of harmful cyanobacterial blooms. *Environ. Microbiol. Rep.* **2009**, *1*, 27–37.

8. El-Shehawy, R.; Gorokhova, E.; Piñas, F.F.; del Campo, F.F. Global warming and hepatotoxin production by cyanobacteria: What can we learn from experiments? *Water Res.* **2012**, *46*, 1420–1429.

9. Reichwaldt, E.S.; Ghadouani, A. Effects of rainfall patterns on toxic cyanobacterial blooms in a changing climate: Between simplistic scenarios and complex dynamics. *Water Res.* **2012**, *46*, 1372–1393.

10. Paerl, H.W.; Paul, V.J. Climate change: Links to global expansion of harmful cyanobacteria. *Water Res.* **2012**, *46*, 1349–1363.

11. Tsuji, K.; Masui, H.; Uemura, H.; Mori, Y.; Harada, K. Analysis of microcystins in sediments using MMPB method. *Toxicon* **2001**, *39*, 687–692.

12. Babica, P.; Kohoutek, J.; Blaha, L.; Adamovsky, O.; Marsalek, B. Evaluation of extraction approaches linked to ELISA and HPLC for analyses of microcystin-LR, -RR and -YR in freshwater sediments with different organic material contents. *Anal. Bioanal. Chem.* **2006**, *385*, 1545–1551.

13. Mez, K.; Beattie, K.A.; Codd, G.A.; Hanselmann, K.; Hauser, B.; Naegeli, H.; Preisig, H.R. Identification of a microcystin in benthic cyanobacteria linked to cattle deaths on alpine pastures in Switzerland. *Eur. J. Phycol.* **1997**, *32*, 111–117.

14. Chen, W.; Song, L.; Peng, L.; Wan, N.; Zhang, X.; Gan, N. Reduction in microcystin concentrations in large and shallow lakes: Water and sediment-interface contributions. *Water Res.* **2008**, *42*, 763–773.

15. Montagnolli, W.; Zamboni, A.; Luvizotto-Santos, R.; Yunes, J.S. Acute effects of *Microcystis aeruginosa* from the Patos Lagoon estuary, Southern Brazil, on the microcrustacean *Kalliapseudes schubartii* (Crustacea: Tanaidacea). *Arch. Environ. Contam. Toxicol.* **2004**, *46*, 463–469.

16. Mohamed, Z.A.; El-Sharouny, H.M.; Ali, W.S.M. Microcystin production in benthic mats of cyanobacteria in the Nile River and irrigation canals, Egypt. *Toxicon* **2006**, *47*, 584–590.

17. Wu, X.; Wang, C.; Xiao, B.; Wang, Y.; Zheng, N.; Liu, J. Optimal strategies for determination of free/extractable and total microcystins in lake sediment. *Anal. Chim. Acta* **2012**, *709*, 66–72.

18. Mohamed, Z.; el-Sharouny, H.; Ali, W. Microcystin concentrations in the Nile River sediments and removal of microcystin-LR by sediments during batch experiments. *Arch. Environ. Contam. Toxicol.* **2007**, *52*, 489–495.

19. Ihle, T.; Jähnichen, S.; Jürgen, B. Wax and wane of *Microcystis* (cyanophyceae) and microcystins in lake sediments: A case study in Quitzdorf Reservoir. *J. Phycol.* **2005**, *41*, 479–488.

20. Latour, D.; Salencon, M.-J.; Reyss, J.-L.; Giraudet, H. Sedimentary imprint of *Microcystis aeruginosa* (cyanobacteria) blooms in Grangent reservoir (Loire, France). *J. Phycol.* **2007**, *43*, 417–425.

21. Wörmer, L.; Cirés, S.; Quesada, A. Importance of natural sedimentation in the fate of microcystins. *Chemosphere* **2011**, *82*, 1141–1146.

22. Munusamy, T.; Hu, Y.-L.; Lee, J.-F. Adsorption and photodegradation of microcystin-LR onto sediments collected from reservoirs and rivers in Taiwan: A laboratory study to investigate the fate, transfer, and degradation of microcystin-LR. *Environ. Sci. Pollut. Res. Int.* **2012**, *19*, 2390–2399.

23. Song, H.; Reichwaldt, E.S.; Ghadouani, A. Contribution of sediments in the removal of microcystin-LR from water. *Toxicon* **2014**, *83*, 84–90.

24. Miller, M.J.; Critchley, M.M.; Hutson, J.; Fallowfield, H.J. The adsorption of cyanobacterial hepatotoxins from water onto soil during batch experiments. *Water Res.* **2001**, *35*, 1461–1468.

25. Wang, H.X.; Ho, L.; Lewis, D.M.; Brookes, J.D.; Newcombe, G. Discriminating and assessing adsorption and biodegradation removal mechanisms during granular activated carbon filtration of microcystin toxins. *Water Res.* **2007**, *41*, 4262–4270.

26. Liu, G.; Qian, Y.; Dai, S.; Feng, N. Adsorption of microcystin LR and LW on suspended particulate matter (SPM) at different pH. *Water Air Soil Pollut.* **2008**, *192*, 67–76.

27. Wu, X.; Xiao, B.; Li, R.; Wang, C.; Huang, J.; Wang, Z. Mechanisms and factors affecting sorption of microcystins onto natural sediments. *Environ. Sci. Technol.* **2011**, *45*, 2641–2647.

28. Arnold, T.N.; Oldham, C.E. Trace-element contamination of a shallow wetland in Western Australia. *Mar. Freshwater Res.* **1997**, *48*, 531–539.

29. Bailey, M.C.; Hamilton, D.P. Wind induced sediment resuspension: A lake-wide model. *Ecol. Model.* **1997**, *99*, 217–228.

30. Kemp, A.; John, J. Microcystins associated with *Microcystis* dominated blooms in the southwest wetlands, Western Australia. *Environ. Toxicol.* **2006**, *21*, 125–130.

31. Reichwaldt, E.S.; Song, H.; Ghadouani, A. Effects of the distribution of a toxic *Microcystis* bloom on the small scale patchiness of zooplankton. *PLoS One* **2013**, *8*, e66674.

32. Sinang, S.C.; Reichwaldt, E.S.; Ghadouani, A. Spatial and temporal variability in the relationship between cyanobacterial biomass and microcystins. *Environ. Monit. Assess.* **2013**, *185*, 6379–6395.

33. Ho, L.; Hoefel, D.; Saint, C.P.; Newcombe, G. Isolation and identification of a novel microcystin-degrading bacterium from a biological sand filter. *Water Res.* **2007**, *41*, 4685–4695.

34. Cao, H.S.; Kong, F.X.; Luo, L.C.; Shi, X.L.; Yang, Z.; Zhang, X.F.; Tao, Y. Effects of wind and wind-induced waves on vertical phytoplankton distribution and surface blooms of *Microcystis aeruginosa* in Lake Taihu. *J. Freshwater Ecol.* **2006**, *21*, 231–238.

35. Donati, C.; Drikas, M.; Hayes, R.; Newcombe, G. Microcystin-LR adsorption by powdered activated carbon. *Water Res.* **1994**, *28*, 1735–1742.

36. Rapala, J.; Lahti, K.; Sivonen, K.; Niemela, S.I. Biodegradability and adsorption on lake sediments of cyanobacterial hepatotoxins and anatoxin-A. *Lett. Appl. Microbiol.* **1994**, *19*, 423–428.

37. Lam, A.K.Y.; Prepas, E.E.; Spink, D.; Hrudey, S.E. Chemical control of hepatotoxic phytoplankton blooms: Implications for human health. *Water Res.* **1995**, *29*, 1845–1854.

38. Lambert, T.W.; Holmes, C.F.B.; Hrudey, S.E. Adsorption of microcystin-LR by activated carbon and removal in full scale water treatment. *Water Res.* **1996**, *30*, 1411–1422.

39. Morris, R.J.; Williams, D.E.; Luu, H.A.; Holmes, C.F.B.; Andersen, R.J.; Calvert, S.E. The adsorption of microcystin-LR by natural clay particles. *Toxicon* **2000**, *38*, 303–308.

40. Grützmacher, G.; Wessel, G.; Klitzke, S.; Chorus, I. Microcystin elimination during sediment contact. *Environ. Sci. Technol.* **2010**, *44*, 657–662.

41. Barrington, D.J.; Ghadouani, A.; Sinang, S.C.; Ivey, G.N. Development of a new risk-based framework to guide investment in water quality monitoring. *Environ. Monit. Assess.* **2014**, *186*, 2455–2464.

42. Nang, S.C.S. Spatial and Temporal Dynamics of Cyanobacteria and Microcystins in Freshwater Systems: Implications for the Management of Water Resources. Ph.D. Thesis, the University of Western Australia, Crawley, WA, Australia, 2012.

43. Yen, H.; Lin, T.; Tseng, I.; Tung, S.; Hsu, M. Correlating 2-MIB and microcystin concentrations with environmental parameters in two reservoirs in South Taiwan. *Water Sci. Technol.* **2007**, *55*, 33–41.

44. Bowman, G.M.; Hutka, J. Particle size analysis. In *Soil Physical Measurement and Interpretation for Land Evaluation*; McKenzie, N.J., Coughlan, K.J., Cresswell, H.P., Eds.; CSIRO Publishing: Collingwood, VIC, Australia, 2002; pp. 224–239.

45. Heiri, O.; Lotter, A.; Lemcke, G. Loss on ignition as a method for estimating organic and carbonate content in sediments: Reproducibility and comparability of results. *J. Paleolimnol.* **2001**, *25*, 101–110.

46. Lawton, L.A.; Edwards, C.; Codd, G.A. Extraction and high-performance liquid chromatographic method for the determination of microcystins in raw and treated waters. *Analyst* **1994**, *119*, 1525–1530.

47. Ghadouani, A.; Smith, R.E.H. Phytoplankton distribution in Lake Erie as assessed by a new *in situ* spectrofluorometric technique. *J. Great. Lakes Res.* **2005**, *31*, 154–167.

48. Beutler, M.; Wiltshire, K.H.; Meyer, B.; Moldaenke, C.; Luring, C.; Meyerhofer, M.; Hansen, U.P.; Dau, H. A fluorometric method for the differentiation of algal populations *in vivo* and *in situ*. *Photosynth. Res.* **2002**, *72*, 39–53.

49. APHA, AWWA, and WEF. *Standard Methods for the Examination of Water and Wastewater*, 20th ed.; American Public Health Association: Washington, DC, USA, 1998.

Chapter 2:
Human Health Risk Assessment

Cyanobacteria and Algae Blooms: Review of Health and Environmental Data from the Harmful Algal Bloom-Related Illness Surveillance System (HABISS) 2007–2011

Lorraine C. Backer, Deana Manassaram-Baptiste, Rebecca LePrell and Birgit Bolton

Abstract: Algae and cyanobacteria are present in all aquatic environments. We do not have a good sense of the extent of human and animal exposures to cyanobacteria or their toxins, nor do we understand the public health impacts from acute exposures associated with recreational activities or chronic exposures associated with drinking water. We describe the Harmful Algal Bloom-related Illness Surveillance System (HABISS) and summarize the collected reports describing bloom events and associated adverse human and animal health events. For the period of 2007–2011, Departments of Health and/or Environment from 11 states funded by the National Center for Environmental Health (NCEH), Centers for Disease Control and Prevention contributed reports for 4534 events. For 2007, states contributed 173 reports from historical data. The states participating in the HABISS program built response capacity through targeted public outreach and prevention activities, including supporting routine cyanobacteria monitoring for public recreation waters. During 2007–2010, states used monitoring data to support196 public health advisories or beach closures. The information recorded in HABISS and the application of these data to develop a wide range of public health prevention and response activities indicate that cyanobacteria and algae blooms are an environmental public health issue that needs continuing attention.

Reprinted from *Toxins*. Cite as: Backer, L.C.; Manassaram-Baptiste, D.; LePrell, R.; Bolton, B. Cyanobacteria and Algae Blooms: Review of Health and Environmental Data from the Harmful Algal Bloom-Related Illness Surveillance System (HABISS) 2007–2011. *Toxins* **2015**, *7*, 1048-1064.

1. Introduction

Algae and cyanobacteria are present in all aquatic environments, and these organisms produce some of the most potent natural toxins known. We do not have a good sense of the extent of human and animal exposures to these organisms or their toxins, nor do we understand the public health impacts from acute exposures associated with recreational activities or chronic exposures associated with drinking water. To support public health decision-making about health risks from exposure to cyanobacteria and algae blooms and associated toxins, various efforts have been undertaken to collect and assess data describing the blooms, exposures, and associated human and animal health outcomes.

Efforts to understand algae and cyanobacteria blooms and the full spectrum of public health effects were initially supported by the Centers for Disease Control and Prevention's Cooperative Agreements (Program Announcement Number 98019 (1998); Program Announcement Number 03102 (2003); CDC-RFA-EH08-801 (2009)). This funding was intended to support state responses to the purported adverse human health and ecologic effects associated with the presence of the dinoflagellate, *Pfistieria psicicida* in the Chesapeake Bay [1]. Specifically, original goals for the

NCEH funding were to develop a case definition for disease associated with exposure to *P. piscicida* and any toxins it produced, conduct health surveillance, conduct analytic studies, and develop a biomarker of exposure/effect.

Eventually, it was determined that *P. piscicida* did not pose a substantive, definable human health threat, e.g., [2]. However, states identified potential public health issues associated with exposures to toxins produced by other types of algae (e.g., brevetoxins produced by the marine dinoflagellate *Karenia brevis*, the organism responsible for Florida red tides, and microcystins produced by several species of cyanobacteria, the organisms responsible for many green scums on fresh waters). In response, state activities supported by CDC funding expanded to include human and animal morbidity and mortality associated with exposure to any cyanobacteria or harmful algae bloom.

During this time, the National Center for Environmental Health (NCEH), CDC created, in collaboration with state partners, the Harmful Algal Bloom-related Illness Surveillance System (HABISS). The goals for HABISS were: (1) Describe the temporal and geographic distribution of cyanobacteria and algae blooms and (2) Describe the suspected human and animal morbidity and mortality associated with bloom events. HABISS was uniquely designed to capture, in one database, information describing suspected adverse human and animal health effects and environmental information about blooms as potential sources of exposure. A review of the HABISS data collection system was published by Glynn and Backer [3].

Various other efforts captured the public health consequences associated with cyanobacteria and algae blooms. Reports of health events associated with exposure to cyanobacteria, algae, and related toxins have been captured in CDC's National Outbreak Reporting System (NORS) [4]. Hilborn *et al.* [5] compiled a summary of 11 outbreaks involving 58 persons reported to NORS between 2009 and 2010.

Animal morbidity and mortality is an indicator for human health. To summarize what is currently known about cyanobacteria poisonings of pet dogs, Backer *et al.* [6] reviewed information collected from the following sources: HABISS; retrospective case files from a large, regional veterinary hospital in California; and publicly available information including scientific and medical manuscripts; written media; and web-based reports from pet owners, veterinarians, and other individuals. The authors summarized 231 discreet events and identified 368 cases of cyanotoxin poisonings of pet dogs throughout the U.S. between the late 1920s and 2012.

In the present paper, we describe HABISS and summarize the collected reports describing bloom events and suspected adverse health effects associated with exposure to freshwater cyanobacteria blooms or marine HABs and their associated toxins. We also discuss other public health promotion activities conducted by states that received funding from NCEH to address cyanobacteria and algae blooms.

2. Materials and Methods

2.1. HABISS

2.1.1. Partners

NCEH partnered with state representatives from the 11 funded states (FL, IA, MD, MA, NC, NY, OR, SC, VA, WA, WI; note that not all states were funded for the entire period from 1998 to 2013) and representatives from the University of Miami and Wright State University to develop the initial data collection instruments for HABISS. Data collection ended in 2013 when funding ended.

2.1.2. Electronic Platform

HABISS was an active surveillance system that operated on NCEH's secure platform, the Rapid Data Collector (RDC) [3]. The RDC tool was designed by NCEH specifically for rapid survey design and data collection; and HABISS was the first RDC tool supported for long-term surveillance. Protected by a secure data network (SDN), state users could choose to enter, edit, and save data for subsequent sessions.

2.1.3. HABISS Surveillance

HABISS was a passive surveillance activity for tracking reports of human and animal morbidity and mortality from exposures to cyanobacteria and algae blooms. Reports often triggered active surveillance activities, including direct follow-up on events or reports of morbidity/mortality in the media.

2.1.4. Data Elements

HABISS allowed contributors to input several key indicators (e.g., dates, agency contact information, state codes, route of exposure, patient's chief complaint). HABISS prompted users to report data elements to describe suspected or confirmed human or animal illnesses. The data elements were parallel for reporting adverse health effects for humans and animals and included contact location with the HAB or cyanobacteria bloom, identifying information for the potential case (which was not shared with CDC), demographics of the potential case, environmental information describing the water body, exposure information, signs and symptoms, medical review, laboratory analyses, and case assessment and follow-up. We worked with our state partners to ensure they did not enter duplicate cases into the system.

HABISS contributors were requested to report key data elements for a bloom report, which included water sample collection methods, analytic methods and test results, taxonomy, toxin identification and concentration, and geographic coordinates via a live link to Google Maps©. Human and animal morbidity and mortality reports were linked to each other and linked to data collected on relevant blooms.

There were few established case definitions to use for this surveillance effort see, for example, [7,8]. State contributing data used categories of confidence that the case or outbreak was bloom-related defined as follows: (1) A *suspect* case had exposure to water or seafood with a confirmed bloom AND onset of associated signs and symptoms within a reasonable time after exposure AND without identification of another cause of illness; (2) A *probable* case met criteria for suspect case AND there is laboratory documentation of bloom toxins in the water; and (3) A *confirmed* case met criteria for probable case combined with a professional judgment based on medical review. Also, a case may be defined as confirmed by meeting criteria for a probable case AND having documentation of a bloom-related toxin in a clinical specimen.

2.1.5. Contributors

The 11 funded states (FL, IA, MD, MA, NC, NY, OR, SC, VA, WA, and WI) and four additional states (CA, KS, MN, and MT) contributed data to HABISS.

2.1.6. Data Sources

The states used various methods to gather data describing cyanobacteria and harmful algae blooms and associated health effects. Many states previously identified cyanobacteria and harmful algae blooms as an ongoing public health issue and had established continual or seasonal monitoring programs. Environmental data, which may include water samples, captured in HABISS were categorized as follows: (1) Routine monitoring at public water bodies used for recreational purposes or water bodies with a history of blooms to monitor conditions that could be used to predict blooms; (2) Health event response, *i.e.*, collection of data in response to a human or animal illness or death following exposure to that water body, even in absence of a visible bloom; (3) Bloom report response, *i.e.*, collection of data from a water body reported to be blooming. The bloom could be reported by residents after noticing an unusual appearance or odor emanating from a community water body, local health officials, environmental regulatory agency staff, local or state park staff, watershed organizations, or other community groups; or (4) Fish kill response, *i.e.*, collection of data in response to a report of sick or dead fishes in or around the shoreline of a water body.

All contributing states conducted investigations if there was a case or outbreak of illness reported after exposure to recreational waters. These follow-up investigations included gathering environmental data (sometimes from established monitoring programs), water sample collection and analysis, and interviewing potential cases, when possible, by telephone or in person to ascertain exposure and health effects information. Owners whose pet dog or other domestic animal became ill or died after exposure to water with a suspected bloom or veterinarians who treated these animals provided health-related data during telephone interviews with investigators.

Several other sources of information for bloom-related health effects contributed to HABISS. NCEH monitored the National Poison Data System for reports of specific diseases, such as ciguatera fish poisoning and shared these alerts with appropriate states for follow-up. Other sources of data included the national and state notifiable disease reporting systems [9]. NCEH monitored media reports using Google Alerts©, and states conducted relevant follow-up activities when bloom-related cases of illness were identified.

2.1.7. Data Access and Download

Data contributors had access to their state's data as well as to data from other states with which they had established data sharing agreements. Data could be exported into Access©, Excel©, or XML© for analysis.

3. Results

For the period of 2007–2011, Departments of Health and/or Environment from 11 states funded by NCEH (Florida, Iowa, Maryland, Minnesota, New York, North Carolina, Oregon, Virginia, Washington, and Wisconsin) contributed reports for 4534 events. For 2007, states contributed 173 reports from historical data. The states also reported 458 cases of suspected and confirmed human bloom-associated illnesses and 175 animal morbidity and mortality events.

Although most of the contributing states conducting routine monitoring of public recreation waters for blooms, other states collected and documented bloom events only if there were reports of visible blooms, blooms with harmful algae or cyanobacteria identified, fish mortalities, or illnesses in people or animals following exposure to the water body.

The majority of reports (4245, 94%) represented routine monitoring. A summary of the number of reports and the reasons for the associated data collection by year is in Table 1.

Table 1. The number of reports recorded in Harmful Algal Bloom-related Illness Surveillance System (HABISS) from 2007 to 2011, by year, and the reason why the data were collected.

| Year | Reason for Bloom-Related Data Collection (Percent by Year) | | | | |
	Routine Monitoring	Bloom Report Response	Health Event Response	Fishkill Response	Total Reports
2007	167 (96)	1 (<1)	5 (3)	0	173
2008	509 (90)	7 (1)	41 (7)	8 (1)	565
2009	1344 (93)	55 (4)	28 (19)	23 (2)	1450
2010	977 (94)	25 (2)	19 (2)	16 (2)	1037
2011	1248 (95)	31 (2)	20 (52)	10 (1)	1309
Total Reports	4245	119	113	57	4534

3.1. Environmental Reports

Freshwater sources, which included lakes, rivers, streams, and ponds, were the most frequently reported type of water body ($n = 3499$, or 77% of the reports). Of the remaining reports, brackish (*i.e.*, a mixture of marine and fresh water) water bodies were identified in 973 (21%); marine waters in 82 (2%) and unknown water bodies in 172 (4%) of the reports.

3.2. Cyanobacteria, Algae, and Toxin Testing

Contributors identified cyanobacteria, the most common type of organism reported, in 1690 of 2323 (73%) samples analyzed for organism taxonomy. States most commonly reported *Anabaena* spp. (454, 20% of samples) followed by *Aphanizomenon* spp. (164, 7% of samples), and *Microcystis* spp. (165 or 7% of samples). Cyanobacteria cell counts ranged from 12,060 cells/mL of water (*Aphanizomenon* spp.) in a sample collected in response to a health event to 40,106,667 cells per mL of water (*Anabaena flos-aquae*) in a sample collected for routine monitoring (Table 2).

Table 2. Maximum and mean cell counts for cyanobacteria species listed by reason for sample collection. Samples collected in response to fish kills were not analyzed for *Microcystis* spp.

Species	Reason for Sample Collection (Cells/mL)			
	Monitoring	Health Event Response	Bloom Response	Fish Kill
Anabaena spp.	Max: 40,107,000	Max: 731,000	Max: 4,231,000	Max: 472,000
	Mean: 516,000	Mean: 96,000	Mean: 294,000	Mean: 267,000
	$N = 360$	$N = 12$	$N = 22$	$N = 4$
Aphanizomenon spp.	Max: 16,912,000	Max: 12,000	Max: 172,000	Max: 19,146,000
	Mean: 533,000	Mean: 6300	Mean: 85,500	Mean: 4,939,000
	$N = 102$	$N = 6$	$N = 14$	$N = 4$
Microcystis spp.	Max: 6,742,000	Max: 614,000	Max: 230,000	Max: NA
	Mean: 212,000	Mean: 194,000	Mean: 60,000	Mean: NA
	$N = 117$	$N = 14$	$N = 9$	$N = 4$

Other identified species included diatoms, dinoflagellates, prorocetrales, and raphidophyceans. Thirty-nine (2%) samples contained multiple species, and 367 (16%) of samples were not analyzed for cyanobacteria or algae species.

States reported toxin testing in 3301 reports (Table 3). Microcystins were the most common toxin and were identified in 2629 (80%) samples followed by saxitoxins (311 samples, 9%) anatoxin-a (246 samples, 7%). Domoic acid was the most commonly reported marine toxin (31 samples, 1%). The toxins maitotoxin and prymnesin were not found in any samples.

HABISS contributors recorded data related to cyanobacteria blooms in fresh waters for 439 water samples collected in response to a report of an ongoing bloom and 120 water samples collected in response to an adverse health event involving people or animals. Contributors also recorded data for 97 water samples collected in response to fish kills that occurred in fresh or brackish waters. A summary of cyanobacteria cell counts and toxin concentrations for samples collected in response to these events is in Table 4.

3.3. Animal Health Events

Animal illness reports included individual case reports for domestic animals and wildlife and case reports involving flocks of birds or schools of fish. During 2007–2011, states reported 175 events of animal morbidity or mortality. Of these, 93 (53%) were described as probable or suspected, and 7 (4%) were described as confirmed bloom-related events. There were 95 reports of fish mortalities; however, fewer than half ($n = 35$, 37%) were reported as bloom-related. Low dissolved oxygen concentration was the cause of fish mortalities in 30 (32%) events. Among the 11 reported cases of livestock mortalities, nine were cows that died in a single event in Montana after drinking water from a lake with a visible bloom. However, no water testing confirmed the presence of harmful algae, cyanobacteria, or toxins. There was one case report describing bird mortalities, but no environmental data were collected during the event.

Table 3. Toxins identified in the first water sample collected (2007–2011) by type of water sample.

Toxin	Fresh	Brackish	Marine	Unknown	Total (%)
			Water Type		
Anatoxin	243	2	0	1	246 (7)
Azaspiracid	0	0	1	0	1 (<1)
Brevetoxoins	0	3	0	0	3 (<1)
Cylindrospermopsin	4	0	0	0	4 (<1)
Domoic Acid	0	0	31	0	31 (1)
Karlotoxins	0	3	1	0	4 (<1)
Microcytins Total	2629	35	2	10	2676 (81)
Microcytsin LR	21	0	0	0	21 (1)
Okadaic Acid	1	2	0	0	3 (<1)
Saxitoxins	296	1	11	3	311 (9)
Unidentified Toxin	0	1	0	0	1 (<1)
Total	3194	47	46	14	3301

Table 4. Cyanobacteria cell counts and toxin concentrations in water samples collected in response to a health event, fish kill, or report of an ongoing bloom. Values are median (range).

Water Sample Parameter	Reason for Water Sample Collection		
	Response to a Human or Animal Health Event	Response to a Fish Kill	Response to a Report of a Bloom
Cyanobacteria Cell Counts (cells/mL)			
Anabaena spp.	12,700 (251–7,600,000) (N = 13)	34,000 (184–190,000) (N = 14)	19,000 (87–4,231,033) (N = 79)
Aphanizomenon spp.	NR [1]	41,000 (9000–9,500,000) (N = 7)	26,000 (230–172,000) (N = 61)
Cylindrospermopsis spp.	1700 (N = 1)	NR	14,017 (34–28,000) (N = 2)
Lyngbya spp.	206 (N = 1)	98,400 (N = 1)	NR
Microcystis spp.	27,000 (81–6,100,000) (N = 16)	8000 (1200–614,000) (N = 4)	14,300 (60–253,849) (N = 36)
Oscillatoria spp.	NR	32,000 (6500–521,000) (N = 5)	NR
Planktothrix spp.	140 (26–245) (N = 2)	NR	NR
Pseudoanabaena spp.	119 (28–210) (N = 2)	930 (105–116,000) (N = 3)	NR
Woronichia spp.	NR	NR	13,000 (11,000–23,000) (N = 3)
Toxin Concentrations (µg/L)			
Anatoxin	0.75 (0–500) (N = 12)	NR	0.05 (0–3,302,000) (N = 15)
Brevetoxins	NR	0.0 (0.0–1.0) (N = 7) [2]	NR
Cylindrospermopsin	0.5 (0–0.5) (N = 6)	NR	0.1 (0–9.0) (N = 5)
Microcystins total	15 (0–700) (N = 19)	0.06 (0.0–307) (N = 22)	0.9 (0–1385) (N = 140)
Microcystin-LR	1.3 (1–249) (N = 9)	NR	0.8 (0.2–1,120,000) (N = 16)

[1]: Not reported; [2]: *Chatonella* spp. identified but not quantified.

Among domestic animal reports, canine poisonings were the most frequent (n = 67, 38%). Thirty-eight (57%) of the canine poisonings were fatal. Common reported routes of exposure for dogs included dermal contact (n = 36, 54%) and inhalation/ingestion from swimming in water with an ongoing bloom (n = 15, 22%). Gastrointestinal symptoms (e.g., vomiting, foaming at the mouth) were most frequently reported symptoms in dogs (n = 29, 43%), followed by lethargy (n = 12, 18%) and neurologic symptoms such as stumbling and behavior changes (n = 6, 9%).

The majority of canine-related reports (58% of 67% or 87%), the 11 cattle mortality reports, and the single bird mortality report were associated with exposures to fresh waters. Most of the fish-kill-related reports (61% of 95%, or 64%) were associated with brackish waters.

Water samples were collected in response to 74 (42%) animal morbidity or mortality reports; however, 37 (50%) of these events were reported as cyanobacteria- or algae-related even though no cells or toxins were identified. The presence of cyanobacteria in water samples was reported for 24 (32%) events. Of the events accompanied by data on water samples, anatoxin-a was identified in 14 (19%) samples and microcystins were identified in 13 (18%) samples. Of the 67 canine mortalities, anatoxin exposure was implicated in 12 (18%), microcystin poisoning was identified in 3 (4%), and no specific toxin was noted for 5 (7%) cases. For the canine poisonings, toxin levels were measured in water samples collected in response to the event.

3.4. Human Health Events

During the period 2007–2011, states contributed 584 case reports of human illnesses associated with exposures to cyanobacteria or algae. Of these, 253 (40%) were described as probable or suspect and 219 (38%) met the criteria for confirmed cases. Of the 456 case reports with relevant data (two reports did not provide source of exposure), food was identified as the source of exposure in 273 (60%) reports and water was identified as the source of exposure in 183 (40%) reports. Of the reports identifying water-related exposures, freshwaters 176 (96%) were the most common, followed by marine waters (4, 2%) and brackish water (1, <1%).

Of the reports identifying food as the source of exposure, 248 (91%) reported ciguatera fish poisoning or poisoning by other toxins in seafood, including saxitoxin (13, 5%) and brevetoxin (2, <1%). The first or primary symptom was noted for only 74 (27%) food-related human cases and included gastrointestinal symptoms for 35 (47%) cases and neurologic symptoms for 22 (28%) cases. For the 207 reports in which the food was specified, the source of exposure was finfish for 185 (89%) cases and shellfish for 22 (11%) cases.

The majority of ciguatera fish poisoning cases (211, 85%) met the confirmed case definition, and the remaining 37 (15%) cases were reported as suspect or probable. Confirmed cases that occurred in states where physicians are required to report ciguatera fish poisoning (e.g., Florida and Washington) met the reporting state's case definitions. Confirmed cases that occurred in other states met the HABISS case definition: symptoms compatible the ciguatera fish poisoning (e.g., neurologic symptoms, including paresthesias of the extremities or metallic taste; gastrointestinal distress; hypotension with bradycardia), acute onset of illness within hours after eating a suspect fish (e.g., grouper, barracuda), and either verification of the toxin in a leftover meal remnant or professional medical judgment following medical review. A recent review provides an update of ciguatera signs and symptoms, treatments, and long-term sequelae [10].

Contributors reported 181 probable and confirmed cases of illness related to sources other than food. The reported health effects included 89 (49%) reports of rash from exposure to unknown toxin, 28 (16%) reports of microcystin poisoning, and other reports (27, 14%) of gastrointestinal or respiratory illness for which there were no confirmed toxin exposures (see Table 5). The primary or first symptom reported by probable and confirmed non-food-related cases (181 reports) included dermatologic effects such as rash, itching, and blisters ($n = 93$, 51%); gastrointestinal symptoms such as nausea and vomiting ($n = 25$, 19%); neurologic effects such as weakness and confusion ($n = 11$, 6%); and other general symptoms such as fatigue and fever ($n = 10$, 6%). For the subgroup of cases ($n = 174$) where non-food exposure was reported, most ($n = 157$, 90%) exposures occurred during recreational activities such as swimming, using personal water craft, or boating; and 17 (10%) cases occurred during occupational activities, such as water sample collection. Dermal contact ($n = 119$, 66%) and inhalation ($n = 51$, 28%) were the most common routes of non-food related exposures for these cases.

Table 5. Suspected and confirmed cases of human illnesses following exposure to cyanobacteria or algae (2007–2011).

Human Illness	Number of Cases (%)
Ciguatera fish poisoning	248 (54)
Rash from unknown organism or toxin	89 (19)
Illness from unknown organism or toxin	49 (11)
Microcystin poisoning	28 (6)
Other cyanobacteria- or algae-related illness not specified in HABISS	27 (6)
Paralytic shellfish poisoning (saxitoxins)	13 (3)
Neurotoxic shellfish poisoning (brevetoxins)	2 (<1)
Anatoxin poisoning	1 (<1)
Amnesic shellfish poisoning (domoic acid)	1 (<1)
Total	458

Of the 181 reports of non-food related human illness reports, 80 (44%) were linked to environmental data, for which 55 (40%) included water sample analysis for cyanobacteria, algae and/or toxins. Of the 52 case reports associated with exposure to cyanobacteria, 28 (54%) water samples contained *Microcystis spp.*, 20 (38%) contained *Anabaena spp.*, and 4 (8%) contained *Aphanizomenon spp.* Toxin test results were included in 27 of these reports; anatoxin, microcystins, and cylindrospermopsins were found in 22 (81%), 4 (15%), and 1 (4%) samples, respectively.

3.5. Public Health Actions Supported by the HABISS Program

One of the goals of HABISS was to accumulate data to support public health activities to reduce future morbidity and mortality resulting from exposure to harmful algal blooms. States participating in the HABISS program built response capacity through targeted public outreach and prevention activities. Some states also used resources provided by NCEH to increase or implement routine cyanobacteria monitoring for public recreation waters to prevent human and animal exposures to potentially hazardous blooms. During 2007–2010, states used these monitoring data to support decisions to issue 196 public health advisories or beach closures.

A sick or dead animal may be the first indication that a water body has an ongoing cyanobacteria or algae bloom. NCEH used information from HABISS to create a tool kit of materials (e.g., veterinary reference card, animal health alert poster) to raise awareness among veterinarians and the public about risks to pets from cyanobacteria. Between 2009 and 2010, NCEH distributed 2000 fact cards and 1500 posters to state partners. The tool kit also includes a physician reference card. Materials will be available as part of the updated CDC Drinking Water Advisory Communication Toolbox [11].

Examples of state activities, partnerships, and protocols developed using resources provided by HABISS is in Table 6.

Table 6. State activities, partnerships, and protocols that were developed using resources provided by HABISS. URL links to websites and materials are provided when available.

State Entity that Received Funding from HABISS	Activities, Partnerships, and Protocols Supported by HABISS
Florida Department of Health (FDOH)	•Supplemented ongoing public health surveillance (*i.e.*, reportable conditions using a system called MERLIN, foodborne disease surveillance, and events identified through the Poison Information Center) via the Aquatic Toxins Disease Prevention Program (ATDPP). Case reports and complaints associated with exposure to cyanobacteria blooms and reports of respiratory illnesses associated with exposures to airborne brevetoxins during Florida red tide events were recorded in HABISS. •Used the Electronic Surveillance System for Early Notification of Community Epidemics (ESSENCE) to provide early warning of cyanobacteria- and algae-related illness outbreaks, rapidly detect and report cyanobacteria and algae blooms, and identify bloom events with potential public health significance. •Made information available on website: http://www.floridahealth.gov/environmental-health/aquatic-toxins/index.html.
Iowa: Harmful Algal Bloom Program, Iowa Department of Public Health (IHAB)	•Implemented a cyanobacteria bloom advisory for Iowa during the 2011 monitoring season, and the IDPH temporarily designated suspected or confirmed exposures to microcystins as a reportable condition. The designation will continue to be used during future bloom seasons. •In 2010, collaborated with IDNR to launch an improved version of their interactive mapping application to allow visitors to the site to view current swimming advisories and water quality information, including the most recent sample analyzed for microcystins, for state park beaches. The website allows the public to contact IDPH with questions about beach water quality and to report a bloom or suspected bloom exposure.
Massachusetts Bureau of Health, Massachusetts Department of Public Health BEH/MDPH	•Used active surveillance to improve bloom-related symptom and illness reporting. •Provided bloom data that served as guidance for local health officials, other government officials, and community members to address health concerns related to blooms. For example, during the 2009 and 2010 bloom seasons, BEH used HABISS data to support issuing 23 and 24 health advisories, respectively, for public recreational waters affected by cyanobacteria blooms.

Table 6. *Cont.*

State Entity that Received Funding from HABISS	Activities, Partnerships, and Protocols Supported by HABISS
Maryland Department of Health and Mental Hygiene MDHMH)	•Expanded a web-based bloom outreach program to health care professionals through a series of Grand Rounds. •Linked monitoring data with the MD Healthy Beaches program as part of risk communication and public outreach efforts. •Conducted outreach activities to expand knowledge and awareness of harmful cyanobacteria and algae blooms. •http://www.dec.ny.gov/outdoor/64824.html •http://www.nyhealth.gov/environmental/water/drinking/bluegreenalgae.htm
New York State Department of Health	•Provided park rangers, lifeguards, and victims of cyanobacteria exposures information, fact sheets, water sampling and analysis, and guidance for bloom response. •Collaborated with the Citizen Statewide Lake Assessment Program, a citizen-based monitoring program run by the NYS Department of Environmental Conservation and the NYS Federation of Lake Associations.
North Carolina	•Provided information on website: http://epi.publichealth.nc.gov/oee/a_z/algae.html
Oregon: Oregon Harmful Algae Bloom Surveillance Program, Oregon Health Authority (OR-HABS)	•Improved the quality of information provided to various audiences and to better respond to requests for guidance in developing policy and responding to events. •http://www.oregon.gov/DHS/ph/hab/index.html •Collaborated with the state Drinking Water Program to develop a HAB Communications Plan for public water systems, and other program partners and stakeholders to develop permanent HAB advisory signage that can provide general HAB messages to the public as well as cautionary messages related to specific HABs. •Supported a website with outreach and education materials: •http://www.vdh.virginia.gov/epidemiology/DEE/HABS/
Virginia Department of Health (VDOH)	•Created the VDOH Algal Bloom Monitoring Network that is active during the summer and fall. The network covers 44 recreational beaches and 60 shellfish harvesting sites; and responds to fish kills and request for water sample analysis. •Collaborated with Washington State Department of Ecology and local health jurisdictions to provide resources and technical assistance for Washington's passive Harmful Algae Bloom (HAB) surveillance system. •http://www.doh.wa.gov/CommunityandEnvironment/Contaminants/BlueGreenAlgae •http://www.ecy.wa.gov/programs/wq/plants/algae/monitoring/index.html
Washington State Department of Health (WSDOH)	•Strengthened its work on the Regional Examination of Harmful Algae Blooms (REHAB) which involves the monitoring of 30 lakes in three Washington counties through the active bloom months of June-October. Developed public access to cyanotoxin data: •https://www.nwtoxicalgae.org/ •Developed recreational guidance values for microcystins, anatoxin-a, cylindrospermopsins and saxitoxins which are incorporated into a protocol for local health jurisdictions, lake managers, and other agencies to follow in the case of toxic blooms.
Wisconsin Department of Health Services (WI DOHS)	•Collected and disseminated harmful algae-related illness data and environmental data. Specifically, resources supported the redesign of an interactive website that citizens and local health departments can use to report human or animal illnesses related to algal blooms in Wisconsin. This has resulted in the investigation of 102 human illness reports, and nine animal illness reports to date. •http://www.dhs.wisconsin.gov/eh/bluegreenalgae •Conducted active surveillance using an interactive website through a partnership with Poison Control Centers.

4. Discussion

Addressing the potential public health issues associated with the presence of toxin-producing cyanobacteria and algae in our drinking and recreational waters is an ongoing challenge because the risks associated with exposure vary across organisms, toxins, and routes of exposure. HABISS represented the first broad-scale attempt to conduct surveillance for human and animal health events and collect associated environmental data describing cyanobacteria and algae blooms in the U.S.

One of the key accomplishments of the HABISS program was the creation of partnerships among state-level health and environment departments. To complete HABISS data entry, NCEH's public health partners needed access to environmental data typically collected by another entity, such as the department of environmental protection or environmental quality. Existing relationships across various departments were strengthened in some states, while others had to build new relationships to access the needed environmental data.

HABISS-related data collection allowed states to begin to understand the public health burden from human and animal exposures to cyanobacteria and algae blooms. For 2007–2011, 11 states reported over 4500 bloom events, 458 cases of suspected and confirmed human bloom-associated illnesses, and 175 animal morbidity and mortality events. Over half (248 of 458) of the human illnesses were ciguatera fish poisonings (CFP). CFP cases from outbreaks should be captured by CDC's ongoing Foodborne Disease Outbreak Surveillance System (FDOSS) [4]. Individual CFP cases would not be captured in FDOSS; however, they could be captured in HABISS.

We anticipated many reports of adverse health outcomes (e.g., respiratory irritation, asthma exacerbations) associated with Florida red tides based on the work of the Red Tide Research Group [12–14]. However, thousands of beach-goers may be adversely affected by aerosolized toxins generated during Florida red tides, and it is not possible to accurately record the number of people with health-related complaints. Further, we understand the mechanism of the biological response to brevetoxins [15] and Florida has developed outreach and education materials to help beach-goers understand the risks associated with visiting the beach or bathing while there is an ongoing Florida red tide (see the website of the Florida Fish and Wildlife Conservation Commission [16]). Rather than marine waters, fresh waters were the source of exposure in nearly all (176 of 183, 96%) the adverse human health outcomes reported to HABISS.

There are few clinical data describing adverse health effects from exposure to cyanobacteria and associated toxins, making the clinical differential diagnosis difficult. The human and animal modules of HABISS were designed to collect specific information about signs and symptoms from exposure to cyanobacteria, including self-reported data. About half of the human cases reported dermatologic symptoms following exposure to cyanobacteria blooms, while much smaller numbers reported gastrointestinal or neurologic symptoms. This makes sense as over 90% of the exposures occurred during recreational activities involving direct contact with the water, such as swimming, *i.e.*, dermal contact could produce rashes, and swallowing water during swimming could induce gastrointestinal and/or neurologic effects. However, in reviewing the HABISS data, no clear clinical picture of cyanobacteria- and cyanotoxin-related illnesses emerged. Additional epidemiologic and detailed clinical information describing the health effects associated with exposure to freshwater cyanobacteria and algae is needed to create more specific case definitions.

Although we cannot specifically identify which cyanobacteria produced the toxins reported in HABISS, the cyanobacteria cell counts and concentrations provide some interesting findings (Table 4). For *Anabaena* spp., the cell counts in waters associated with a health event, a fish kill, or a bloom event were all of the same order of magnitude (tens of thousands of cells/mL). However, the median concentration of anatoxin-a (produced by *Anabaena flos-aquae* and *A. lemmermannii* [17]) was an order of magnitude greater in samples collected in response to a health event when compared with the concentrations in water samples collected in response to a sighted bloom. Our results are consistent with the fact that not all cyanobacteria blooms produce toxin and the idea that an *Anabaena* bloom may be visible before it produces enough toxin to be a health threat.

There were few samples collected in response to an event that were analyzed for *Cylindrospermopsis* spp., perhaps because this species does not form floating scums, but tends to concentrate well below the water surface [18]. Six samples were collected in response to a health event and 5 were collected in response to a bloom report. These samples were analyzed for cylindrospermopsins, which are produced by *Anabaena*, *Aphanizomenon*, and *Cylindrospermopsis* spp. A higher median concentration of cylindrospermopsins was found in samples collected in response to a health threat than in samples collected in response to a bloom report.

Cell counts from 63 samples were reported for *Microcystis*, *Plantothrix*, and *Oscillatoria* spp., all of which can produce microcystins [18]. The median concentrations for total microcystins and microcystin L-R were higher in samples collected in response to a health event than for those collected in response to a bloom report, but the maximum concentration (120,000 µg/L) was much higher for the bloom response samples. While there are some trends in the cell counts and toxin concentrations, more data are needed to begin to extrapolate from these values to potential adverse health outcomes from specific blooms.

An electronic system to capture new cyanobacteria and algae bloom-related human and animal health and environmental data will be available through CDC's NORS. Although NORS is a passive surveillance activity, CDC requires all states to report all disease "outbreaks" (defined as more than one case of a disease epidemiologically linked in space and time). Several states have attempted to enter HAB-related outbreak data using existing NORS forms but encountered difficulties in entering toxin concentrations and relevant symptoms because the system is currently designed to report infectious disease outbreaks. We expect improved HAB-related illness outbreak reporting for both people and animals from all states once the module specifically designed to capture these data becomes available.

In addition to access to a standardized surveillance system, the HABISS program provided resources to state partners to mitigate the public health impacts from cyanobacteria and algae blooms. States had a number of challenges in creating outreach and education materials about the potential risks from cyanobacteria and algae for the public. Many popular lakes experience blooms every summer; and it was difficult to craft prevention messages warning about risks from an event that has occurred and been observed many times without apparent associated illness outbreaks. Signs warning the public about blooms caused confusion when they are placed to identify a toxin-producing bloom occurring near, but not affecting, a swimming beach. Warnings are sometimes ignored by swimmers and others using waterbodies for recreational activities. Citizen groups that support monitoring activities caused confusion if they reported the presence of toxins found only in visible scums that are typically avoided by people. By contrast, people who live near lakes that bloom often may have a history of experiencing health symptoms, such as respiratory or eye irritation, and stay away from the water during blooms.

The data in HABISS reflects recreational exposures for humans and domestic pets. However, large surface waters that provide drinking water to towns and cities are also at risk for cyanobacteria blooms that could result in disease outbreaks. For example, the 2014 *Microcystis aeruginosa* bloom in Lake Erie resulted in measurable, but low, levels of microcystins in Toledo, Ohio's drinking water. Nearly 500,000 people were affected by the Ohio EPA's "Do not boil, do not drink" order. Toledo was able to quickly restore water to its distribution system, however, smaller community drinking water systems may lack resources needed to prevent or respond quickly to a large bloom in their water source [19].

People continue to ask local health and environmental experts the following questions about the risks associated with using a waterbody with an ongoing bloom: Can I swim in the water during a bloom?, Is my drinking water safe?, Can I eat the fish I catch?, Can I let my child or dog play in the water?, Why does my lake stink?, and "I bought this house so I could enjoy lakeside living--how do I clean up my lake? Answers to these questions comprise public and environmental health considerations, and many states have developed guidelines for informing the public about risks from cyanobacteria blooms, including risks from direct water contact, swallowing untreated water, and eating fish [20]. These efforts demonstrate that exposure to cyanobacteria blooms and associated toxins is a national public health issue needing ongoing attention.

Despite increasing awareness of HABs we can assume that there is under-reporting of possible cyanobacteria- and algae-related illnesses. Under-reporting is an issue with public health surveillance in general because ill people may not report the event to a health care practitioner, or the practitioner may not make the correct diagnosis. Even with a correct diagnosis, diseases are not typically reported to local or state public health departments for surveillance unless specific legislation requires reporting [1]. Reporting of illnesses suspected or confirmed to be associated with an environmental exposure is even less likely to occur because many state health departments lack resources to identify and follow up these events to collect and analyze appropriate environmental samples.

In addition to the problem of under-reporting, there are a number of other limitations with HABISS data. The system was available for data entry for a short time. The number of reports tended to increase over time, partly because public health practitioners established links with environmental health practitioners, allowing them to exchange environmental and health information about these events and partly because outreach activities encouraged reporting. HABISS collected data on acute events, and we were not able to capture cases with chronic effects. One way to address this would be to create a data-sharing partnership with another state or national system, such as the National Poison Data System (NPDS), which receives calls from people with chronic complaints as well as those with acute illnesses. As part of outreach efforts, State Health Departments can encourage physicians to report cases involving chronic health outcomes, such as neurologic effects sometimes associated with ciguatera fish poisoning or liver toxicity associated with exposure to microcystins, to the HAB module of NORS. Finally, clinical data are needed to inform and improve case definitions. Many of these limitations will be addressed by new data collected as part of the updated NORS. For example, NORS is a familiar surveillance system and contributing data to a new module of an existing system would be less burdensome than contributing to an independent surveillance system such as HABISS. Because of our experience with HABISS, the HAB module in NORS comprises variables that reflect data, such as exposure location, exposure routes, and signs and symptoms of exposure, available to state health departments.

5. Summary and Conclusions

Although potential health hazards associated with the toxins produced by cyanobacteria and algae have been known for decades or more, identifying individual cases of many of the illnesses produced by exposure to these toxins remains a diagnosis of exclusion accompanied by detailed information about the patient's recent exposure history. States entered 458 suspected or confirmed human illnesses and 175 animal morbidity and mortality cases into HABISS associated with bloom events during 2007–2011. The information recorded in HABISS and the application of these data to develop a wide range of public health prevention and response activities indicate that cyanobacteria and algae blooms are an environmental public health issue that needs continuing attention at local, state, and national levels. Going forward, we will use the NORS module to track the frequency and geographic extent of cyanobacteria and algae blooms that affect public health.

Acknowledgments

The authors would like to acknowledge the contributions to HABISS data collection efforts by all of our state partners.

Author Contributions

Lorraine Backer was PI and had primary responsibility for the project and manuscript. Deana Manassaram-Baptiste, maintained the surveillance system and data bases, interacted with state partners, and summarized data from the HABISS dataset. Rebecca LePrell and Birgit Bolton maintained the surveillance system, interacted with state partners, and contributed to the manuscript.

Conflicts of Interest

The authors declare no conflict of interest.

Disclaimer

References

1. Glasgow, H.B.; Burkholder, J.M.; Schmechel, D.E.; Tester, P.A.; Rublee, P.A. Insidious effects of a toxic estuarine dinoflagellate on fish survival and human health. *J. Toxicol. Environ. Health* **1995**, *46*, 501–522.

2. Morris, J.G., Jr. *Pfiesteria*, "Cell from hell" and other toxic algal nightmares. *Clin. Infect. Dis.* **1999**, *28*, 1191–1198.

3. Glynn, M.K.; Backer, L.C. Collecting public health surveillance data: Creating a surveillance system. In: *Principles and Practice of Public Health Surveillance*; Lee, L., Teutsch, S., Thacker, S., St. Louis, M., Eds.; Oxford University Press: New York, NY, USA, 2010; pp. 44–64.

4. Gould, L.H.; Walsh, K.A.; Vieira, A.R.; Herman, K.; Williams, I.T.; Hall, A.J.; Cole, D. Surveillance for foodborne disease outbreaks—United States, 1998–2008. *MMWR* **2013**, *62*, 1–34.

5. Hilborn, E.D.; Roberts, V.A.; Backer, L.; DeConno E.; Egan, J.S.; Hyde, J.B.; Nicholas, D.C.; Viegert, E.J.; Billing, L.M.; DiOrio, M.; *et al.* Algal bloom-associated disease outbreaks among users of freshwater lakes—United States, 2009–2010. *MMWR* **2014**, *63*, 11–15.

6. Backer, L.C.; Landsberg, J.H.; Miller, M.; Keel, K.; Taylor, T.K. Canine cyanotoxin poisonings in the United States (1920s–2012): Review of suspected and confirmed cases from three data sources. *Toxins* **2013**, *5*, 1597–1628.

7. Backer, L.C.; Fleming, L.E.; Rowan, A.D.; Baden, D.G. Epidemiology and public health of human illnesses associated with harmful marine algae. In *IOC Manual on Harmful Marine Microalgae*; Cembella, H.A., Ed.; UNSECO: Paris, France, 2003; Chapter 26.

8. Fleming, L.E.; Kirkpatrick, B.; Backer, L.C.; Bean, J.A.; Wanner, A.; Reich, A.; Zaias, J.; Cheng, Y.S.; Pierce, R.; Naar, J.; *et al.* Aerosolized red tide toxins (Brevetoxins) and asthma. *Chest* **2006**, *131*, 187–194.

9. Centers for Disease Control and Prevention. Summary of notifiable diseases. *MMWR* **2014**, *61*, 1–122.

10. Friedman, M.A.; Fleming, L.E.; Fernandez, M.; Bienfang, P.; Schrank, K.; Dickey, R.; Bottein, M.-Y.; Backer, L.; Ayyar, R.; Weisman, R.; *et al.* Ciguatera fish poisoning: Treatment, prevention, and management. *Mar. Drugs* **2008**, *6*, 456–479.

11. CDC. Drinking water advisory communication toolbox. Available online: http://www.cdc.gov/healthywater/emergency/dwa-comm-toolbox/index.html (accessed on 25 March 2015).

12. Backer, L.C.; Fleming, L.E.; Rowan, A.; Cheng, Y.-S.; Benson, J.; Pierce, R.H.; Zaias, J.; Bean, J.; Bossart, G.D.; Johnson, D.; *et al.* Recreational exposure to aerosolized brevetoxins during florida red tide events. *Harmful Algae* **2003**, *2*, 19–28.

13. Backer, L.C.; Kirkpatrick, B.; Fleming, L.E.; Cheng, Y.-S.; Pierce, R.; Bean, J.A.; Clark, R.; Johnson, D.; Wanner, A.; Tamer, R.; *et al.* Occupational exposure to aerosolized brevetoxins during florida red tide events: impacts on a healthy worker population. *Environ Health Perspect.* **2005**, *113*, 644–649.

14. Fleming, L.E.; Kirkpatrick, B.; Backer, L.C.; Bean, J.A.; Wanner, A.; Dalpra, D.; Tamer, R.; Zaias, J.; Cheng, Y.-S.; Pierce, R.; *et al.* Initial evaluation of the effects of aerosolized florida red tide toxins (Brevetoxins) in persons with asthma. *Environ. Health Perspect.* **2005**, *113–115*, 650–657.

15. Abraham, W.M.; Bourdelais, A.J.; Ahmed, A.; Serebriakoy, I.; Baden, D.G. Effects of inhaled brevetoxins in allergic airways: Toxin-allergen interactions and pharmacologic intervention. *Environ Health Perspect.* **2005**, *113*, 632–637.

16. Florida Fish and Wildlife Conservation Commission. Red Tide. Available online: http://myfwc.com/research/redtide (accessed on 25 March 2015).

17. Humpage, A. Toxin types, toxicokinetics, and toxicodynamics. In *Cyanobacterial Harmful Algal Blooms State of the Science and Research Needs*; Hudnell, K., Ed.; Springer: New York, NY, USA, 2008; Chapter 16, pp. 384–415.

18. Kuiper-Goodman, T.; Falconer, I.; Fitzgerald, J. Human health aspects. In *Toxic Cyanobacteria in Water. A Guide to Their Public Health Consequences, Monitoring, and Management*; Chorus, I., Bartram, J., Eds.; E & FN SPON: London, UK, 1999; Chapter 4, pp. 115–153.

19. Rose, J.D. What happened to Toldedo's drinking water: Understanding microcytsins. Available online: http://www.waterandhealth.org/happened-toledos-drinking-water-understanding-microcystins (accessed on 25 March 2015).

20. Hudnell, H.K.; Backer, L.C.; Anderson, J.; Dionysiou, D.D. United States of America: Historical review and current policy addressing cyanobacteria. In *Current Approaches to Cyanotoxin Risk Assessment, Risk Management and Regulations in Different Countries*; Chorus, I., Ed.; Federal Environmental Agency (Umweltbundesamt): Dessau-Roßlau, Germany, 2013; pp. 137–147.

Human Illnesses and Animal Deaths Associated with Freshwater Harmful Algal Blooms—Kansas

Ingrid Trevino-Garrison, Jamie DeMent, Farah S. Ahmed, Patricia Haines-Lieber, Thomas Langer, Henri Ménager, Janet Neff, Deon van der Merwe and Edward Carney

Abstract: Freshwater harmful algal bloom (FHAB) toxins can cause morbidity and mortality in both humans and animals, and the incidence of FHABs in the United States and Kansas has increased. In 2010, the Kansas Department of Health and Environment (KDHE) developed a FHAB policy and response plan. We describe the epidemiology of FHAB-associated morbidity and mortality in humans and animals in Kansas. Healthcare providers and veterinarians voluntarily reported FHAB-associated cases to KDHE. An investigation was initiated for each report to determine the source of exposure and to initiate public health mitigation actions. There were 38 water bodies with a confirmed FHAB in 2011. There were 34 reports of human and animal FHAB-associated health events in 2011, which included five dog deaths and hospitalization of two human case patients. Five confirmed human illnesses, two dog illnesses and five dog deaths were associated with one lake. Four human and seven dog cases were exposed to the lake after a public health alert was issued. Public health officials and FHAB partners must ensure continued awareness of the risks to the public, educate healthcare providers and veterinarians on FHAB-related health events and encourage timely reporting to public health authorities.

Reprinted from *Toxins*. Cite as: Trevino-Garrison, I.; DeMent, J.; Ahmed, F.S.; Haines-Lieber, P.; Langer, T.; Ménager, H.; Neff, J.; van der Merwe, D.; Carney, E. A New Nanometer-Sized Ga(III)-Oxyhydroxide Cation. *Toxins* **2015**, *7*, 353-366.

1. Introduction

Cyanobacteria, also known as blue-green algae, are found throughout the world in a variety of aquatic environments. This ancient class of microorganisms includes multiple species that produce some of the most powerful toxins known to man [1]. When environmental conditions are favorable, cyanobacteria can proliferate to dominate the phytoplankton within a body of water and form a bloom [2]. The cyanobacteria within the bloom can produce toxins that adversely affect human and animal health. The majority of freshwater cyanobacteria toxins are classified into two categories; hepatotoxins (toxins that target the liver) and neurotoxins (toxins that target the nervous system) [3]. Microcystin, a hepatotoxin, is produced by multiple species of cyanobacteria within the genera *Microcystis, Planktothrix, Anabaena* and *Oscillatoria* [3]. Microcystins are the most frequently occurring and widespread cyanotoxin throughout the world and the most commonly found cyanotoxin in Kansas lakes [4,5]. The effects of microcystin poisoning depend on the route of exposure (e.g., ingestion, inhalation, direct contact) and the amount of toxin to which the human, or animal, has been exposed. The onset of signs and symptoms can occur within minutes to hours of exposure. Clinical signs and symptoms of acute microcystin poisoning, in both animals and humans, are non-specific and can include; nausea, vomiting, diarrhea, cough, sore throat, rash and liver damage [4,6–8]. Most people with recreational water exposure to cyanobacteria recover without sequelae; however, the outcome for most dogs is death [4,6–8].

The incidence of freshwater harmful algal blooms (FHABs) has increased over the last three decades. In the United States, there were three FHAB-associated outbreaks from 1978 to 2008 compared to 11 outbreaks from 2009 to 2010 reported to the Waterborne Disease Outbreak Surveillance System (WBDOSS) and the Harmful Algal Bloom-Related Illness Surveillance System (HABISS) [8]. An outbreak must meet the following criteria; two or more people linked epidemiologically and the epidemiologic evidence must implicate recreational water as the probable source of illness [8]. Ten states (Florida, Iowa, Maryland, Massachusetts, New York, Oregon, South Carolina, Virginia, Washington, and Wisconsin) received grants to participate in HABISS; however, any state could report FHAB-associated outbreaks to the system. Although HABISS has been discontinued, voluntary reports of FHAB-associated outbreaks can be made to WBDOSS through the National Outbreak Reporting System (NORS) [8]. Anecdotal case reports and case studies have provided information on a wide range of acute illnesses associated with recreational exposure to cyanobacteria and their toxins; however, there is limited availability of epidemiological data [2].

By 2010, the Kansas Department of Health and Environment had received reports of and tested water bodies for FHABs for more than 25 years. However, there was no formal policy in place to protect public health. No U.S. Federal policy, regulations or guidelines exist for FHABs in recreational waters, although several states have developed their own policies [1,9,10]. In 2010, the Kansas Department of Health and Environment established a policy and response plan for FHABs in public waters. The public health Advisory and Warning levels were based on World Health Organization recommendations for recreational water use [4]. The policy included an active response to reports of human or animal illness or death potentially associated with a FHAB. The response included a case investigation and collection of water samples from the implicated body of water. Here, we describe the epidemiology of human and animal morbidity and mortality associated with freshwater harmful algal blooms in Kansas.

2. Results

2.1. FHAB Identification and Water Sampling

Public water bodies were sampled for FHAB when: (1) a report of a FHAB in a public body of water was received, or (2) a suspected FHAB-related illness in animals or humans was identified and reported to KDHE. A public water body was defined as those waters referred to as reservoirs, community lakes, state fishing lakes or were waters managed or owned by federal, state, county or municipal authorities. Also included were all privately-owned lakes that served as a public drinking water supply or were open to the general public for primary or secondary contact recreation [11]. In 2011, there were 42 water bodies reported to KDHE with a suspect harmful algal bloom; 38 water bodies were confirmed with a FHAB. A report of FHAB-associated human illness, Case 1, triggered sampling of one water body.

Between March 18 and October 31, 2011, 16 water bodies met the criteria for the Warning level ($\geq$100,000 cyanobacteria cells/mL, $\geq$20 µg/L microcystin toxin or visible cyanobacteria surface accumulation) and four water bodies met the Advisory level (20,000 to <100,000 cyanobacteria cells/mL or detectable to <20 µg/L microcystin toxin) classification for at least one week due to a high cell concentration, elevated microcystin toxin or a combination of both.

We report the water sample results for Milford Lake, the largest man-made lake in Kansas, with 15,700 surface acres of water and 163 miles of shoreline [12]. Five locations were sampled at Milford Lake weekly beginning July 18 through October 10, 2011, for a total of 55 samples. We report the maximum, minimum, median and mean for cyanobacteria cell concentration (Table 1) and microcystin toxin level each week (Table 2). Milford Lake was issued a public health alert for FHAB conditions for 12 consecutive weeks (July 18–October 13, 2011). The highest maximum cyanobacteria cell concentration (5,576,000/mL) and microcystin toxin level (1,600 µg/L) occurred in samples taken August 22, 2011. The maximum total cyanobacteria cell concentration corresponded to the maximum microcystin enzyme-linked immunosorbent assay (ELISA) in all samples; however, the minimum cell concentration did not correspond to the minimum microcystin ELISA in two samples taken on August 29 and September 19. The predominant cyanobacteria type was *Microcystis* spp. in 82% (45/55) of the samples. *Anabaena* spp. was the predominant cyanobacteria type in four samples taken on or after September 26.

Table 1. Milford Lake cyanobacteria cell concentration, 2011 *.

Date of Collection (2011)	Maximum Total Cyanobacteria Cell Concentration * (No./mL)	Minimum Total Cyanobacteria Cell Concentration * (No./mL)	Median Cyanobacteria Cell Concentration * (No./mL)	Mean Cyanobacteria Cell Concentration * (No./mL)
July 18	1,825,000	6000	104,000	458,000
July 25	98,000	3000	28,000	28,000
August 1	335,000	31,000	252,000	189,000
August 8	60,000	4000	60,000	43,000
August 22	5,576,000	132,000	830,000	1,536,000
August 29	171,000	13,000	31,000	56,000
September 6	1,096,000	176,000	231,000	388,000
September 12	1,530,000	159,000	414,000	577,000
September 19	19,000	2,000	7000	9000
September 26	560,000	0	11,000	117,000
October 10	2000	0	300	700

* The data presented are a composite of all five sample sites from the same date.

2.2. Trend Analysis

We evaluated water sample data collected from 1989 to 2009 and assigned a public health alert to each water body based on the criteria set forth in the KDHE 2010 FHAB Policy and Response Plan. Between 1989 and 2009, there were 413 water bodies that met the public health alert criteria (274 advisories and 139 warnings) [13]. We compared the median number of public health alerts that would have been issued based on the 2010 FHAB alert levels. We grouped the data into seven-year increments (1989–1995, 1996–2002 and 2003–2009). The median number of FHABs increased between each increment; 13 (1989–1995), 18 (1996–2002) and 25 (2003–2009). KDHE did not receive reports of human or animals cases associated with FHABs prior to 2011; however, a review of canine cyanotoxin poisonings in the United States by Backer *et al.*, found two media reports of FHAB-associated deaths of four dogs in Kansas in 2007 and 2008 [6]. Veterinarians play a key role in the detection of FHABs, as they may be the first healthcare provider to recognize signs of FHAB-illness in animals [6]. Timely reporting of FHABs to public health officials is crucial to prevent human morbidity and additional animal mortality.

Table 2. Milford Lake microcystin toxin level, 2011 *.

Date of Collection (2011)	Maximum ELISA * (µg/L)	Minimum ELISA * (µg/L)	Median ELISA * (µg/L)	Mean ELISA * (µg/L)
July 18	110	1	9	30
July 25	60	<1	3	15
August 1	60	6	35	30
August 8	9	6	6	7
August 22	1600	25	250	441
August 29	150	15	15	38
September 6	20	5	12	13
September 12	1000	12	180	322
September 19	6	2	2	3
September 26	60	0	2	13
October 10	0	0	0	<1

* The data presented are a composite of all five sample sites from the same date.

2.3. Outreach to Physicians and Veterinarians

Harmful algal bloom-related illnesses in humans are not considered reportable conditions in Kansas. However, any outbreak of any disease or condition is required to be reported to KDHE per Kansas statute. Similarly, FHAB-related illnesses and deaths among animals are not required to be reported to the Kansas Department of Agriculture.

Human and animal cases could be reported via phone call to KDHE or through the KDHE Harmful Algal Bloom website (http://www.kdheks.gov/algae-illness/index.htm). No cases of human or animal illness were reported in 2010. During 2011, KDHE sent letters to physicians and veterinarians to increase awareness of FHAB-related illness and encourage reporting of cases. A survey was administered to veterinarians and physicians during 2012 to evaluate the effectiveness of the messaging campaign and knowledge of public health advisories and warnings in or near their area of practice [14]. Although respondents displayed an increase in awareness of the adverse health effects caused by exposure to FHABs from 2010 to 2011, the majority were not aware of FHABs that had occurred in their county of practice or the surrounding counties [14]. KDHE and all FHAB stakeholders must continue to educate both human and animal healthcare providers regarding diagnosis and reporting of FHAB-related illnesses and deaths throughout the FHAB season each year.

2.4. Human Cases

KDHE received 25 reports of human illnesses potentially associated with FHABs in 2011. Three reports were anonymous complaints, and we were unable to complete an investigation. Of the 25 reports, nine were classified as not a case, primarily due to the healthcare provider failing to rule out other potential causes of illness. The remaining 13 cases were classified as suspect ($n = 1$), probable ($n = 5$) and confirmed ($n = 7$). Of the seven confirmed human illnesses, the median age was 40 years (range: 17–63 years); 71% (5/7) were male, and 29% (2/7) were hospitalized (Table 3). All human cases survived. Primary symptoms included: 71% (5/7) eye and upper respiratory tract irritation, 29% (2/7) rash and 14% (1/7) gastrointestinal. The most common primary route of exposure included direct contact, 100% (7/7), followed by ingestion, 43% (3/7), and inhalation, 14% (1/7). The median time from exposure to symptom onset was 24 h, with a range of 3–48 h.

Case 2, a 17-year-old male, presented to an emergency department on July 23, 2011. His symptoms included; sore throat, cough, malaise, headache and a fever of 104.1 °F. He did not report a rash. His symptoms began approximately 24 h after swimming at Milford Lake on July 20, 2011. He was diagnosed with pneumonia and hospitalized for three days for supportive care. A report of a potential FHAB at Milford Lake was reported to KDHE on July 18, 2011, and five water samples from high-traffic public access points were taken the same day. The water sample testing confirmed high cyanobacteria cell concentrations and microcystin toxin levels at a public health Warning level, and a press release was issued on July 22, 2011.

Table 3. Confirmed human freshwater harmful algal bloom-associated cases, Kansas, 2011.

Case	Sex	Age (Years)	Exposure Date	Time to Symptom Onset (h)	Primary Route of Exposure	Primary Symptoms	Recreational Water Activity
1	Male	63	06/15/11	7.5	Direct Contact	Rash	Fishing
2 *	Male	17	07/20/11	24	Direct Contact, Ingestion	Eye and Upper Respiratory Tract Irritation	Swimming
3	Female	52	07/21/11	48	Direct Contact	Eye and Upper Respiratory Tract Irritation	Swimming
4	Female	42	07/26/11	24	Direct Contact, Ingestion, Inhalation	Eye and Upper Respiratory Tract Irritation	Knee Boarding
5	Male	38	07/30/11	48	Direct Contact	Eye and Upper Respiratory Tract Irritation	Swimming
6 *	Male	38	08/05/11	3	Direct Contact, Ingestion	Eye and Upper Respiratory Tract Irritation and Rash	Water Skiing
7	Male	40	08/12/11	24	Direct Contact, Ingestion	Gastrointestinal	Jet Skiing

* Case 2 and Case 6 were hospitalized.

Case 6, a 38-year-old male, presented to an emergency department on August 8, 2011, with symptoms that included headache, joint pain, fatigue, sore throat, fever (102.5 °F), chills and diaphoresis. Healthcare providers initially suspected meningitis, but this, and other infectious diseases, were ruled out. He reported swallowing water when he fell in the lake while water skiing at Milford Lake on August 5, 2011. Milford Lake was under a public health Warning due to high cyanobacteria cell concentrations and microcystin toxin levels. He was diagnosed with cyanobacteria toxicosis. He was hospitalized for three days for supportive care.

In 2012, KDHE investigated five probable and two suspected cases. In 2013, there was one suspected case of FHAB-related morbidity in humans.

2.5. Canine Cases

In 2011, there were seven reports of FHAB-associated illnesses and deaths in dogs: one suspected, one confirmed illness and fiver confirmed deaths. One dog illness was classified as not a case. Of the six confirmed dog illnesses and deaths, the median age was 1.3 years (range: four months–six years), and 50% (3/6) were male (Table 4); the median weight was 51 pounds (range: 40–60 pounds). The median time from exposure to onset of clinical signs was 3.5 h (range: 1–48 h). Clinical signs included vomiting, diarrhea, lethargy, staggering, seizures and death.

All six confirmed canine cases had at least one alanine aminotransferase (ALT) test performed (Table 4). ALT is a serum liver enzyme biomarker that can be measured to determine the presence of injury to the liver. The largest increases in ALT develop with hepatocellular necrosis and inflammation [15]. The highest ALT level is reported for those dogs with multiple tests. The median ALT (13,958 µ/L) was higher than the reference range of ALT for dogs (10–109 µ/L).

Cases 3, 4, 5 and 6 were treated at the Kansas State University Animal Health Center in Manhattan, Kansas. *Microcystis* spp. was identified on hair samples from Case 4 and in vomitus from Case 6 [16]. No cyanobacteria were found on hair from Case 5; however, the dog was bathed prior to testing of the hair [16]. The stomach contents of Case 4 were examined for the presence of cyanobacteria; the dog vomited numerous times prior to death; therefore, no cyanobacteria were identified. A necropsy was performed on Cases 3, 4, and 6. All three dogs had massive, diffuse, acute hepatic necrosis consistent with microcystin toxicity. Case 5 developed liver failure and had the highest ALT level (60,585 µ/L); this dog survived with intensive supportive care [17].

In 2012, there was one suspected case, and in 2013, there were two suspected cases of FHAB-related morbidity reported to KDHE in dogs. There was one canine FHAB-associated fatality due to exposure to Milford Lake in 2013.

Table 4. Confirmed canine freshwater harmful algal bloom-associated cases, Kansas, 2011.

Case	Sex	Age	Breed	Date of Exposure	Time to Onset of Signs (h)	Route of Exposure	Initial Signs	Outcome	Maximum ALT Level (µ/L); Ref. Range: 10–109 µ/L	Toxicology	Pathology
1 †	Female	7 months	German Shepherd	08/12/11	48	Direct Contact, Ingestion, Inhalation	Lethargy	Died 08/16/11	>6,000	N/A	N/A
2 †	Male	4 months	German Shepherd	08/12/11	48	Direct Contact, Ingestion	Vomiting	Survived	5,889	N/A	N/A
3 ‡	Male	3 years	Vizsla	08/17/11	3	Direct Contact, Ingestion	Vomiting Lethargy	Died 08/18/11	21,916	N/A	Hepatocellular necrosis, massive, acute and renal tubular epithelial necrosis, diffuse severe
4 ‡	Male	5 months	Vizsla	08/17/11	3	Direct Contact, Ingestion	Vomiting Lethargy	Died 08/18/11	3,378	*Microcystis* spp. on hair.	Hepatocellular necrosis, massive, acute
5	Female	2 years	Weimaraner	08/25/11	1	Direct Contact, Ingestion	Vomiting Lethargy Weakness	Survived	60,585	No cyanobacteria on hair	N/A
6	Female	6 years	Briard	09/24/11	4	Ingestion	Vomiting	Died 09/26/11	39,326	*Microcystis* spp. in vomitus	Hepatocellular necrosis, massive, acute and renal proximal tubular necrosis, acute

† Case 1 and 2 from the same household; ‡ Case 3 and 4 from the same household.

Recently, a case report was published by Rankin *et al.*, who described the use of oral cholestyramine to successfully treat a dog with acute cyanobacterial toxicosis [18]. Cholestyramine is a bile acid sequestrant; it adsorbs and combines with bile acids in the intestine, where it forms an insoluble complex that is excreted in the feces [19]. This prevents enterohepatic recirculation of bile acids and any associated bound substances, such as microcystin toxins [18]. In addition, cholestyramine has been used to treat human patients with possible estuary-associated syndrome (PEAS), caused by an estuarine dinoflagellate that produces a neurotoxin [20]. Veterinarians and physicians should consider the use of cholestyramine, in addition to supportive care, for patients with suspected cyanobacterial toxicosis.

3. Experimental Section

3.1. FHAB Identification and Water Sampling

Water samples were collected in accordance with the KDHE Bureau of Environmental Field Service's Lake Monitoring Protocol [21]. This protocol has been in place for the last thirty years to standardize monitoring of lakes to protect public health. Sample locations included areas identified as the most frequently used points of public access, such as swimming beaches, boat docks and ramps, marinas and public drinking water intakes. Water samples were collected by trained field staff using a beaker on a telescopic pole. The beaker was submerged approximately 1–2 inches below the water's surface. Two collections were made, and the contents of the beaker were transferred to a one-liter cubitainer. The cubitainer was marked with the sample location identification number, collection time, collection date and the collector's name. The cubitainer was placed in a cooler with ice to keep the sample cool, but not frozen. All samples were transported to the Kansas Health and Environmental Laboratories within twenty-four hours. Analysis of the samples included cyanobacteria cell concentrations and microcystin toxin analysis via enzyme-linked immunosorbent assay (ELISA). A public health Advisory was issued if the water test results had cyanobacteria cell concentrations of 20,000 to <100,000 cells/mL or microcystin toxin that was detectable to <20 µg/L. The water body would be re-tested within 4 weeks. The Advisory remained in effect until cyanobacteria concentrations were <20,000 cyanobacteria cells/mL and microcystin toxin concentrations were no longer detectable at all sample sites. A public health Warning was issued if the water test results had cyanobacteria cell concentrations ≥100,000 cells/mL, microcystin toxin ≥20 µg/L or visible cyanobacteria surface accumulation. The water body would be re-tested within one week. The Warning remained in effect until the cyanobacteria concentrations were <100,000 cyanobacteria cells/mL and the microcystin toxins <20 µg/L for two consecutive weeks at all sample sites. Bodies of water that fell below these levels would still be within an Advisory level and remain on a public health alert.

The Kansas Department of Health and Environment updated the Harmful Algal Bloom Policy and Response plan in April, 2012. A public health Advisory was issued when microcystin toxin levels were ≥4 to <20 µg/L; the other conditions that required issuing a public health alert remained the same.

3.2. Outreach to Physicians and Veterinarians

A letter was sent to healthcare providers and veterinarians to alert them of the signs and symptoms of FHAB-related health events and to encourage them to report cases to KDHE. A letter, written by the KDHE Secretary of Health, was mailed to members of the Kansas Academy of Family Physicians on May 23, 2011. This letter was also distributed electronically through the Kansas Health Alert Network. An article written by the State Public Health Veterinarian was distributed to veterinarians via e-mail to members of the Kansas Veterinary Medical Association on July 20, 2011.

Table 5. CDC proposed case definitions for algal toxin-related diseases. FHAB, freshwater harmful algal bloom.

Case	Suspect	Probable	Confirmed
Animal	Exposure to water or to seafood with a confirmed algal bloom AND onset of associated signs within a reasonable time after exposure AND without identification of another cause of illness.	Meets criteria for *Suspect Case* AND there is laboratory documentation of HAB toxin(s) in the water.	Meets criteria for a *Probable Case* combined with professional judgment based on medical review. or Meets criteria for a *Probable Case* and documentation of a HAB toxin(s) in a clinical specimen, provided appropriate testing is available.
Human	Same as animal *Suspect Case.*	Same as animal *Probable Case.*	Meets criteria for a *Probable Case* combined with professional judgment based on medical review.

3.3. Case Reports and Investigations

FHAB-related illness reports were made by phone or through an online reporting system available on the Kansas Department of Health and Environment website. Each report was reviewed by an epidemiologist, and KDHE Environmental Field Services staff collected water samples for testing. The Centers for Disease Control and Prevention's (CDC) proposed case definitions for algal toxin-related diseases were used to classify animal and human cases (Table 5). Suspect, probable and confirmed human and animal cases were submitted to the Harmful Algal Bloom-related Illness Surveillance System (HABISS) of the National Center for Environmental Health (NCEH), Centers for Disease Control and Prevention.

4. Discussion

In 2011, all confirmed FHAB-associated illnesses and deaths in dogs and 70% (5/7) of confirmed FHAB-associated illnesses in humans were exposed at Milford Lake. KDHE sampled Milford Lake on July 20, 2011. All animal and human cases (Cases 2, 3, 5, 6 and 7) were exposed at Milford Lake between July 20 and September 24. Milford Lake has an estimated 500,000 visitors each year [12]. The majority of these visits likely included some form of recreational water use that placed people, and animals, at risk for exposure to the harmful algal bloom. Due to the high cyanobacteria cell concentrations, level of microcystin and duration of the FHAB, it is surprising that there were not more cases of FHAB-related illnesses reported. Shoreline areas were closed, and there were intensive outreach efforts to educate the general public on FHABs through weekly media releases, website updates, printed brochures and informational signs posted at the lake. Despite these efforts, four confirmed human cases of FHAB-associated illness and all dog deaths occurred after a public health alert was issued for Milford Lake. There are many people who visit from outside the local area and may not be familiar with the appearance of a FHAB or local news media stations that would report public health alert messages. We recommend all FHAB-related case investigations include questions on the knowledge of FHABs and public health alerts, as applicable. This will allow public health officials to determine the effectiveness of messaging and to determine the best use of limited resources for education and outreach to prevent FHAB-associated morbidity and mortality.

The demographic data from our cases differ from national freshwater FHAB-associated outbreak cases. From 2009 to 2010, 11 waterborne disease outbreaks associated with freshwater algal blooms were reported to CDC [8]. These outbreaks caused at least 61 illnesses and two hospitalizations [8]. Demographic information was available for 34 ill persons; 38 (66%) were aged ≤ 19 years of age. The median age of confirmed human cases during our study period was 40 years; there was only one pediatric case reported (Case 2). If we expand our case-patient analysis to include suspect ($n = 1$) and probable ($n = 5$) cases, there were only two additional FHAB-related illnesses in children (two years old and 19 years old) This is surprising, as children are more sensitive to FHAB toxins than adults and have a penchant for risky behaviors, such as drinking lake water [7].

FHAB-related illness can be mild and self-limiting; however, the spectrum of illness can be severe. We report the first detailed information of two hospitalized case patients with recreational exposure to a confirmed freshwater harmful algal bloom in the United States. FHAB-related illness is a diagnosis of exclusion; although microcystin toxin can be identified in biological specimens (e.g., blood, vomitus), these tests are not readily available. A healthcare provider may find it difficult to confirm that FHAB toxins are the cause of a patient's illness based on symptoms alone [7]. The hospitalized case patients relayed information on their exposure to a FHAB during the initial consultation with their healthcare provider. An accurate exposure history provided by the case patient, the healthcare provider's ability to rule-out other likely causes of the patient's illness and the healthcare provider's report of the cases to public health authorities were crucial components to confirm a FHAB-related health event. Each report of human or animal illness potentially associated with a FHAB should be reported to public health authorities. An investigation of the implicated water body and subsequent testing for cyanobacteria and toxins is needed to confirm the presence of a FHAB and to classify a patient as a case. Case reports and epidemiological information on FHAB outbreaks should be published to add to the knowledge of this emerging public health threat. Reports of FHAB-associated outbreaks can be made through the National Outbreak Reporting System (NORS), as the Harmful Algal Bloom-Related Illness Surveillance System (HABISS) has been discontinued [8].

We collected five water samples weekly at Milford Lake and monitored cyanobacteria cell concentration and microcystin toxin levels. Variations in wind speed and direction, in part, may account for variations in cyanobacteria cell concentrations and microcystin at the five sample locations in Milford Lake [16]. Animal behavior may also contribute to risk, particularly in dogs that are prone to exploring shorelines and may seek out and ingest small pockets of accumulated algal scum that are present along the shoreline, but are not apparent from water test results. In addition, there was a delay of up to several days between exposure and when the case patient was reported to public health authorities. Ideally, water samples should be collected at the time and location of exposure.

Two human case patients reported exposure to Milford Lake in 2012, and one dog was reported to be exposed at Milford Lake in 2013. Milford Lake was under a public health alert for a FHAB for five weeks during 2012 and four weeks in 2013. The reduction in case reports is likely due to at least two factors. First, although Milford Lake experienced a FHAB in both 2012 and 2013, the duration of the FHAB was significantly shorter, reducing the amount of time humans, and animals, could be exposed. Second, an aggressive education and outreach effort by FHAB partners, including the media, to recreational water users, healthcare providers and veterinarians likely contributed to the reduction in case reports. However, an evaluation of FHAB public health messaging to recreational water users is needed to validate and quantify this hypothesis.

This study is subject to at least two limitations. First, under-reporting of human and animal cases to public health authorities may have occurred. Human healthcare providers and veterinarians must first recognize that a patient's symptoms or clinical signs may be due to exposure to a FHAB, rule-out other likely causes of illness and then report the case to public health authorities. KDHE requests that human healthcare providers and veterinarians report FHAB-related cases; however, it is not mandatory. Second, case misclassification of FHAB-related cases may have occurred. The majority of human cases classified as "not a case" were due to the absence of laboratory testing for other etiologies that may explain a patient's symptoms.

No U.S. Federal policy, regulations or guidelines exist for FHABs in recreational waters; however, several states have developed their own policies [1,9,10]. The state of Nebraska demonstrated a robust public health response to reports of two dog deaths from cyanobacterial toxicosis in 2004 [9]. The implicated lake was sampled for total microcystins; levels exceeded 15 μg/L, and a health alert was issued. Due to the short amount of time between the alert and the weekend, when the lake was heavily patronized, numerous people were exposed, and more than 50 cyanobacteria health-related complaints were documented. Currently, the Nebraska Department of Environmental Quality conducts weekly or bi-weekly sampling at 47 public lakes from May through September, and results are updated weekly on their website (http://deq.ne.gov/NDEQProg.nsf/Beaches2014.xsp). A lake is placed on a public health alert if the microcystin concentration is ≥20 μg/L.

5. Conclusions

The incidence of freshwater harmful algal blooms has increased in Kansas and caused human illnesses, including two hospitalized case patients and several dog deaths. The Kansas Department of Health and Environment, in conjunction with their local and national partners, developed a Harmful Algal Bloom Policy and Response Plan based on historical lake water sample data and incorporated human and veterinary case reports as a part of its core surveillance activities. Voluntary reports of FHAB-related cases by human and veterinary healthcare providers and investigation of each report by public health officials were critical components to the FHAB surveillance system. The annual review of the water sample data and human and veterinary surveillance data guided changes to the policy and response plan.

The Kansas experience, as described in this article, demonstrates the importance of a systematic data collection system to document the impact of FHABs on human and animal health. States without a formal FHAB program should consider the development of a policy to address this emerging issue to prevent morbidity and mortality, among humans and animals, at public recreational water venues. In addition, public health officials and FHAB partners must ensure continued awareness of the risks to the public, educate healthcare providers and veterinarians on FHAB-related illness and encourage timely reporting to public health authorities each year.

Acknowledgments

The authors would like to acknowledge all healthcare providers and veterinarians who reported FHAB-related health events.

Author Contributions

Ingrid Trevino-Garrison's contributions to this article include: development of the 2010 Kansas Department of Health and Environment Harmful Algal Bloom Policy and Response Plan, the descriptive epidemiologic analysis of the human and dog health event data and writing this report.

Jamie DeMent's contributions to this article include: case investigation for reports of FHAB-related health events (2011) and management of the FHAB-related health event database. DeMent completed this work while employed by the Kansas Department of Health and Environment.

Farah S. Ahmed's contributions to this article include: investigation of reports of FHAB-related health events (2012–2014) and creation of the survey, which was administered to veterinarians and physicians during 2012.

Patricia Haines-Lieber's contributions to this article include: development of the 2010 Kansas Department of Health and Environment Harmful Algal Bloom Policy and Response Plan, content contribution to the KDHE Harmful Algal Bloom website, development, along with the KDHE Geographic Information Systems section, of the KDHE Harmful Algal Bloom Data Management Program.

Thomas Langer's contributions to this article include: development of the 2010 Kansas Department of Health and Environment Harmful Algal Bloom Policy and Response Plan, the analysis of lake water sample data during the bloom period and stakeholder communication throughout the 2011 HAB season. Langer completed this work while employed by the Kansas Department of Health and Environment.

Henri Ménager's contributions to this article include: investigation of reports of FHAB-related health events (2012–2014), writing summary reports of lake-water testing activities and documenting the public health alert status of tested lakes.

Janet Neff's contributions to this article include: coordination of the KDHE Harmful Algal Bloom Outreach and Communication Plan and coordination of HAB partnerships and conferences.

Deon van der Merwe's contributions to this article include: investigations of FHAB-related poisoning in animals.

Edward Carney's contributions to this article include: development of the of the 2010 Kansas Department of Health and Environment Harmful Algal Bloom Policy and Response Plan, development of the Freshwater Harmful Algal Bloom sampling protocols and serving as the principle algal taxonomist, limnologist and lake ecologist at KDHE (1984–2014). Carney completed this work while employed by the Kansas Department of Health and Environment.

Disclaimer

The findings and conclusions in this report are those of the author(s) and do not necessarily represent the official position of the Kansas Department of Health and Environment.

Conflicts of Interest

The authors declare no conflict of interest.

References

1. Hudnell, H.K. The state of U.S. freshwater harmful algal blooms assessments, policy and legislation. *Toxicon* **2010**, *55*, 1024–1034.
2. Stewart, I.; Webb, P.M.; Schluter, P.J.; Shaw, G.R. Recreational and occupational field exposure to freshwater cyanobacteria—A review of anecdotal and case reports, epidemiological studies and the challenges for epidemiologic assessment. *Environ. Health* **2006**, *5*, 1–13.
3. Briand, J.; Jacquet, S.; Bernard, C.; Humbert, J. Health hazards for terrestrial vertebrates from toxic cyanobacteria in surface water ecosystems. *Vet. Res.* **2003**, *34*, 361–377.
4. World Health Organization. Coastal and fresh waters. In *Guidelines for Safe Recreational Water Environments*; World Health Organization: Geneva, Switzerland, 2003; Volume 1.
5. Dodds, W.K. *Assessment of Blue-Green Algal Toxins in Kansas*; Kansas Water Resources Research Institute: Manhattan, KS, USA, 1996; Report no. G202–02.
6. Backer, L.C.; Landsberg, J.H.; Miller, M.; Keel, K.; Taylor, T. Canine cyanotoxin poisonings in the United States (1920s–2012): Review of suspected and confirmed cases from three data sources. *Toxins* **2013**, *5*, 1597–1628.
7. Weirich, C.A.; Miller, T.R. Freshwater harmful algal blooms: Toxins and children's health. *Curr. Probl. Pediatr. Adolesc. Health Care* **2014**, *44*, 2–24.
8. Hilborn, E.D.; Roberts, V.A.; Backer, L.; DeConno, E.; Egan, J.S.; Hyde, J.B.; Nicholas, D.C.; Wiegert, E.J.; Billing, L.M.; DiOrio, M.; *et al.* Algal bloom-associated disease outbreaks among users of freshwater lakes—United States, 2009–2010. *MMWR* **2014**, *63*, 11–15.
9. Walker, S.R.; Lund, J.C.; Schumacher, D.G.; Brakhage, A.P.; McManus, C.B.; Miller, D.J.; Augustine, M.M.; Carney, J.J.; Holland, S.R.; Hoagland, D.K.; *et al.* Nebraska experience. *Adv. Exp. Med. Biol.* **2008**, *619*, 139–152.
10. Stone, D.; Bress, W. Addressing public health risks for cyanobacteria in recreational freshwaters: The Oregon and vermont framework. *Integr. Environ. Assess. Manag.* **2007**, *3*, 137–143.

11. Haines-Lieber, P. Kansas department of health and environment's harmful algal bloom response plan. Proceedings of the Kansas Harmful Algal Bloom Workshop, Topeka, KS, USA, 15 May 2012.

12. U.S. Army Corps of Engineers. Available online: http://www.nwk.usace.army.mil/Locations/ DistrictLakes/MilfordLake.aspx (accessed on 12 November 2014).

13. Carney, E. Kansas Integrated Water Quality Assessment Report. Kansas Department of Health and Environment. 1989–2014. Available online: http://www.kdheks.gov/befs/resources_ publications.html (accessed on 15 October 2014).

14. Moser, K. *The Blue, the Green, and the Toxic: Knowledge, Attitudes, and Practices of Physicians and Veterinarians Regarding Harmful Algal Blooms*; Kansas State University: Manhattan, KS, USA, 2012.

15. The Merck Veterinary Manual. Available online: http://www.merckmanuals.com/vet/digestive_ system/hepatic_disease_in_small_animals/enzyme_activity_in_hepatic_disease_in_small_anima ls.html (accessed on 12 November 2014).

16. Van der Merwe, D.; Seebag, L.; Nietfeld, J.C.; Aubel, M.T.; Foss, A.; Carney, E. Investigation of a *Microcystis aeruginosa* cyanobacterial freshwater harmful algal bloom associated with acute microcystin toxicosis in a dog. *J. Vet. Diagn. Invest.* **2012**, *24*, 679–687.

17. Seebag, L.; Smee, N.; van der Merwe, D.; Schmid, D. Liver failure in a dog following suspected ingestion of blue-green algae (*Microcystis* spp.): A case report and review of the toxin. *J. Am. Anim. Hosp. Assoc.* **2013**, *49*, 342–346.

18. Rankin, K.A.; Alroy, K.A.; Kudela, R.M.; Oates, S.C.; Murray, M.J.; Miller, M.A. Treatment of cyanobacterial (microcystin) toxicosis using oral cholestyramine: Case report of a dog from Montana. *Toxins* **2013**, 5, 1051–1063.

19. Physicians' Desk Reference. Available online: http://www.pdr.net/drug-summary/prevalite? druglabelid=1938 (accessed 7 January 2015).

20. Hudnell, H.K. Chronic biotoxin-associated illness: Multiple-system symptoms, a vision deficit, and effective treatment. *Neurotoxicol. Teratol.* **2005**, *27*, 733–743.

21. Division of Environment, Kansas Department of Health and Environment. Quality Management Plan, Part III, Lake and Westland Water Quality Monitoring Program Quality Assurance Management Plan. Revision 4. 2014. Available online: http://www.kdheks.gov/environment/ qmp/qmp.htm#BOW (accessed 9 October 2014).

One Health and Cyanobacteria in Freshwater Systems: Animal Illnesses and Deaths Are Sentinel Events for Human Health Risks

Elizabeth D. Hilborn and Val R. Beasley

Abstract: Harmful cyanobacterial blooms have adversely impacted human and animal health for thousands of years. Recently, the health impacts of harmful cyanobacteria blooms are becoming more frequently detected and reported. However, reports of human and animal illnesses or deaths associated with harmful cyanobacteria blooms tend to be investigated and reported separately. Consequently, professionals working in human or in animal health do not always communicate findings related to these events with one another. Using the One Health concept of integration and collaboration among health disciplines, we systematically review the existing literature to discover where harmful cyanobacteria-associated animal illnesses and deaths have served as sentinel events to warn of potential human health risks. We find that illnesses or deaths among livestock, dogs and fish are all potentially useful as sentinel events for the presence of harmful cyanobacteria that may impact human health. We also describe ways to enhance the value of reports of cyanobacteria-associated illnesses and deaths in animals to protect human health. Efficient monitoring of environmental and animal health in a One Health collaborative framework can provide vital warnings of cyanobacteria-associated human health risks.

Reprinted from *Toxins*. Cite as: Hilborn, E.D.; Beasley, V.R. One Health and Cyanobacteria in Freshwater Systems: Animal Illnesses and Deaths Are Sentinel Events for Human Health Risks. *Toxins* **2015**, *7*, 1374-1395.

1. Introduction

1.1. Freshwater Cyanobacteria

Freshwater cyanobacteria and their toxins (cyanotoxins) pose risks to human and animal health via contamination of water sources and aquatic communities globally. Dense accumulations of cyanobacterial cells, or colonies are termed 'blooms' and these occur most commonly, but not exclusively, in nutrient-rich, warm, bodies of water with little movement or mixing among layers [1]. When cyanotoxins are produced, or when cyanobacterial biomass and/or cyanotoxins disrupt ecological processes, the events are loosely termed 'harmful algal blooms' (HABs). The World Health Organization has developed guidelines based upon cyanobacterial cell densities in water, and advises that the presence of dense scums near bathing areas may indicate substantial human health risks [2]. Although cyanobacteria are naturally-occurring, anthropogenic activities now contribute to increased occurrence of HABs globally [3]. Nutrient pollution from human and animal wastes that wash into surface waters, fertilizer applications, atmospheric nutrient deposition, burning of plant material, overgrazing, warmer weather, drought conditions that reduce terrestrial plant uptake of nutrients as well as reduce the depth and flow of water bodies all contribute to bloom formation [4]. Conditions that promote cyanobacteria occurrences are expected to increase based upon model projections of future human population growth, land use patterns and climate change [5].

Many genera of cyanobacteria produce potent toxins as secondary metabolites, some of which are released before, and others largely after, cyanobacterial lysis. The evolutionary value of cyanotoxins to their producers is not fully characterized, although benefits may include: quorum sensing, grazer deterrence, a potential competitive advantage in aquatic environments via allelopathy toward other cyanobacteria, and improved regulation of intracellular phosphate or electrolyte concentrations [6–8]. Cyanobacteria often produce foul taste and odor compounds such as geosmin and 2-methylisoborneol during their life cycle, senescence and decomposition [9,10]. These taste and odor compounds are not believed to present major health risks, but their potential toxicity has been little studied [11]. Importantly, these odorous compounds can indicate the need to prevent human and animal exposure to water that may also contain potentially lethal cyanotoxins [9].

During the 19th and most of the 20th century, the toxicity of water samples was assessed primarily by the use of the animal bioassay. Francis, in 1878 authored one of the first reports of the toxicological assessment of a harmful cyanobacterial bloom and the intentional use of an animal as an indicator of human health risk [12]. During the last 100 years, advances in investigative and diagnostic tools have helped characterize cyanobacteria and cyanotoxins, including: light microscopy with increasingly refined phycology and cyanobacterial taxonomy; and the identification and characterization of some cyanotoxins using molecular, chemical and biochemical assays [13,14]. During the latter part of the 20th century, over 100 unique cyanotoxins have been identified, and new compounds continue to be isolated, and structurally characterized. Multiple functional classes of cyanotoxins have now been described, including: hepatotoxins, neurotoxins, dermatotoxins and cytotoxins [15–18]. Examples of hepatotoxins include the cyclic peptides: microcystins and nodularins, although their effects are broader than liver toxicity alone. Cylindrospermopsin is a potent sulfated tricyclic guanidine cytotoxin with bioactive metabolites. Cyanobacterial neurotoxins include saxitoxin and neosaxitoxin, which are complex alkaloid sodium channel blockers, the cyclic alkaloid nicotinic agonists anatoxin-a and homoanatoxin-a, and the organophosphorus cholinesterase inhibitor anatoxin-a(s). Lyngbyatoxins are cyanobacterial dermatotoxins that occur in fresh, brackish, and marine waters. Cyanobacteria also produce lipopolysaccharides, which are general irritants [18]. No cyanotoxins are fully characterized for toxicity, for geographic occurrence, or for the environmental conditions necessary and sufficient for their production. Concerted research efforts are underway in many countries to characterize the occurrence of harmful cyanobacteria and their effects on ecosystem functions as well as human and animal health. However, the number of cyanotoxins and combinations of cyanotoxin mixtures in the environment complicates risk assessments focused on potentially harmful cyanobacterial exposures.

1.2. The Concept of "One Health"

"One Health" is a term that is increasingly being used in the early 21st century to convey how health rests upon interdependent collaborations among professionals in human and animal health, and wildlife and environmental sciences [19,20]. Nevertheless, the concept of One Health as a more inclusive and holistic way to study and maintain health within a cross-species continuum is ancient. Zinsstag *et al*. (2011) provided overviews of the origins, scope, systems thinking, and value of One Health, including how China's Zhou Dynasty (11th–13th century) organized public health systems involving both medical doctors and veterinarians [21]. In the 1960s, Rachel Carson made connections between the application of highly toxic pesticides and adverse effects on human, domestic animal, and terrestrial and aquatic wildlife health. A One Health approach would have benefitted all of those involved in an incident of methylmercury intoxication in Japan in the 1950s [22]. A prolonged industrial release of methylmercury into waters off the coast of Minamata poisoned first fish and then birds; later cats and thousands of humans were sickened as the toxin spread throughout the food web. One Health insights relevant to infectious diseases were relied upon by such scientists as Edward Jenner, when, in developing a vaccine against smallpox (a human disease), he demonstrated the cross reactivity of human antibodies between smallpox and the less pathogenic cowpox (an animal disease). Countless other scientists, clinicians and public health practitioners have operated in a One Health paradigm in the pursuit of control of zoonotic disease, in food and water safety, as well as in environmental protection to optimize the health and wellbeing of earth's biota. In short, One Health is a paradigm that recognizes the interdependence of human, animal, plant, microbial, and ecosystem health [23]. Effective multidisciplinary research, surveillance, and stewardship are essential for synchronous improvements in the health of humans, other animals, plants and ecosystems [19]. Recently, funding for public health from public and private sources has declined [24,25]. Unfortunately, this has coincided with reductions in essential public health services provided by functional ecosystems [26]. The One Health framework offers an interdisciplinary paradigm that seeks to optimize health by leveraging existing resources and capabilities among human, veterinary and ecosystem health experts to address some of the most the complex, multidisciplinary challenges that define the 21st century.

Reports of human health and animal health tend to be published separately and are discussed separately. However, harmful cyanobacteria impact both humans and animals. Animals often experience direct, high-intensity exposures to harmful cyanobacteria which result in illnesses and deaths. Cyanobacteria-associated animal illnesses or deaths can therefore be used to warn of risks and if heeded, action may be implemented to avoid adverse human health effects [27]. Our goal is to provide a representative overview of the adverse effects of harmful freshwater cyanobacteria on humans and other vertebrates and to comprehensively review reports that include incidents where animal illnesses and deaths have served as sentinel events to warn of potential or actual human health risks.

2. Selected Human Health Reports

Human health may be adversely impacted by harmful cyanobacteria from many sources, and via multiple routes of exposure. The highest impact outbreaks of cyanobacteria-associated intoxications and deaths have been reported when patients requiring hemodialysis were directly exposed to cyanotoxins intravenously via dialysate prepared from contaminated water [28,29]. This route of exposure to cyanotoxins resulted in toxic hepatitis, multi-organ damage and death [28–31].

People are most frequently exposed to harmful cyanobacteria via contaminated water. People may be exposed orally, dermally and occasionally by aspiration to aquatic microbial communities containing cyanobacterial cells and mixtures of cyanotoxins during recreational activities on or in untreated surface waters [32–36]. Occasionally, these exposures have resulted in severe respiratory impairment characterized by pneumonia and adult respiratory distress syndrome [32,35]. Less severe effects include fever, other respiratory illness, signs and symptoms of respiratory and dermal allergy, and dermatologic, gastrointestinal, neurologic, otic, and ocular signs and symptoms [33,34,36–43]. Occupational exposures to harmful cyanobacteria have been reported after routine work on an incidentally contaminated surface water body, in relation to investigation of a cyanobacterial bloom, and following an investigation of cyanobacteria-associated animal illnesses and deaths [34].

Drinking water contaminated with harmful cyanobacteria has been associated with liver and kidney damage [44,45], and rarely, severe illness, extended hospitalizations and deaths have occurred [45–47]. Acute health effects such as gastroenteritis, muscle pain and dermatitis associated with home use of contaminated drinking water have been reported [43,48]. When municipal systems have been contaminated, large numbers of people may be exposed and become ill [49–53]. The International Agency for Research on Cancer has determined that, while current data on microcystins and nodularins are inconclusive in regard to human carcinogenesis, promotion of liver tumors by these toxins is plausible [54]. Zhou [55] reported that use of potentially microcystin-contaminated drinking water supplies was associated with higher rates of colorectal cancer in human populations in parts of China. Conventional drinking water treatment involving filtration, flocculation, and disinfection reduces, but does not always eliminate cyanobacteria and cyanotoxins. More sophisticated methods may be required to reduce cyanotoxins in finished drinking water to acceptable concentrations [56]. However, drinking water treatment processes may become impaired or ineffective when large quantities of cyanobacterial biomass enter the source water intake.

Some poorly characterized human health risks include: repeated voluntary exposure to cyanotoxins through ingestion of cyanobacteria (blue green algae) as food or as supplements [57,58]; involuntary exposure via inhalation of cyanotoxins during activities on or in contaminated waters, and ingestion of contaminated aquatic animal foods or vegetables grown with contaminated irrigation water [59–62].

3. Selected Animal Health Reports

HABs and associated adverse animal health impacts have been recorded for over 180 years. The first published report believed to document a harmful cyanobacteria bloom was by Hald to the Danish government in 1833. Hald described cattle and fish deaths associated with 'sick' lakes where green material covered the surface of the water. The bloom material itself was uncharacterized. Hald wrote that he did not know if the green substance was "…caused by water plants, insects or minerals…" [63].

Most early reports of animal deaths associated with harmful blooms were circumstantial. Waters were initially suspected of being harmful because of the temporal and spatial proximity of dead and dying animals observed in and around a bloom. Although the toxicity of these aquatic 'plant' materials was surmised by observation of associated animal deaths, the toxigenic organisms and the toxic principles themselves were uncharacterized. Francis was the first to scientifically investigate the toxic effects of a cyanobacterial bloom [12]. After mass livestock deaths in Lake Alexandrina in Australia, he administered a sample of the *Nodularia spumigena* bloom material from the lake to a sheep. He then compared necropsy results of the animal experimentally exposed with sheep that had died following natural exposure to the bloom and concluded that cyanobacteria were the source of the toxic effects.

Harmful cyanobacteria adversely affect wildlife, livestock and companion animals. Schwimmer and Schwimmer [64] compiled and summarized over 65 wildlife, livestock and domestic animal mortality events associated with cyanobacteria during 1878–1960. Animal deaths associated with harmful cyanobacteria have been reported from Europe, North America, South America, Australia, Africa and Asia [12,65–69]. Stewart, *et al.* [70] provided a selective review of published reports of cyanobacteria-associated animal morbidity and mortality events from around the world, with representative case studies of livestock, companion animal and wildlife deaths.

Reports of livestock deaths following exposures to cyanobacteria under field conditions have been reported from every inhabited continent and involved ruminants, hogs, horses, fowl, cultured fish and even honeybees [65,66,71–75]. Livestock with access to farm ponds and portions of lakes may be at risk of exposure during a bloom, especially when wind-driven surface blooms accumulate at the site of animals' water access. Overflow of bloom material from farm ponds that contaminates animals' pasture can also be a source of poisoning for livestock [76]. Antemortem signs of intoxication vary and are dependent upon the cyanotoxins, the dose and time frames involved, the therapeutic interventions employed and individual characteristics of the exposed animals. Acute effects often include: hypersalivation, agitation, anorexia, pale mucus membranes, weakness, dyspnea, recumbancy, depression, ataxia, diarrhea, muscle tremors and fasciculations, convulsions, apparent blindness and sudden death [77–79]. Birds may display weakness and neurologic signs such as ataxia, and hyperextended necks (opisthotonos) prior to death. Cyanobacteria have been associated with mass mortality events in catfish and carp cultured in ponds; microcystins in water were accompanied by clinical signs of illness and gross lesions in the liver [73,75]. Because of microcystin residues, the latter authors (Singh and Asthana) cautioned against human consumption of the tissues of contaminated fish.

Reports of cyanobacteria-associated companion animal illnesses and deaths have most often involved dogs. Dogs have been observed consuming scums of cyanobacteria that accumulate near the shore, drinking contaminated water, and licking bloom material from their hair coats after wading or swimming [80]. A recent summary of cyanobacteria-associated dog deaths in the United States compiles over 100 reports over the last 80 years [81]. The frequency of reporting of these events has greatly increased since the 1970s, however, reporting, attribution and detection biases were all factors that influenced the number of events that were confirmed as being associated with cyanobacteria during the study period. Deaths among other companion animal deaths such as cats are rarely reported [77]. Acute effects among companion animals include: vomiting, diarrhea, profuse salivation, weakness, convulsions, hemorrhage and sudden death [82,83].

Wildlife deaths associated with harmful freshwater cyanobacterial blooms are commonly reported, but undoubtedly many occur and are unreported because of the lack of human observation of the event. Multiple types of vertebrates may be harmed, from fish to birds to mammals [84–86]. In some instances it is not always possible to attribute wildlife deaths to harmful cyanobacteria because when the affected animals are found, they are too decomposed for reliable pathological and toxicological analyses. Fish and water birds are at especially high risk of harmful c yanobacteria-associated effects, and mass mortality events have been reported from most continents [66,68,85,87,88]. Cyanobacteria blooms may have direct and indirect adverse effects on fish and water birds. Direct intoxication may occur after exposure to harmful cyanobacteria, or cyanotoxin-contaminated food and water. Indirect effects of cyanobacterial blooms include a decrease in dissolved oxygen and the proliferation of *Clostridium botulinum* [89]. Large mortality events have occurred when birds are poisoned by botulinum toxin in aquatic environments [90,91].

4. Results: Animal Illnesses and Deaths that Served as Sentinel Events for Cyanobacteria-Associated Human Health Risks

Our search of the scientific literature yielded 18 reports describing at least 29 events where there were actual or potential cyanobacteria-associated human health risks accompanied by observations of sick or dead animals that were exposed to harmful cyanobacteria (Table 1). These episodes of human health risks have occurred among drinking water consumers, among workers investigating mass mortality events, and among recreational users of water bodies that were contaminated with cyanobacteria. Eleven of 18 reports describe animal illnesses or deaths that alerted authorities to the presence of contaminated water and warnings were issued and/or action was taken to prevent human exposure.

In multiple instances, reports of animal deaths prompted investigations that led to the initial isolation and structural characterization of cyanotoxins from a water body without a specified use for drinking or recreation. One such report is Devlin *et al.* [103], who isolated and cultured a cyanobacterium associated with cattle deaths and determined the structure of anatoxin-a for the first time. In some instances, the toxic mechanism of action was first deduced in studies conducted after animals died in the field, and those mechanisms later were used for toxin isolation and structural elucidation. For example, after dog and other animal deaths were observed in a lake in South Dakota, United States, Mahmood *et al.* [104] detected a cholinesterase-inhibiting cyanotoxin for the first time. Subsequent studies based upon that biochemical mechanism led to characterization of anatoxin-a(s), the only known naturally occurring organophosphorous cholinesterase-inhibiting toxin [105].

Table 1. Reports of animal illnesses and deaths that served as sentinel events for cyanobacteria-associated human health risks.

Location; reference	Year	Number events	Cyanobacteria	Toxin	Animal illness	Human illness, exposure route	Interagency coordination
Lake Alexandrina, Australia; [92]	1878	>1	*Nodularia spumigena* identified in water	Unknown	Several hundred livestock deaths	Undescribed illness in one individual after drinking contaminated water	Investigation, warnings issued prior to human illness
Elk River, Kanawha River, Ohio River, West Virginia; Ohio River Ohio; Ohio River, Kentucky, United States; [50]	1930–1931	>6	*Anabaena flos-aquae* identified in water	Unknown	Fish deaths Kanawha River	Gastrointestinal illness among thousands of people receiving drinking water from rivers	Investigation, no known warnings issued
Storm Lake, Iowa, United States; [85]	1948	>1	*Anabaena flos-aquae* identified in water	Unknown	Fish, dogs died	None reported	Investigation, warnings issued
Lake Dauphin, Manitoba, Canada; [77]	1951	1	*Aphanizomenon flos-aquae* identified in water	Unknown	Horse, dogs died	None reported	Investigation, warnings issued
Echo Lake, Qu'Appelle Lake, other lakes in Saskatchewan, Canada; [93,94]	1959	>2	*Anabaena circinalis* (identified in stool sample)	Unknown	Multiple livestock, fish, geese, dogs died	Gastrointestinal illness among individuals with recreational exposure to lakes	Investigation, warnings issued prior to human illness
Hegman Reservoir, Montana, United States; [95]	1977	1	*Anabaena* spp. and *Aphanizomenon flos-aquae* identified in water	Unknown	Cattle, dogs died	None reported	Investigation, warnings issued
Lakes in Pennsylvania, United States; [40]	1979	2	*Anabaena* spp. identified in water	Unknown	Dog illness	None reported	Investigation, warnings issued before dog illness
Lake in Montana, United States; [96]	1984	1	Unspecified bloom identified in water	Unknown	Cattle deaths	None reported	Investigation, warnings issued
Lake in Alberta, Canada; [97]	1985	1	Unspecified bloom identified in water	Unknown	Bats, ducks died	None reported	Investigation, warnings issued
Guandiana River in Portugal; [98]	1987	1	*Aphanizomenon flos-aquae* bloom identified in water	Unknown	Fish deaths	Gastroenteritis, dermatitis among those who consumed drinking water	None known

Table 1. *Cont.*

Location; reference	Year	Number events	Cyanobacteria	Toxin	Animal illness	Human illness, exposure route	Interagency coordination
Lake—Rutland Water in Leicestershire, United Kingdom; [99]	1989	1	*Microcystis aeruginosa* bloom identified in water	Microcystin-LR	Dog and sheep deaths	Gastroenteritis, dermatitis among those who recreated in water	Investigation, no known warnings issued
Zeekoevlei Lake, and others, near or in Western Cape Province, South Africa; [100,101]	1994	4	*Nodularia spumigena* and *Microcystis aeruginosa* bloom identified in water	Nodularin, Microcystin-LR	Dog and livestock deaths	None reported	Investigation, warnings issued
Pond in Mymensingh, Bangladesh; [74]	2002	1	*Anabaena flos-aquae* and *Microcystis aeruginosa* bloom identified in water	Unknown	Fish and goat deaths	Rash, eye and ear irritation	Investigation, no known warnings issued
River Meuse, Venlo Municipality, Netherlands; [102]	2003	1	Unspecified cyanobacteria	Unknown	Fish and bird deaths	Rash	Investigation, no known warnings issued
Buccaneer Bay Lake, multiple other lakes, Eastern Nebraska, United States; [42]	2004	>3	*Anabaena, Microcystis, Oscillatoria, Aphanizo-menon*	Microcystin-LR and microcystins	Dog, livestock, wildlife deaths	More than 50 reports of rash, skin lesions, headache and/or gastroenteritis	Investigation, warnings issued
Lakes, Ohio, United States; [36]	2010	2	*Anabaena* spp., *Cylindro-spermopsis raciborskii, Aphanizomenon* spp., *Planktolyngbya limnetica*	Microcystins, Anatoxin-a cylindrospermopsin, saxitoxins	Dog, fish deaths, bird illness	Multiple effects including dermatologic, respiratory, neurologic illness and/or gastroenteritis	Investigation, no known warnings issued

Animal deaths have also been the trigger for the first regional detections of harmful cyanobacteria and specific cyanotoxins. Skulberg [87] raised awareness of problems from harmful cyanobacteria in Europe's eutrophic waters by summarizing the findings of a 1980 survey performed in 26 European countries. At that time, eleven countries reported outbreaks of blue-green algae-associated animal intoxications. James [106] reported detecting anatoxin-a in Irish lakes for the first time during the summers of 1994 and 1995; the investigations followed reports of potentially toxic cyanobacteria-associated dog deaths at lakes during 1992 and 1993. Multiple reports of dog deaths in Scotland, New Zealand and France led to the finding of anatoxin-a in the absence of surface blooms; instead, the cyanotoxin was found to be associated with benthic cyanobacteria [83,107,108]. Mez et al. [109] reported isolation of microcystins from Swiss oligotrophic water for the first time after observing a pattern of cattle deaths.

5. Discussion

We found 18 reports of 29 or more events where animal illnesses and deaths served as potential sentinel events for human health risks related to harmful cyanobacteria [36,40,42,50,74,77,85,92–102]. Among 15 of 18 reports describing 25 or more events, cyanobacteria-associated animal illness clearly preceded any reports of human illness [36,42,50,77,85,92–97,99–102]. Among 11 of 18 reports describing 15 or more events, cyanobacteria-associated animal illness or death was recognized, authorities were alerted to the presence of contaminated water, and action was taken to warn people of the risk associated with exposure to potentially toxic water [42,77,85,92–97,100,101]. We found that among the instances where sentinel events were used to warn of the potential for human health risks there was effective communication among environmental, wildlife and health officials.

We selectively described multiple additional reports of animal deaths that alerted investigators to the potential presence of harmful cyanobacteria, some even in the absence of an apparent surface bloom. These bodies of water were not reported as being used for human recreation or drinking water, so the risk for adverse human health effects was unclear [83,103,104,106–109]. However, the animal illnesses and deaths acted as sentinel events that warned of potential cyanobacteria-associated water toxicity.

Dogs, livestock and fish were most frequently cited as animals involved in sentinel events that warned of harmful cyanobacteria. Dogs in particular may be exposed to surface water bodies as they accompany people during recreation and some outdoor types of work. Dogs are likely to drink water they encounter and may ingest algal scums that are present. Dogs acted as sentinels of human health risk in 17 or more events, these events involved primarily recreational water sources, and one event described a poisoning at a potential drinking water source [36,40,42,77,85,93–95,99,100]. Livestock historically have been given access to ponds or lakes that people may use for recreation or drinking water. Types of livestock reportedly involved in sentinel events included primarily cattle and horses; fewer reports involved pigs and smaller ruminants. Livestock acted as sentinels of human health risks in 15 or more events, nine of these were described at recreational water sources, and at least two were described at potential drinking water sources [42,74,77,92–96,99,101]. Fish are raised in ponds as livestock, but also are free-living in lakes, rivers, and other water bodies. Fish acted as sentinels of human health risks in at least 14 events, seven of these were described at recreational waters, and seven were described at drinking water sources [36,50,74,85,93,98,102].

History has shown that the presence of dead or moribund animals in and around a body of water has served as a warning of potential human health risk associated with the water [63]. However, animal illnesses and deaths only effectively warn of human health risks if they are actually seen and the risk recognized. Therefore, it is important for animal deaths potentially associated with harmful cyanobacteria to be investigated and warnings to be issued to potential water users in a timely manner. Ideally, information should be transmitted from those who first encounter dead or dying animals, to wildlife or environmental stewards, veterinarians and public safety personnel. Samples of water and affected animals should be evaluated by laboratory and veterinary professionals. People with health effects should be referred to health care providers. The results of clinical and laboratory analyses should be communicated to investigators and primary reporters as well as to regulatory officials. Regulatory officials should develop monitoring programs and incident response protocols in concert with water and wildlife agencies, and develop and distribute educational materials and perform outreach to those potentially impacted by harmful cyanobacteria with the goal of risk reduction. Clinical care providers should be provided with information on sources and health impacts of harmful cyanobacteria as well as any established diagnostic methods and criteria. Therefore, wildlife, veterinary, medical, water management, laboratory and public health officials may all be potentially involved in a successful response to the occurrence of harmful cyanobacteria (Figure 1) [77,85,93,94].

Unfortunately, communication among these groups is not always frequent or timely, suggesting that there may be significant professional, structural and institutional barriers to adopting the widespread use of sentinel events to protect human health [110]. Auf der Heide notes that in smaller communities, where few public professionals are employed, professionals from multiple disciplines may actually interact more frequently and perform more efficiently and cohesively in the face of unusual or emergent health events [110]. In larger communities with frequent cyanobacterial blooms, providing the opportunity for intentional communication and collaboration activities among these groups before concerted action is needed may be rewarded by more efficient human, animal and environmental health protection.

The One Health initiative provides a framework for multidisciplinary interaction and cooperation among specialists in human, animal and environmental health [19]. This approach has most frequently been applied to the identification and control of zoonotic diseases, but there is a need for coordination among professionals who normally focus solely on human, domestic animal, or wildlife/ecological toxicology as well [111,112]. Commonly-occurring environmental contaminants such as harmful cyanobacteria are human health hazards for which a One Health approach is being successfully applied. A number of the reports of integrated surveillance and preventive measures mentioned above attest to the value of attention to multiple species groups, but these are largely "after-the-fact" responses, when what is needed is to be more proactive.

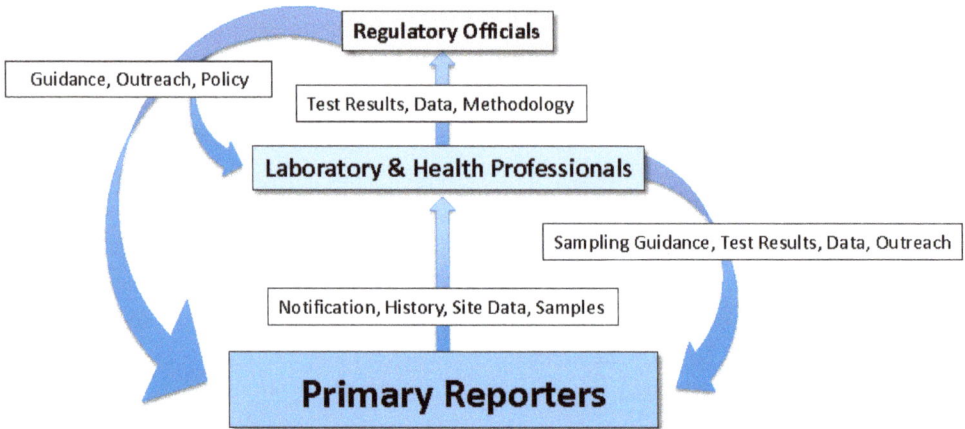

Figure 1. Functional groups and flow of information in a model One Health approach to harmful cyanobacteria identification, risk characterization and response. **Primary Reporters** include: Those who live, recreate or work on or near cyanobacteria-impacted water bodies such as: residents of water front homes; animal owners; lake and waterkeepers; environmental professionals; wildlife professionals; water management and utility personnel; fishermen; public safety personnel. **Laboratory and Health Professionals** include: Chemists, phycologists, wildlife biologists, agricultural specialists, toxicologists, veterinary pathologists, veterinarians and human health care providers. **Regulatory Officials** include: Public health, environmental health, environmental management, wildlife and agricultural personnel.

Nations in Europe have developed One Health guidelines to reduce health risks associated with harmful cyanobacteria. For example, in Scotland, a set of guidelines for risk assessment of cyanobacteria-impacted waters has been developed and updated with the goal of protecting both human and animal health [113]. The responsibility to initially assess the potential risks to human and animal health from harmful cyanobacteria has been assigned to water quality officials and workers, public and environmental health officials and interested individuals. Guidelines for incident investigation, reporting and deployment of warnings to the public have been developed. France has developed the SAGIR (*surveiller les maladies de la faune sauvage pour agir*), a surveillance network for zoonotic disease and environmental toxins which includes the *Fédérations des chasseurs* and *l'Office national de la chasse et de la faune sauvage*. Hunters report wildlife mortality events to SAGIR, which then prompts wildlife personnel to investigate the animal death(s) and accompanying environmental conditions. This helps to maximize the early detection of emerging health threats, informs risk assessment and ultimately contributes to the protection of animal and human health [114].

In the United States, the Centers for Disease Control and Prevention (CDC), National Center for Environmental Health had historically provided funding to states to collect reports of cyanobacteria-associated human and animal health, but funding has ended and not all member states are able to continue related activities [81]. Currently, efforts are underway to incorporate reports of animal and human illness associated with harmful algal blooms into the CDC National Outbreak

Reporting System (NORS), a voluntary national system that receives reports of food-borne, waterborne and other outbreaks of human illness [115]. Although the incorporation of human and animal-related illnesses and deaths into NORS will raise general awareness about harmful cyanobacteria among some state health officials, it is currently too early to see if these efforts will be successful in fostering integration and communication among human, animal and environmental health specialists that will lead to a One Health collaborative framework for integrated health protection.

Limitations and Sources of Uncertainty

Cyanobacteria blooms do not always produce toxins, and cyanobacteria and cyanotoxin concentrations are heterogeneous spatially and temporally [116]. Acute animal illnesses and deaths are useful as indicators of human health risks, but harmful cyanobacterial blooms may exist in the absence of dead or impaired animals [117]. Therefore, the absence of animal illness and death at a water body should not be interpreted that no risk, or minimal human health risk exists.

Published reports of cyanobacteria-associated animal death and illness are relatively uncommon. Many events are inaccessible to the public as they remain in the notes and files of wildlife officials, public and environmental health personnel, and veterinarians. Many cases of suspected cyanotoxin poisoning are not confirmed because of the limited availability and cost of cyanotoxin analyses. An expanded review and report of all data sources including those: presented through the broadcast media, published in print, on-line and in newsletters, and stored in medical (human health and veterinary) records, and records of public, environmental health and wildlife officials would likely augment the total number of recognized events where animals have acted as sentinels for cyanobacteria-associated human health risks.

For an animal death to serve as a sentinel event of cyanobacteria-associated risk, people must observe the animal's remains in a timely manner. Carcasses of smaller species will not necessarily persist in the environment. Such deaths, especially if few animals are involved, may often be missed by human observers. Conversely, large numbers of smaller animals that are obvious to the observer, large animals whose carcasses persist in the environment, and human-affiliated animals such as companion animals or livestock are more likely to be observed and recorded.

When dead animals are observed, prompt notification of veterinary, wildlife or health officials is needed to determine a cause for the deaths. However, a prompt post-mortem examination alone is insufficient to conclude that a death is associated with harmful cyanobacteria [118]. Chen *et al.* suggested that analysis of the contents of the gastrointestinal tract may provide a useful indication of the recent composition of cyanobacteria at the collection site [119]. Animals appear to bioaccumulate cyanotoxins at different rates so that tissue concentrations evaluated at the time of death may not reflect current environmental conditions at the collection site [120]. Animals of different species also vary in susceptibility to certain cyanotoxins, but the basis of this variation remains to be well characterized [121].

Cyanobacteria may persist in water bodies and may recur at a given site. However, a previous mass mortality event correctly attributed to cyanobacteria and cyanotoxins, does not mean that a subsequent event at the same site has the same causation. For example, mass bird and fish mortality events in Donaña National Park, Spain in 2001 were confirmed to be associated with microcystins [122], but mass bird deaths at the same site in 2003 were eventually attributed to an infectious etiology, *Pasteurella* spp. [123].

Some freshwater biotoxins have not been included in this review due to insufficient information about human health risks. These include: emerging toxins such as β-methylamino-L-alanine (BMAA), or toxins that are currently only associated with animal toxicity such as the recently reported causative agent of avian vacuolar myelinopathy (AVM) [124,125]. However, these contaminants may potentially play a larger role in future reports of outbreaks of illness that involve both animals and humans.

6. Conclusions

This report illustrates how the recognition of and response to cyanobacteria-associated animal illnesses and deaths may be used to reduce the risks associated with human exposures to harmful cyanobacteria. Using a One Health approach is an efficient way to manage an environmental risk that involves multiple disciplines and professional specialties. Currently, barriers to maximizing the value of animals as sentinels in this context include: under reporting; limited resources for surveillance and investigation of events; and the potential lack of routine means of communication among potential One Health partners in environmental health, environmental management, human and veterinary medicine [111]. To enhance the value of animal sentinel events for harmful cyanobacteria-associated human health risk, we recommend:

- Engaging public health, domestic animal health, wildlife and ecosystem health personnel in group training and communication exercises.
- Developing improved methods to support identification and quantification of harmful cyanobacteria in water sources and analyses of cyanotoxins in cyanobacteria, water, and biological samples from exposed animals and humans.
- Including reports of harmful algal blooms and associated human and animal illness in health and environmental surveillance systems.
- Using successful models such as the Scottish risk assessment reporting guidelines and SAGIR to improve harmful cyanobacteria recognition and response in other nations around the world [113,114].

Such actions, combined with greater global awareness of harmful algal blooms as a multidisciplinary problem should increase the utility of reports of animal illnesses and deaths to inform the characterization of human health risks.

7. Materials and Methods

We searched PubMed and Web of Science databases for the terms: "(cyanobacter* AND animal)"; "(blue-green algae AND animal)"; "(cyanobacter* AND human)"; "(blue-green algae AND human)"; "(cyanobacter* AND health)"; "(blue-green algae AND health)". We restricted these records to: (1) reports of animal exposures to cyanobacteria, cyanotoxins or uncharacterized freshwater blooms and evaluated these to determine if there was a human health or ambient human exposure component also described; (2) among reports of cyanobacteria-associated human illness, we assessed if there was animal death or illness also reported from the site of exposure. When more than one report described a single event, we chose the most comprehensive report(s) of human health exposure and effects. References of all reports were examined to identify other applicable reports to include in the review.

Acknowledgments

We thank librarians and staff members of the US Environmental Protection Agency's library at Research Triangle Park, North Carolina for technical assistance and for access to reference material. We thank Madeleine LaRue and Whitney Krueger, ORISE Participants, funded by the Environmental Protection Agency, for their thoughtful review.

Author Contributions

Elizabeth D. Hilborn and Val R. Beasley conceived of and wrote the paper.

Conflicts of Interest

The authors declare no conflict of interest.

Disclaimer

The views expressed in this report are those of the individual authors and do not necessarily reflect the views and policies of the U.S. Environmental Protection Agency. Mention of trade names or commercial products does not constitute endorsement or recommendation for use.

References

1. Mur, L.R.; Skulberg, O.M.; Utkilen, H. Cyanobacteria in the environment. In *Toxic Cyanobacteria in Water: A Guide to Their Public Health Consequences, Monitoring, and Management*; Chorus, I., Bartram, J., Eds.; E & FN Spon, for World Health Organization, Routledge: London, UK, 1999; pp. 15–40.
2. World Health Organization. *Guidelines for Safe Recreational Water Environments. Volume 1: Coastal and Fresh Waters*; World Health Organization: Geneva, Switzerland, 2003. Available online: http://whqlibdoc.who.int/publications/2003/9241545801.pdf (accessed on 26 March 2015).
3. Paerl, H.W.; Hall, N.S.; Calandrino, E.S. Controlling harmful cyanobacterial blooms in a world experiencing anthropogenic and climatic-induced change. *Sci. Total Environ.* **2011**, *409*, 1739–1745.
4. Davis, T.W.; Berry, D.L.; Boyer, G.L.; Gobler, C.J. The effects of temperature and nutrients on the growth and dynamics of toxic and non-toxic strains of Microcystis during cyanobacteria blooms. *Harmful Algae* **2009**, *8*, 715–725.

5. Paerl, H.W.; Paul, V.J. Climate change: Links to global expansion of harmful cyanobacteria. *Water Res.* **2012**, *46*, 1349–1363.

6. Wiegand, C.; Pflugmacher, S. Ecotoxicological effects of selected cyanobacterial secondary metabolites a short review. *Toxicol. Appl. Pharmacol.* **2005**, *203*, 201–218.

7. Holland, A.; Kinnear, S. Interpreting the possible ecological role(s) of cyanotoxins: Compounds for competitive advantage and/or physiological aide? *Mar. Drugs* **2013**, *11*, 2239–2258.

8. Freitas, E.C.; Printes, L.B.; Rocha, O. Acute effects of *Anabaena spiroides* extract and paraoxon-methyl on freshwater cladocerans from tropical and temperate regions: Links between the ChE activity and survival and its implications for tropical ecotoxicological studies. *Aquat. Toxicol.* **2014**, *146*, 105–114.

9. Graham, J.L.; Loftin, K.A.; Meyer, M.T.; Ziegler, A.C. Cyanotoxin Mixtures and Taste-and-Odor Compounds in Cyanobacterial Blooms from the Midwestern United States. *Environ. Sci. Technol.* **2010**, *44*, 7361–7368.

10. Jüttner, F.; Watson, S.B. Biochemical and ecological control of geosmin and 2-methylisoborneol in source waters. *Appl. Environ. Microbiol.* **2007**, *73*, 4395–4406.

11. Burgos, L.; Lehmann, M.; de Andrade, H.H.R.; de Abreu, B.R.R.; de Souza, A.P.; Juliano, V.B.; Dihl, R.R. *In vivo* and *in vitro* genotoxicity assessment of 2-MIB taste and odor in water. *Ecotoxicol. Environ. Saf.* **2014**, *100*, 282–286.

12. Francis, G. Poisonous Australian lake. *Nature* **1878**, *18*, 11–12.

13. Lawton, L.; Marsalek, B.; Padisák, J.; Chorus, I. Determination of cyanobacteria in the laboratory. In *Toxic Cyanobacteria in Water: A Guide to Their Public Health Consequences, Monitoring, and Management*; Chorus, I., Bartram, J., Eds.; E & FN Spon, for World Health Organization, Routledge: London, UK, 1999; pp. 347–367.

14. Harada, K.-I.; Kondo, F.; Lawton, L. Laboratory analysis of cyanotoxins. In *Toxic Cyanobacteria in Water: A Guide to Their Public Health Consequences, Monitoring, and Management*; Chorus, I., Bartram, J., Eds.; E & FN Spon, for World Health Organization, Routledge: London, UK, 1999; pp. 369–405.

15. Carmichael, W.W. Health Effects of Toxin-Producing Cyanobacteria: "The CyanoHABs". *Hum. Ecol. Risk Assess.* **2001**, *7*, 1393–1407.

16. Codd, G.A.; Lindsay, J.; Young, F.M.; Morrison, L.F.; Metcalf, J.S. Harmful Cyanobacteria: From mass mortalities to management measures. In *Aquatic Ecology Series*; Huisman, J., Matthijs, H.C.P., Visser, P.M., Eds.; Springer: Berlin, Germany, 2005; Volume 3, pp. 1–23.

17. Valério, E.; Chaves, S.; Tenreiro, R. Diversity and impact of prokaryotic toxins on aquatic environments a review. *Toxins* **2010**, *2*, 2359–2410.

18. Sivonen, K.; Jones, G. Cyanobacterial toxins. In *Toxic Cyanobacteria in Water: A Guide to Their Public Health Consequences, Monitoring, and Management*; Chorus, I., Bartram, J., Eds.; E & FN Spon, for World Health Organization, Routledge: London, UK, 1999; pp. 41–111.

19. King, L.J.; Anderson, L.R.; Blackmore, C.G.; Blackwell, M.J.; Lautner, E.A.; Marcus, L.C.; Meyer, T.E.; Monath, T.P.; Nave, J.E.; Ohle, J.; *et al.* Executive summary of the AVMA One Health Initiative Task Force report. *J. Am. Vet. Med. Assoc.* **2008**, *233*, 259–261.

20. Barrett, M.; Osofsky, S. One Health: Interdependence of People, Other Species, and the Planet. In *Jekel's Epidemiology, Biostatistics, Preventive Medicine, and Public Health*, 4th ed.; Katz, D., Elmore, J., Eds.; Saunders: Philadelphia, PA, USA, 2013; pp. 364–377.

21. Zinsstag, J.; Schelling, E.; Waltner-Toews, D.; Tanner, M. From "one medicine" to "one health" and systemic approaches to health and well-being. *Prev. Vet. Med.* **2011**, *101*, 148–156.

22. Harada, M. Minamata Disease: Methylmercury poisoning in Japan caused by environmental pollution. *Crit. Rev. Toxicol.* **1995**, *25*, 1–24.

23. The One Health Initiative. Available online: http://www.onehealthinitiative.com/about.php (accessed on 26 March 2015).

24. Brinkman, H.-J.; de Pee, S.; Sanogo, I.; Subran, L.; Bloem, M.W. High food prices and the global financial crisis have reduced access to nutritious food and worsened nutritional status and health. *J. Nutr.* **2010**, *140*, 153S–161S.

25. Karanikolos, M.; Mladovsky, P.; Cylus, J.; Thomson, S.; Basu, S.; Stuckler, D.; Mackenbach, J.P.; McKee, M. Financial crisis, austerity, and health in Europe. *Lancet* **2013**, *381*, 1323–1331.

26. World Health Organization, Millennium Ecosystem Assessment. *Ecosystems and Human Well-being, Health Synthesis*; World Health Organization: Geneva, Switzerland, 2005. Available online: http://www.who.int/globalchange/ecosystems/ecosys.pdf (accessed on 26 March 2015).

27. Van der Schalie, W.H.; Gardner, H.S., Jr.; Bantle, J.A.; de Rosa, C.T.; Finch, R.A.; Reif, J.S.; Reuter, R.H.; Backer, L.C.; Burger, J.; Folmar, L.C.; *et al.* Animals as sentinels of human health hazards of environmental chemicals. *Environ. Health Perspect.* **1999**, *107*, 309–315.

28. Jochimsen, E.M.; Carmichael, W.W.; An, J.S.; Cardo, D.M.; Cookson, S.T.; Holmes, C.E.M.; Antunes, M.B.D.C.; Filho, D.A.D.M.; Lyra, T.M.; Barreto, V.S.T.; *et al.* Liver failure and death after exposure to microcystins at a hemodialysis center in Brazil. *N. Engl. J. Med.* **1998**, *338*, 873–878.

29. Soares, R.M.; Yuan, M.; Servaites, J.C.; Delgado, A.; Magalhães, V.F.; Hilborn, E.D.; Carmichael, W.W.; Azevedo, S.M.F.O. Sublethal exposure from microcystins to renal insufficiency patients in Rio de Janeiro, Brazil. *Environ. Toxicol.* **2006**, *21*, 95–103.

30. Pouria, S.; de Andrade, A.; Barbosa, J.; Cavalcanti, R.L.; Barreto, V.T.; Ward, C.J.; Preiser, W.; Poon, G.K.; Neild, G.H.; Codd, G.A. Fatal microcystin intoxication in haemodialysis unit in Caruaru, Brazil. *Lancet* **1998**, *352*, 21–26.

31. Hilborn, E.D.; Soares, R.M.; Servaites, J.C.; Delgado, A.G.; Magalhães, V.F.; Carmichael, W.W.; Azevedo, S.M. Sublethal microcystin exposure and biochemical outcomes among hemodialysis patients. *PLoS One* **2013**, *8*, e69518, doi:10.1371/journal.pone.0069518.

32. Turner, P.C.; Gammie, A.J.; Hollinrake, K.; Codd, G.A. Pneumonia associated with contact with cyanobacteria. *Br. Med. J.* **1990**, *300*, 1440–1441

33. Rapala, J.; Robertson, A.; Negri, A.P.; Berg, K.A.; Tuomi, P.; Lyra, C.; Erkomaa, K.; Lahti, K.; Hoppu, K.; Lepistö, L. First report of saxitoxin in Finnish lakes and possible associated effects on human health. *Environ. Toxicol.* **2005**, *20*, 331–340.

34. Stewart, I.; Webb, P.M.; Schluter, P.J.; Shaw, G.R. Recreational and occupational field exposure to freshwater cyanobacteria—A review of anecdotal and case reports, epidemiological studies and the challenges for epidemiologic assessment. *Environ. Health* **2006**, *5*, 1–13.

35. Giannuzzi, L.; Sedan, D.; Echenique, R.; Andrinolo, D. An acute case of intoxication with cyanobacteria and cyanotoxins in recreational water in Salto Grande Dam, Argentina. *Mar. Drugs* **2011**, *9*, 2164–2175.

36. Hilborn, E.D.; Roberts, V.A.; Backer, L.; Deconno, E.; Egan, J.S.; Hyde, J.B.; Nicholas, D.C.; Wiegert, E.J.; Billing, L.M.; Diorio, M.; Centers for Disease Control and Prevention; *et al.* Algal bloom-associated disease outbreaks among users of freshwater lakes—United States, 2009–2010. *Morb. Mortal Wkly. Rep.* **2014**, *63*, 11–15.

37. Heise, H.A. Symptoms of hay fever caused by algae. *J. Allergy* **1949**, *20*, 383–385.

38. Cohen, S.G.; Reif, C.B. Cutaneous sensitization to blue-green algae. *J. Allergy* **1953**, *24*, 452–457.

39. Pilotto, L.S.; Douglas, R.M.; Burch, M.D.; Cameron, S.; Beers, M.; Rouch, G.J.; Robinson, P.; Kirk, M.; Cowie, C.T.; Hardiman, S.; *et al.* Health effects of exposure to cyanobacteria (blue-green algae) during recreational water activities. *Aust. N. Zeal. J. Public Health* **1977**, *21*, 562–566.

40. Billings, W.H. Water-associated human illness in Northeastern Pennsylvania and its suspected association with blue-green algae blooms. In *The Water Environment: Algal Toxins and Health Environmental Science Research*; Carmichael, W., Ed.; Plenum Press: New York, NY, USA, 1981; pp. 243–255.

41. Soong, F.S.; Maynard, E.; Kirke, K.; Luke, C. Illness associated with blue-green algae. *Med. J. Aust.* **1992**, *156*, 67.

42. Walker, S.R.; Lund, J.C.; Schumacher, D.G.; Brakhage, P.A.; McManus, B.C.; Miller, J.D.; Augustine, M.M.; Carney, J.J.; Holland, R.S.; Hoagland, K.D.; *et al.* Nebraska experience. *Adv. Exp. Med. Biol.* **2008**, *619*, 139–152.

43. Lévesque, B.; Gervais, M.C.; Chevalier, P.; Gauvin, D.; Anassour-Laouan-Sidi, E.; Gingras, S.; Fortin, N.; Brisson, G.; Greer, C.; Bird, D. Prospective study of acute health effects in relation to exposure to cyanobacteria. *Sci. Total Environ.* **2014**, *466–467*, 397–403.

44. Falconer, I.R.; Beresford, A.M.; Runnegar, M.T. Evidence of liver damage by toxin from a bloom of the blue-green alga, *Microcystis aeruginosa. Med. J. Aust.* **1983**, *1*, 511–514.

45. Byth, S. Palm Island mystery disease. *Med. J. Aust.* **1980**, *2*, 40–42.

46. Teixera, M.; Costa, M.; Carvalho, V.; Pereira, M.; Hage, E. Gastroenteritis epidemic in the area of the Itaparica Dam, Bahia, Brazil. *Bull. PAHO* **1993**, *27*, 244–253.

47. Hawkins, P.R.; Runnegar, M.T.; Jackson, A.R.; Falconer, I.R. Severe hepatotoxicity caused by the tropical cyanobacterium (blue-green Alga) *Cylindrospermopsis raciborskii* (Woloszynska) seenaya and subba raju isolated from a domestic water supply reservoir. *Appl. Environ. Microbiol.* **1985**, *50*, 1292–1295.

48. El Saadi, O.; Esterman, A.J.; Cameron, S.; Roder, D.M. Murray River water, raised cyanobacterial cell counts, and gastrointestinal and dermatological symptoms. *Med. J. Aust.* **1995**, *162*, 122–125.

49. Tisdale, E.S. Epidemic of intestinal disorders in Charleston, W. Va. occurring simultaneously with unprecedented water supply conditions. *Am. J. Public Health* **1931**, 198–200.

50. Veldee, M.V. Epidemiological study of suspected water-borne gastroenteritis. *Am. J. Public Health* **1931**, *21*, 1227–1235.

51. Lippy, E.C.; Erb, J. Gastrointestinal illness at Sewickley, Pa. *J. Am. Water Work Assoc.* **1976**, *68*, 606–610.

52. Bourke, A.T.C.; Hawes, R.B.; Neilson, A.; Stallman, N.D. An outbreak of hepato-enteritis (the Palm Island mystery disease) possibly caused by algal intoxication. *Toxicon* **1983**, *21* (Suppl. 3), 45–48.

53. Annadotter, H.; Cronberg, G.; Lawton, L.; Hansson, H.; Göthe, U.; Skulberg, O. An extensive outbreak of gastroenteritis associated with the toxic cyanobacterium *Planktothrix agardhii* (Oscillatoriales, Cyanophyceaea) in Scania, South Sweden. In *Cyanotoxins: Occurrence, Causes, Consequences*; Chorus, I., Ed.; Springer: Berlin, Germany, 2001; pp. 200–208.

54. World Health Organization. International Agency for Research on Cancer (IARC). *IARC Monographs on the Evaluation of Carcinogenic Risks to Humans. Volume 94, Ingested Nitrate and Nitrite, and Cyanobacterial Peptide Toxins*; IARC: Lyon, France, 2010; pp. 360–362. Available online: http://monographs.iarc.fr/ENG/Monographs/vol94/mono94.pdf (accessed on 26 March 2015).

55. Zhou, L.; Yu, H.; Chen, K. Relationship between microcystin in drinking water and colorectal cancer. *Biomed. Environ. Sci.* **2002**, *15*, 166–171.

56. Westrick, J.A.; Szlag, D.C.; Southwell, B.J.; Sinclair, J. A review of cyanobacteria and cyanotoxins removal/inactivation in drinking water treatment. *Anal. Bioanal. Chem.* **2010**, *397*, 1705–1714.

57. Carmichael, W.W.; Gorham, P.R. Freshwater cyanophyte toxins: Types and their effects on the use of micro algae biomass. In *Algae Biomass: Production and Use*; Shelef, G., Soeder, C.J., Eds.; Elsevier/North-Holland Biomedical Press: Amsterdam, The Netherlands, 1980; pp. 437–448.

58. Gilroy, D.J.; Kauffman, K.W.; Hall, R.A.; Huang, X.; Chu, F.S. Assessing Potential Health risks from microcystin toxins in blue-green algae dietary supplements. *Environ. Health Perspect.* **2000**, *108*, 435–439.

59. Soares, R.M.; Magalhães, V.F.; Azevedo, S.M.F.O. Accumulation and depuration of microcystins (cyanobacteria hepatotoxins) in *Tilapia rendalli* (Cichlidae) under laboratory conditions. *Aquat. Toxicol.* **2004**, *70*, 1–10.

60. Codd, G.A.; Metcalf, J.S.; Beattie, K.A. Retention of *Microcystis aeruginosa* and microcystin by salad lettuce (*Lactuca sativa*) after spray irrigation with water containing cyanobacteria. *Toxicon* **1999**, *37*, 1181–1185.

61. Chen, J.; Song, L.; Dai, J.; Gan, N.; Liu, Z. Effects of microcystins on the growth and the activity of superoxide dismutase and peroxidase of rape (*Brassica napus* L.) and rice (*Oryza sativa* L.). *Toxicon* **2004**, *43*, 393–400.

62. Genitsaris, S.; Kormas, K.A.; Moustaka-Gouni, M. Airborne algae and cyanobacteria: Occurrence and related health effects. *Front. Biosci.* **2011**, *3*, 772–787.

63. Moestrup, Ø. Toxic blue-green algae (cyanobacteria) in 1833. *Phycologia* **1996**, *35*, 5.

64. Schwimmer, M.; Schwimmer, D. Medical aspects of phycology. In *Algae, Man, and the Environment*, Proceedings of the Algae, Man, and the Environment, Syracuse, NY, USA, 18–30 June 1967; Jackson, D.F., Ed.; Syracuse University Press: Syracuse, NY, USA, 1968.

65. Porter, E.M. Fourth biennial report of board of regents of university of Minnesota, supplementary I. In *Investigation of Supposed Poisonous Vegetation in the Waters of Some of the Lakes of Minnesota*; Department of Agriculture: Minneapolis, MN, United States, 1886; Volume 9, pp. 5–96.

66. Steyn, D.G. Poisoning of animals and human beings by algae. *S. Afr. J. Sci.* **1945**, *41*, 243–244.

67. Gunn, G.J.; Rafferty, A.G.; Rafferty, G.C.; Cockburn, N.; Edwards, C.; Beattie, K.A.; Codd, G.A. Fatal canine neurotoxicosis attributed to blue-green algae (cyanobacteria). *Vet. Rec.* **1992**, *130*, 301–302.

68. Matsunaga, H.; Harad, K.I.; Senma, M.; Ito, Y.; Yasuda, N.; Ushida, S.; Kimura, Y. Possible cause of unnatural mass death of wild birds in a pond in Nishinomiya, Japan: Sudden appearance of toxic cyanobacteria. *Nat. Toxins* **1999**, *7*, 81–86.

69. Chellappa, N.T.; Costa, M.A.M.; Marinho, I.D.R. Harmful cyanobacterial blooms from semiarid freshwater ecosystems of Northeast Brazil. Australia. *Aust. Soc. Limnol.* **2000**, *38*, 45–49.

70. Stewart, I.; Seawright, A.A.; Shaw, G.R. Cyanobacterial poisoning in livestock, wild mammals and birds—An overview. *Adv. Exp. Med. Biol.* **2008**, *619*, 613–637.

71. Gillam, W.G. The effect on livestock of water contaminated with freshwater algae. *J. Am. Vet. Med. Assoc.* **1925**, 780–784.

72. May, V.; McBarron, E.J. Occurrence of the blue-green alga, *Ansbaena circinuiis* Rabenh., in New South Wales and toxicity to mice and honey bees. *J. Aust. Inst. Agric. Sci.* **1973**, *39*, 264–266.

73. Zimba, P.V.; Khoo, L.; Carmichael, W.W.; Gaunt, P. Confirmation of catfish mortalities resulting from microcystin produced during *Microcystis* blooms. *J. Phycol.* **2000**, *36*, 72–73.

74. Jewel, M.A.S.; Affan, M.A.; Khan, S. Fish mortality due to a cyanobacterial bloom in an aquaculture pond in Bangladesh. *Pak. J. Biol. Sci.* **2003**, *6*, 1046–1050.

75. Singh, S.; Asthana, R.K. Assessment of microcystin concentration in carp and catfish: A case study from Lakshmikund Pond, Varanasi, India. *Bull. Environ. Contam. Toxicol.* **2014**, *92*, 687–692.

76. Galey, F.D.; Beasley, V.R.; Carmichael, W.W.; Kleppe, G.; Hooser, S.B.; Haschek, W.M. Blue-green algae (*Microcystis aeruginosa*) hepatotoxicosis in dairy cows. *Am. J. Vet. Res.* **1987**, *48*, 1415–1420.

77. McLeod, J.A.; Bondar, G.F. A case of suspected algal poisoning in Manitoba. *Can. J. Public Health* **1952**, *43*, 347–350.

78. Codd, G.A.; Bell, S.G. Eutrophication and toxic cyanobacteria in freshwaters. *Water Pollut. Control* **1985**, *84*, 225–232.

79. Beasley, V.R.; Cook, W.O.; Dahlem, A.M.; Lovell, R.A.; Valentine, W.M. Algae intoxications in livestock and waterfowl. *Vet. Clin. N. Am. Food Anim. Pract.* **1989**, *5*, 345–361.

80. Codd, G.A.; Edwards, C.; Beattie, K.A.; Barr, W.M.; Gunn, G.J. Fatal attraction to cyanobacteria? *Nature* **1992**, *359*, 110–111.

81. Backer, L.C.; Landsberg, J.H.; Miller, M.; Keel, K.; Taylor, T.K. Canine cyanotoxin poisonings in the United States (1920s–2012): Review of suspected and confirmed cases from three data sources. *Toxins* **2013**, *5*, 1597–1628.

82. Corkill, N.; Smith, R.; Seckington, M.; Pontefract, R. Poisoning at Rutland Water. *Vet. Rec.* **1989**, *125*, 356.

83. Hamill, K.D. Toxicity in benthic freshwater cyanobacteria (blue-green algae): First observations in New Zealand. *N. Zeal. J. Mar. Freshw. Res.* **2001**, *35*, 1057–1059.

84. Olsen, T.A. Toxic plankton. In Proceedings of the Inservice Training Course in Water Works Problems, the University of Michigan, School of Public Health, Ann Arbor, MI, USA, 15–16 February 1951; The University of Michigan: Ann Arbor, MI, USA, 1951; pp. 86–95.

85. Rose, E.T. Toxic algae in Iowa lakes. *Proc. Iowa Acad. Sci.* **1953**, *60*, 738–745.

86. Eriksson, J.; Meriluoto, J.; Lindholm, T. Can cyanobacterial peptide toxins accumulate in aquatic food chains? In *Perspectives in Microbial Ecology*, Proceedings of the Fourth International Symposium on Microbial Ecology, Ljubljana, Slovenia, 24–29 August 1986; Megusar, F., Gantar, M., Eds.; Slovene Society for Microbiology: Ljubljana, Slovenia, 1986; pp. 655–658.

87. Skulberg, O.M.; Codd, G.A.; Carmichael, W.W. Toxic blue-green algal blooms in Europe: A growing problem. *Ambio* **1984**, *13*, 244–247.

88. Mancini, M.; Rodriguez, C.; Bagnis, G.; Liendo, A.; Prosperi, C.; Bonansea, M.; Tundisi, J.G. Cianobacterial bloom and animal mass mortality in a reservoir from Central Argentina. *Braz. J. Biol.* **2010**, *70*, 841–845.

89. Bossenmaier, E.F.; Olson, T.A.; Rueger, M.E.; Marshall, W.H. Some field and laboratory aspects of duck sickness at Whitewater Lake, Manitoba. *Trans. N. Am. Wildl. Conf.* **1954**, *19*, 163. Available online: http://www.speciation.net/Database/Journals/Transactions-of-the-North-American-Wildlife-and-Natural-Resources-Conference-;i3358 (accessed on 16 April 2015).

90. Keymer, I.F.; Smith, G.R.; Roberts, T.A.; Heaney, S.I.; Hibberd, D.J. Botulism as a factor in waterfowl mortality at St. James's Park. *Vet. Rec.* **1972**, *90*, 111–114.

91. Murphy, T.; Lawson, A.; Nalewajko, C.; Murkin, H.; Ross, L.; Oguma, K.; McIntyre, T. Algal toxins—Initiators of avian botulism? *Environ. Toxicol.* **1999**, *15*, 558–567.

92. Codd, G.A.; Steffensen, D.A.; Burch, M.D.; Baker, P.D. Toxic blooms of cyanobacteria in Lake Alexandrina: Learning from history. *Aust. J. Mar. Freshw. Res.* **1994**, *45*, 731–736.

93. Dillenberg, H.O.; Dehnel, M.K. Toxic waterbloom in Saskatchewan, 1959. *Can. Med. Assoc. J.* **1960**, *83*, 1151–1154.

94. Senior, V.E. Algal poisoning in Saskatchewan. *Can. J. Comp. Med.* **1960**, *24*, 26–31.

95. Juday, R.E.; Keller, E.J.; Horpestad, A.; Bahls, L.L.; Glasser, S. A toxic bloom of *Anabaena Flos-Aquae* in Hebgen Reservoir Montana in 1977. In *The Water Environment: Algal Toxins and Health*; Carmichael, W.W., Ed.; Plenum Press: New York, NY, USA, 1981; pp. 103–112.

96. Spoerke, D.G.; Rumack, B.H. Blue-green algae poisoning. *J. Emerg. Med.* **1985**, *2*, 353–355.

97. Pybus, M.J.; Hobson, D.P.; Onderka, D.K. Mass mortality of bats due to probable blue-green algal toxicity. *J. Wildl. Dis.* **1986**, *22*, 449–450.

98. Vasconcelos, V.M. Toxic cyanobacteria (blue-green algae) in Portuguese fresh waters. *Arch. Hydrobiol.* **1994**, *130*, 439–451.

99. Codd, G.A.; Beattie, K.A. Cyanobacteria (blue-green algae) and their toxins: Awareness and action in the United Kingdom. *PHLS Microbiol. Dig.* **1991**, *8*, 82–86.

100. Harding, W.R.; Rowe, N.; Wessels, J.C.; Beattie, K.A.; Codd, G.A. Suspected toxicosis of a dog attributed to the cyanobacterial (blue-green algal) hepatotoxin nodularin in South Africa. *J. S. Afr. Vet. Assoc.* **1995**, *66*, 256–259.

101. Van Halderen, A.; Harding, W.R.; Wessels, J.C.; Schneider, D.J.; Heine, E.W.P.; van der Merwe, J.; Fourie, J.M. Cyanobacterial (blue-green algae) poisoning of livestock in the Western Cape Province of South Africa. *J. S. Afr. Vet. Assoc.* **1995**, *66*, 260–264.

102. Pollux, B.J.A.; Pollux, P.M.J. Vis- En Vogelsterfte Door Blauwalgen in de Romeinenweerd. *Natuurhistorisch Maandblad* **2004**, *93*, 207–210.

103. Devlin, J.P.; Edwards, O.E.; Gorham, P.R.; Hunter, N.R.; Pike, R.K.; Stavric, B. Anatoxin-a, a toxic alkaloid from *Anabaena flos-aquae* NRC 44-l. *Can. J. Chem.* **1977**, *55*, 1367–1371.

104. Mahmood, N.A.; Carmichael, W.W.; Pfahler, D. Anticholinesterase poisonings in dogs from a cyanobacterial (blue-green algae) bloom dominated by *Anabaena flosaquae. Am. J. Vet. Res.* **1988**, *49*, 500–503.

105. Matsunaga, H.; Moore, R.E.; Niemczura, W.P.; Carmichael, W.W. Anatoxin-a(s), a potent anthicholinesterase from *Anabaena flos-aquae. J. Am. Chem. Soc.* **1989**, *111*, 8021–8023.

106. James, K.J.; Sherlock, I.R.; Stack, M.A. Anatoxin-a in Irish freshwater and cyanobacteria, using a new fluorimetric liquid chromatographic method. *Toxicon* **1997**, *35*, 963–971.

107. Edwards, C.; Beattie, K.A.; Scrimgeour, C.M.; Codd, G.A. Identification of anatoxin-A in benthic cyanobacteria (blue-green algae) and in associated dog poisonings at Loch Insh, Scotland. *Toxicon* **1992**, *10*, 1165–1175.

108. Gugger, M.; Lenoir, S.; Berger, C.; Ledreux, A.; Druart, J.C.; Humbert, J.F.; Guette, C.; Bernard, C. First report in a river in France of the benthic cyanobacterium *Phormidium favosum* producing anatoxin-a associated with dog neurotoxicosis. *Toxicon* **2005**, *45*, 919–928.

109. Mez, K.; Beattie, K.A.; Codd, G.A.; Hanselmann, K.; Hauser, B.; Naegeli, H.; Preisig, H.R. Identification of a microcystin in benthic cyanobacteria linked to cattle deaths on alpine pastures in Switzerland. *Eur. J. Phycol.* **1997**, *32*, 111–117.

110. Auf Der Heide, E. Inter-agency Communications. In *Disaster Response: Principles for Preparation and Coordination*, Chapter 5. 1989. Available online: ftp://mediccom.org/DISASTER/DR.pdf (accessed on 26 March 2015).

111. Kahn, L.H.; Kaplan, B.; Steele, J.H. Confronting zoonoses through closer collaboration between medicine and veterinary medicine (as "one medicine"). *Vet. Ital.* **2007**, *43*, 5–19.

112. Beasley, V. "'One Toxicology,' 'Ecosystem Health,' and 'One Health.'" *Vet. Ital.* **2009**, *45*, 97–110.

113. Scottish Government Health and Social Care Directorates, Blue-green algae working group. Cyanobacteria (Blue-Green Algae) in Inland and Inshore Waters: Assessment and Minimisation of Risks to Public Health. 2012. Available online: http://www.scotland.gov. uk/resource/0039/00391470.pdf (accessed on 26 March 2015).

114. SAGIR, surveiller les maladies de la faune sauvage pour agir. Available online: http://www.oncfs.gouv.fr/Reseau-SAGIR-ru105 (accessed on 26 March 2015).

115. Roberts, V. Building Health Surveillance Capacity for illnesses and Outbreaks Associated with Harmful Algal Blooms. Available online: http://www2.epa.gov/sites/production/files/2014-12/documents/habs-roberts-12-10-14.pdf (accessed on 26 March 2015).

116. Carmichael, W.W.; Gorham, P.R. The mosaic nature of toxic blooms of cyanobacteria. In *The Water Environment, Algal Toxins and Health. Environmental Science Research*; Carmichael, W.W., Ed.; Plenum Press: New York, NY, USA, 1981; pp. 161–172.

117. Namikoshi, M.; Rinehart, K.L.; Sakai, R.; Stotts, R.R.; Dahlem, A.M.; Beasley, V.R.; Carmichael, W.W.; Evans, W.R. Identification of 12 hepatotoxins from a Homer Lake bloom of the cyanobacteria *Microcystis aeruginosa*, *Microcystis viridis*, and *Microcystis wesenbergii*: Nine new microcystins. *J. Org. Chem.* **1992**, *57*, 866–872.

118. Beasley, V.R.; Dahlem, A.M.; Cook, W.O.; Valentine, W.M.; Lovell, R.A.; Hooser, S.B.; Harada, K.; Suzuki, M.; Carmichael, W.W. Diagnostic and clinically important aspects of cyanobacterial (blue-green algae) toxicoses. *J. Vet. Diagn. Investig.* **1989**, *1*, 359–365.

119. Chen, J.; Zhang, D.W.; Xie, P.; Wang, Q.; Ma, Z.M. Simultaneous determination of microcystin contaminations in various vertebrates (fish, turtle, duck and water bird) from a large eutrophic Chinese lake, Lake Taihu, with toxic Microcystis blooms. *Sci. Total Environ.* **2009**, *407*, 3317–3322.

120. Chen, J.; Xie, P.; Zhang, D.W.; Ke, Z.X.; Yang, H. *In situ* studies on the bioaccumulation of microcystins in the phytoplanktivorous silver carp (*Hypophthalmichthys molitrix*) stocked in Lake Taihu with dense toxic Microcystis blooms. *Aquaculture* **2006**, *261*, 1026–1038.

121. Cook, W.O.; Beasley, V.R.; Dahlem, A.M.; Lovell, R.A.; Hooser, S.B.; Mahmood, N.B.; Carmichael, W.W. Consistent inhibition of peripheral cholinesterases by neurotoxins from the freshwater cyanobacterium *Anabaena flos-aquae*: Studies of ducks, swine, mice, and a steer. *Environ. Toxicol. Chem.* **1989**, *8*, 915–922.

122. Alonso-Andicoberry, C.; Garcia-Villada, L.; Lopez-Rodas, V.; Costas, E. Catastrophic mortality of flamingos in a Spanish national park caused by cyanobacteria. *Vet. Rec.* **2002**, *151*, 706–707.

123. Mateos-Sanz, M.A.; Carrera, D.; López-Rodas, V.; Costas, E. Toxic cyanobacteria and wildlife conservation. *Acta Bot. Malacit.* **2009**, *34*, 5–10.

124. Wilde, S.B.; Murphy, T.M.; Hope, C.P.; Habrun, S.K.; Kempton, J.; Birrenkott, A.; Wiley, F.; Bowerman, W.W.; Lewitus, A.J. Avian vacuolar myelinopathy linked to exotic aquatic plants and a novel cyanobacterial species. *Environ. Toxicol.* **2005**, *20*, 348–353.

125. Holtcamp, W. The Emerging Science of BMAA: Do Cyanobacteria Contribute to Neurodegenerative Disease? *Environ. Health Perspect.* **2012**, *120*, a110–a116.

Chapter 3:
Guideline Development

Health-Based Cyanotoxin Guideline Values Allow for Cyanotoxin-Based Monitoring and Efficient Public Health Response to Cyanobacterial Blooms

David Farrer, Marina Counter, Rebecca Hillwig and Curtis Cude

Abstract: Human health risks from cyanobacterial blooms are primarily related to cyanotoxins that some cyanobacteria produce. Not all species of cyanobacteria can produce toxins. Those that do often do not produce toxins at levels harmful to human health. Monitoring programs that use identification of cyanobacteria genus and species and enumeration of cyanobacterial cells as a surrogate for cyanotoxin presence can overestimate risk and lead to unnecessary health advisories. In the absence of federal criteria for cyanotoxins in recreational water, the Oregon Health Authority (OHA) developed guideline values for the four most common cyanotoxins in Oregon's fresh waters (anatoxin-a, cylindrospermopsin, microcystins, and saxitoxins). OHA developed three guideline values for each of the cyanotoxins found in Oregon. Each of the guideline values is for a specific use of cyanobacteria-affected water: drinking water, human recreational exposure and dog recreational exposure. Having cyanotoxin guidelines allows OHA to promote toxin-based monitoring (TBM) programs, which reduce the number of health advisories and focus advisories on times and places where actual, rather than potential, risks to health exist. TBM allows OHA to more efficiently protect public health while reducing burdens on local economies that depend on water recreation-related tourism.

Reprinted from *Toxins.* Cite as: Farrer, D.; Counter, M.; Hillwig, R.; Cude, C. Health-Based Cyanotoxin Guideline Values Allow for Cyanotoxin-Based Monitoring and Efficient Public Health Response to Cyanobacterial Blooms. *Toxins* **2015**, *7*, 457-477.

1. Introduction

In August of 2009, a series of dog deaths occurred along the South Umpqua River in Douglas County, Oregon. One of those deaths was confirmed to be the result of exposure to a toxin produced by certain genera of photosynthetic cyanobacteria, also called blue-green algae. The deceased dog's stomach contents contained 10 µg/L anatoxin-a. In August of 2010, another dog death was confirmed to be caused by exposure to anatoxin-a. This dog, a healthy six month old black Labrador retriever, was vomiting, staggering, and convulsing within 10 min of drinking and playing in water from an isolated pool along the banks of the same stretch of the South Umpqua River and was dead within an hour. The treating veterinarian reported that her hands were "burning" after handling the dog's body.

A subset of cyanobacterial genera includes member species that are capable of producing toxins, known as cyanotoxins. Cyanotoxin production is not universal or constant even among those species and strains that carry the necessary genes. The conditions that induce cyanotoxin production in capable species have not been elucidated [1]. Under certain environmental conditions that have not been conclusively defined, cyanobacteria can proliferate to form blooms consisting of significant biomass and covering large areas in fresh or marine water [1]. When blooms are dominated by potentially toxigenic genera of cyanobacteria, they are referred to as harmful algae blooms (HABs).

By 2009, HABs composed of genera capable of producing at least four cyanotoxins (anatoxin-a, cylindrospermopsin, microcystins, and saxitoxins) had been identified in fresh bodies of water in Oregon. The anatoxin and saxitoxin families of cyanotoxins are primarily neurotoxic and are structurally described as alkaloids [1]. Anatoxin-a has a molecular weight of 165 daltons and exerts neurotoxicity by binding the neuronal pre-synaptic acetylcholine receptor with higher affinity than either nicotine or acetylcholine [1]. This binding leads to potent and prolonged nerve depolarization, which prevents further impulse transmission and at sufficient doses produces paralysis, asphyxiation, and death [1]. Saxitoxins make up a large family of alkaloids that are all larger than anatoxin-a and are the causative agents in human paralytic shellfish poisoning [1]. Saxitoxins block sodium ion channels in the axonal membranes of nerve cells [1]. This blockage prevents nerve impulse generation and propagation and at sufficient doses can cause paralysis, asphyxiation, and death [1]. Microcystins are a family of structurally related cyclic peptides. All microcystins consist of seven amino acids [1], but there are at least 80 structural variants, or congeners [2]. Microcystins induce cytotoxicity by inhibiting phosphatase activity [1]. Microcystins are primarily hepatotoxic because the cell membrane transporters required for cells to take up microcystins are most abundant in the liver [1]. Cylindrospermopsin is a cyclic guanidine alkaloid with a molecular weight of 415 daltons [1]. In its pure form, cylindrospermopsin primarily targets the liver, but crude extracts from cyanobacteria that produce cylindrospermopsin also affect the kidney, spleen, thymus, and heart [1]. The mechanism of toxicity appears to be inhibition of protein synthesis [1].

At the time of this manuscript's submission, no U.S. federal standards or criteria have been published for any cyanotoxins. The World Health Organization (WHO) has established a suggested drinking water guideline value of 1 µg/L and a recreational exposure guideline value of 10 µg/L for a single variant of microcystin called microcystin-LR [1]. Health Canada has also published a drinking water standard of 1.5 µg/L for microcystin-LR [3].

The Oregon Health Authority (OHA) Public Health Division needed guidelines for meaningful, health-based evaluation of measured cyanotoxin data for all cyanotoxins that occur in Oregon. Drawing from peer-reviewed literature, standard risk assessment methodologies, and efforts of other states and nations, OHA developed provisional guideline values for anatoxin-a, cylindrospermopsin, microcystins and saxitoxins for drinking and recreational water use for humans and recreational water use for dogs. These guidelines allowed for implementation of toxin-based monitoring (TBM) by partner agencies and a more refined public health response.

2. Methods

2.1. Development of Guideline Values

2.1.1. Guideline Derivation and Exposure Assumptions for Humans

OHA independently reviewed toxicity studies in the literature and government reviews of those studies to identify no observable adverse effect levels (NOAELs), lowest observable adverse effect levels (LOAELs) or benchmark doses (BMDs) that could be used as a point of departure (POD) for calculation of a tolerable daily intake (TDI). TDIs were calculated from PODs by applying uncertainty factors (UF) (see Equation (1)).

$$TDI = \frac{POD}{UF} \tag{1}$$

UFs provide a margin of safety in the presence of scientific uncertainties about the applicability of the underlying toxicity studies to the general human population. The most common types of uncertainty that require UFs are interspecies variability, individual variability, and limitations in the toxicological database. Interspecies UFs account for the fact that animals used in toxicity studies may differ from humans in the ways they absorb, distribute, metabolize, or excrete toxins. They may also differ from humans in their ability to repair damage caused by toxins. Individual variability UFs account for the fact that humans could have considerable individual variability in their sensitivity to cyanotoxins. For example, a child may be more sensitive than an adult, or people with particular genetic traits may be more sensitive than the general population. UFs for database limitation indicate a paucity of relevant toxicity studies or toxicological endpoints evaluated in those studies, reflecting the possibility that additional studies or endpoints could identify a lower dose with adverse effect than current studies have characterized.

Once TDIs were established, OHA applied exposure factors to calculate guideline values applicable for drinking water and recreational use in humans and for recreational use in dogs. The exposure factors OHA considered were body weight (BW), oral intake rate (IR) and relative source contribution (RSC), as shown in Equation (2). Government agencies commonly apply RSC when developing drinking water guideline values to account for other sources of a given contaminant, other than drinking water, in an individual's overall exposure.

$$\text{Guideline Value} = \frac{TDI \times BW \times RSC}{IR} \tag{2}$$

Table 1 describes the exposure factors that OHA used to develop drinking water and recreational guideline values for humans. As described above, TDIs are specific to individual cyanotoxins. OHA elected to use the WHO's default BW of 60 kg for drinking water [1] as opposed to the EPA's 70 kg [4] to be more protective of public health. For recreational water use, OHA chose a BW of 20 kg to represent children 4 to 6 years old based on data from the EPA [4]. OHA considered that 4 to 6 year olds would be the youngest age group likely to be swimming up to 2 h per day. OHA selected an RSC of 1, assuming 100% of an individual's cyanotoxin intake would be through water swallowed either as drinking water or incidentally through recreational water use. For drinking water, OHA used EPA's and WHO's default assumption of 2 liters per day for an adult IR [1,4]. For recreational use, OHA used a default IR of 0.05 liters per hour of swimming from the U.S. Agency for Toxic Substances and Disease Registry's (ATSDR) public health assessment guidance manual [5]. OHA further assumed that a child might swim for up to 2 hours per day in affected water, thus, 0.05 liters per hour equals 0.1 liters per day.

Table 1. Exposure factors to calculate human drinking and recreational water guidelines.

Exposure factor name	Drinking water	Recreational water	Units
Tolerable daily intake (TDI)	Cyanotoxin dependent	Cyanotoxin dependent	Micrograms cyanotoxin per kilogram body weight per day (μg/kg-day)
Body weight (BW)	60	20	Kilograms (kg)
Relative source contribution (RSC)	1	1	Unitless
Intake rate	2	0.1	Liters per day (L/day)

2.1.2. Guideline Derivation and Exposure Assumptions for Dogs

OHA calculated dog-specific guideline values using the same TDIs (with the exception of saxitoxins) as for humans but dog-specific exposure factors developed by California's Office of Environmental Health Hazard Assessment (CALOEHHA) [6]. Because BW is so variable among different breeds of dogs, there is no single assumption that could be used with any certainty. CALOEHHA developed a BW-normalized water intake rate of 0.255 L of water per kilogram body weight per day (L/kg-day) for exercising dogs [6]. Therefore, OHA used a BW-normalized water IR (BWIR) of 0.255 L/kg-day in Equation 3 to calculate dog-specific guideline values.

$$\text{Guideline Value} = \frac{\text{TDI}}{\text{BWIR}} \qquad (3)$$

2.2. Derivation of Tolerable Daily Intakes

2.2.1. Anatoxin-a

OHA reviewed available literature on the toxicology of anatoxin-a [1,7–17] as well as accepted and proposed threshold values used in other governmental jurisdictions [18–22]. OHA selected a study conducted by Fawell et al. [13,14] as the critical study for derivation of a TDI. In this study, groups of 10 male and 10 female mice were orally treated with anatoxin-a every day for 28 days at 4 doses (0, 100, 500 and 2500 μg/kg-day). The mice were observed for survival, clinical signs of toxicity or illness, and changes in body weight and food consumption throughout the course of the study. Eye function was evaluated at the beginning and end of the study, and hematology and serum biochemistry were evaluated in the last week of the study. Upon necropsy, Fawell et al. [13,14] examined all mice for gross lesions and examined all tissues from all mice histologically. Mice that died prior to the end of the study were also necropsied for gross lesions, and histological evaluations were performed.

Three animals died during the study. One death, not related to treatment, resulted from animals fighting in their cages. There were two additional deaths, one at 500 μg/kg-day and one at 2500 μg/kg-day. The authors of the study and EPA reviewers indicated that the death at 500 μg/kg-day was not likely associated with treatment [13,14,20]. However, absent any other explanation for the death, OHA decided to assume that the death at 500 μg/kg-day was treatment related and used this as the LOAEL. None of the surviving animals had any observable adverse health effects by the evaluation methods employed, and there were no deaths at the 100 µg/kg-day dose. OHA therefore selected 100 µg/kg-day as the NOAEL and POD for TDI calculation.

OHA applied a total UF of 1000 resulting in a TDI of 0.1 µg/kg-day using the formula shown in Equation 1. This UF is a composite of three types of uncertainty associated with this POD. First, an uncertainty factor of 10 was applied to account for interspecies differences in toxicity between mice and humans. Another UF of 10 was applied to account for individual variability within the human population. Finally, OHA applied an additional UF of 10 due to limitations in the database.

2.2.2. Cylindrospermopsin

OHA selected the EPA's proposed subchronic oral reference dose (RfD) of 0.03 µg/kg-day [23] as the TDI for cylindrospermopsin. EPA's proposed RfD is based on an 11-week study in mice by Humpage, et al. [24] in which groups of male Swiss albino mice were dosed with 0, 30, 60, 120, or 240 µg/kg-day (10 mice per dose group) of purified cylindrospermopsin by daily gavage. Authors monitored food and water consumption and body weights throughout the study. Nine weeks into the study, authors conducted clinical exams with a focus on physiological and behavioral signs of toxicity. An extensive panel of parameters was measured in serum and urine near the end of the study along with hematological endpoints. Upon necropsy, organs were weighed and all tissues were examined histologically. No deaths were reported in the study. The most sensitive endpoint observed was kidney weight, which increased in a dose-dependent manner starting at 60 µg/kg-day [24]. The EPA selected 60 µg/kg-day from this study as the LOAEL and 30 µg/kg-day as the NOAEL [23].

EPA used a linear fit benchmark dose model to calculate a benchmark dose level of 33.1 µg/kg-day using the kidney weight data from all but the highest dose group in the critical study [23]. EPA used 33.1 µg/kg-day as their POD [23]. EPA then applied a total UF of 1000 resulting in an RfD of 0.03 µg/kg-day (with rounding) while noting that application of the same uncertainty factor to the NOAEL of 30 µg/kg-day would have yielded the same RfD [23]. The total UF of 1000 was a composite of an UF of 10 for interspecies variability, 10 for individual variability, and 10 for database limitations [23].

2.2.3. Microcystins

Microcystins are cyclic heptapeptides with approximately 80 known structural variants [2]. These variations have significant influence on the toxicity and physio-chemical properties of the toxin. Microcystin-LR is the only variant for which there is sufficient toxicity data to develop a TDI.

OHA selected a study by Heinze et al. [25] as the critical toxicity study for derivation of a TDI for microcystin-LR. In this study, researchers treated rats with purified microcystin-LR in drinking water for 28 days and then measured body weights and weights of the liver, kidney, adrenal glands, thymus and spleen. Heinze et al. [25] also assessed hematology, measured an extensive list of parameters in serum, and examined all tissues microscopically for histopathology [25]. The Heinze study identified a LOAEL of 50 µg/kg-day for intrahepatic hemorrhage.

OHA used the LOAEL identified in the Heinze study [25] described above (50 µg/kg-day) as the POD to calculate a TDI of 0.05 µg/kg-day by applying a total UF of 1000 (10 for LOAEL to

NOAEL adjustment, 10 for interspecies variability and 10 for individual variability) as described by Equation (1).

2.2.4. Saxitoxins

The saxitoxin family of toxins includes saxitoxin (STX), neosaxitoxin (neoSTX), gonyautoxins, (GTX), C-toxins (C), 11-hydroxy-STX and decarbamoylsaxitoxins (dcSTXs) [17]. Because individual STXs vary in their toxicity, the European Food Safety Authority (EFSA) has developed toxic equivalency factors (TEFs), based on toxicity, in mice, so individual toxin concentrations can be considered relative to the toxicity of STX [26]. The proposed TEFs are: STX = 1, neoSTX = 1, GTX1 = 1, GTX2 = 0.4, GTX3 = 0.6, GTX4 = 0.7, GTX5 = 0.1, GTX6 = 0.1, C2 = 0.1, C4 = 0.1, dc-STX = 1, dc-neoSTX = 0.4, dc-GTX2 = 0.2, GTX3 = 0.4 and 11-hydroxy-STX = 0.3 [26]. OHA adopted these TEFs to develop a TDI for STX-equivalents (STX-eq).

OHA selected a study by the EFSA [26] as the critical study for derivation of a TDI. EFSA established an acute RfD for STX-eq of 0.5 µg STX-eq/kg-day [26]. This acute RfD is based on available intoxication reports in humans across the European population. This acute RfD represents an estimated NOAEL. OHA applied a total UF of 10 for database limitations, since this is the only study of its kind for saxitoxin. For humans, no UF for interspecies variability was needed since the data were from human illnesses. OHA also did not apply an UF for individual variability since the EFSA study covered the general population, which included sensitive individuals. Using the acute RfD (0.5 µg/kg-day) as the POD and applying a total UF of 10 as shown in Equation (1), OHA calculated a human TDI of 0.05 µg/kg-day.

For dogs, OHA applied an additional UF of 10 for interspecies variability since dogs may be more sensitive to saxitoxins than humans. Therefore, using Equation 1 and a total UF of 100 for dogs, OHA calculated a dog-specific TDI of 0.005 µg/kg-day.

2.3. Review of Guideline Values Developed by Other Jurisdictions

For each of the four cyanotoxins, OHA reviewed guideline values developed by other states and nations and the methods used to derive those guidelines. According to the EPA, twenty states, including Oregon, have some kind of program or protocol to respond to HABs [18]. Of these twenty, fifteen include recreational guideline values for cyanotoxins as part of their response protocol [18]. Only three states, including Oregon, have guideline values for cyanotoxins in drinking water [18] and only California and Oregon have guideline values for dogs. The detailed results of this review are presented for each cyanotoxin in the Discussion section.

3. Results

3.1. Guideline Values

Using the exposure assumptions shown in Table 1 and Equations (2) and (3), OHA calculated provisional drinking water and recreational water guideline values for humans and recreational guideline values for dogs for anatoxin-a, cylindrospermopsin, microcystins (microcystin-LR), and saxitoxins (SXT-eq) as summarized in Table 2.

Table 2. Summary of Oregon's tolerable daily intakes and guideline values for four cyanotoxins for use in acute or short-term exposures.

Guideline value	Anatoxin-a	Cylindrospermopsin	Microcystin	Saxitoxin
Human TDI (µg/kg-day)	0.1	0.03	0.05	0.05
Dog TDI (µg/kg-day)	None—used human TDI	None—used human TDI	None—used human TDI	0.005
Drinking Water (µg/L)	3.0	1.0	1.0	1.0
Recreational Water (µg/L)	20.0	6.0	10.0	10.0
Dog-specific (µg/L)	0.4	0.1	0.2	0.02

For drinking water, recreational water, and dog-specific guideline values, OHA rounded calculated results either to the nearest whole number or, if less than or equal to 0.5, to the nearest non-zero, post-decimal digit. Calculated drinking water values for microcystin and saxitoxin were both 1.5 µg/L, and OHA rounded down to 1.0 µg/L for public health protection. OHA used rounding to make the guideline values easier for partners to use and to avoid implying a degree of precision that does not exist.

3.2. Toxin-Based Monitoring Results in Oregon

Health-based guideline values for cyanotoxins allow OHA's recreational HABs advisory program to make use of toxin-based monitoring (TBM) data. The alternatives to TBM in Oregon and in other states involve comparing cyanobacterial cell counts against WHO threshold values or even presence/absence of visible surface scum. Many species of cyanobacteria do not produce toxins, and even those strains that can produce toxins often do not. To be protective of health in the absence of toxin data, public health agencies must assume that potentially toxigenic species over a threshold cell count must be producing toxins at dangerous concentrations. This means that health advisories based on cell count or visible scum alone may often be unnecessary.

Starting in 2012, OHA began encouraging partner agencies to adopt TBM approaches to water bodies that they manage throughout the state. OHA continued to issue health advisories based on cell counts or toxin data, depending on which method the partner agency selected. OHA asked partner agencies using a TBM approach to identify the dominant species in the bloom. This allowed partner agencies to focus testing on those toxins relevant to the species present. Partners sampled every other week throughout the life of the visible bloom. If toxins never exceeded recreational guideline values, OHA did not issue advisories, even if cell counts were over the threshold. If a toxin result exceeded a guideline value, OHA issued an advisory based on the toxin result and partner agencies stopped testing until all visible signs of the bloom were gone. At that point, partners collected confirmatory samples to verify that toxin levels and cell counts were below guideline values, and OHA lifted the advisories.

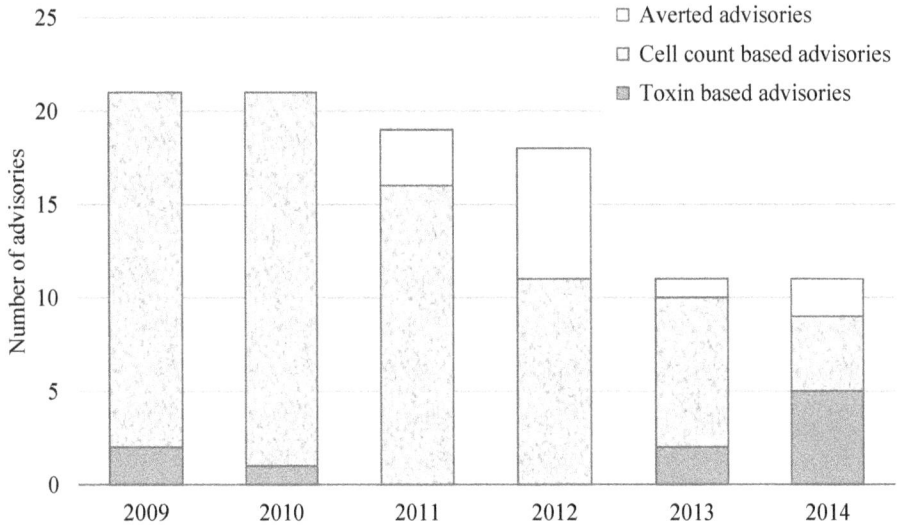

Figure 1. Number of advisories based on cell counts and toxin levels and number of potential advisories with cell counts above threshold that were averted by toxin tests with results below recreational guideline values. Recreational advisory thresholds are 100,000 cells/mL for all toxigenic genera except *Microcystis* and *Planktothrix*, for which the combined threshold is 40,000 cells/mL. Recreational guideline values for cyanotoxins are shown in Table 2.

Prior to the 2012 bloom season, most partner agencies only tested for cell counts and OHA issued advisories when cell counts were above the advisory threshold (100,000 cells/mL for any combination of potentially toxigenic genera or 40,000 cells/mL for any combination of *Microcystis* or *Planktothrix*) [1]. Figure 1 shows Oregon's recreational advisories from 2009 to 2014 by year and basis for advisory (*i.e.*, cell counts *vs.* toxin results). Figure 1 also shows blooms that would have resulted in advisories based on cell count data had TBM not been employed showing toxins below guideline values.

In total, OHA issued 88 recreational HABs advisories from 2009 to 2014. Of those, 78 were based on cell counts and 10 on toxin results. A total of 13 advisories were averted in the same time period where cell counts would have resulted in advisories had toxin results not been below recreational guideline values. Averted advisories shown in Figure 1 include only those HABs where cell counts were above advisory thresholds.

In many cases, monitoring partner agencies noted visible HABs, identified the dominant genera present and went directly to toxin analysis without counting cells. In these cases, toxin levels were frequently below recreational guideline values. By these criteria, additional advisories likely averted by TBM were 12 in 2012, 14 in 2013, and 13 in 2014, though OHA cannot verify that these would have been advisories without cell counts. TBM did not appear to significantly change the mean time under advisory (8.0 weeks for cell count based advisories and 7.8 weeks for toxin based advisories).

TBM also provided a clearer understanding of which cyanobacteria genera and toxins posed the greatest risk in Oregon. Figure 2 shows the number of times, from 2009 to 2014, toxigenic genera of cyanobacteria were counted above recreational advisory thresholds. *Dolichospermum* (formerly *Anabaena*) was the genus most frequently found over threshold, followed by *Microcystis* and more distantly by *Aphanizomenon* and *Gloeotrichia*. Cell counts were found above threshold 117 times during 88 advisories from 2009 to 2014. During 28 of those 88 advisories there were multiple genera counted over the threshold. In 18 out those 28 advisories, two genera were over the threshold. In six advisories, three genera were over the threshold, and in one advisory, four genera were over the threshold.

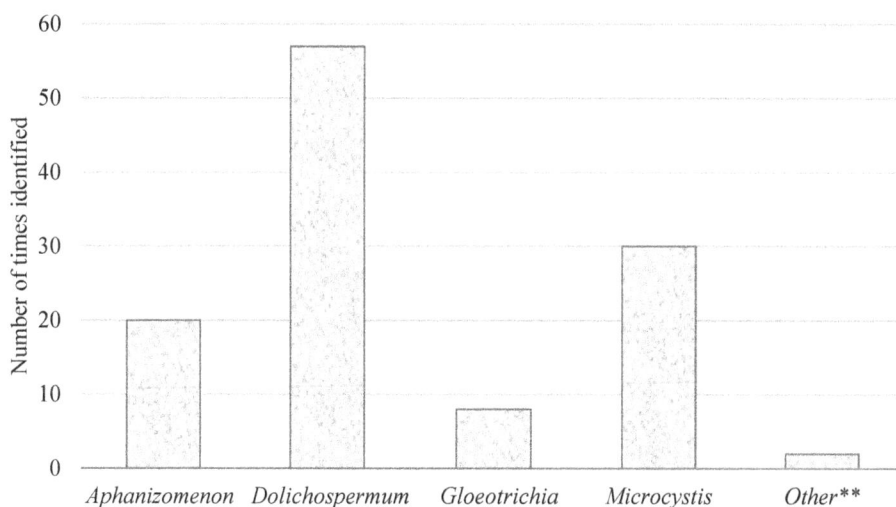

Figure 2. Number of times toxigenic genera of cyanobacteria were identified above cell count thresholds during advisories in monitored waterbodies, 2009–2014. Recreational advisory thresholds are 100,000 cells/mL for all toxigenic genera except *Microcystis* and *Planktothrix*, for which the combined threshold is 40,000 cells/mL. ** Other: *Phormidium* = 1, *Oscillatoria* = 1.

Figure 3 shows the number of times cyanotoxins were detected over the recreational guideline values from 2009 to 2014. Microcystins are the cyanotoxins that most frequently exceed recreational guideline values in Oregon. Microcystins are also the most frequently detected cyanotoxins in Oregon, although all four cyanotoxins have been detected—saxitoxins being the rarest.

In one case, two cyanotoxins (cylindrospermopsin and microcystin) were both measured above their recreational guideline values. In five cases, advisories were issued based on cell count data with toxin data coming in above the recreational guideline value after the advisory had already been established.

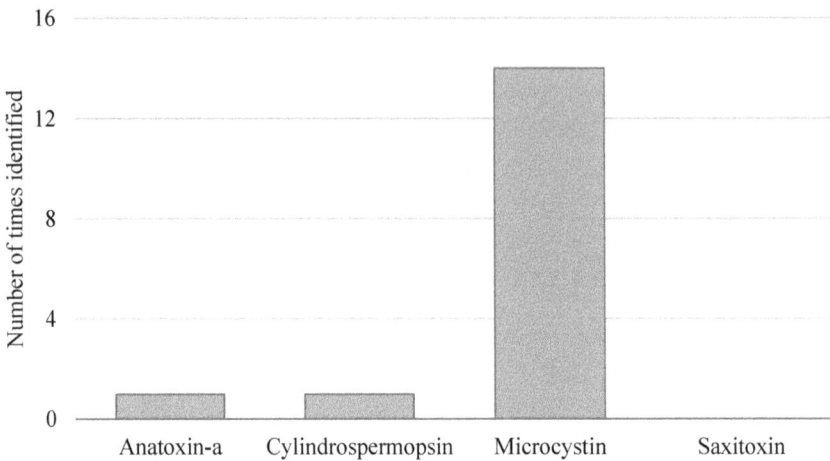

Figure 3. Number of times cyanotoxins were identified over human recreational guidelines during advisories in monitored waterbodies, 2009–2014. Guideline values are shown in Table 2.

In those five cases, multiple genera were counted above their advisory threshold and follow-up cyanotoxin levels were very high. For example, in one case total microcystins were measured at 705 µg/L at the same time *Microcystis*, *Dolichospermum*, and *Aphanizomenon* species were all present over their advisory cell count thresholds.

In another case, total microcystins were measured at 310 µg/L when *Dolichospermum*, *Microcystis*, *Aphanizomenon*, and *Oscillatoria* were all counted above their advisory cell count thresholds. These data suggest that the presence of multiple toxigenic genera over threshold increases the likelihood of cyanotoxins over recreational guideline values and potentially far exceeding those values.

4. Discussion

4.1. Intended Application of Guideline Values

Oregon's cyanotoxin guideline values (summarized in Table 2) are intended to be applied to acute or short-term exposures. All of the studies from which Oregon derived TDIs pertain to exposures that are subchronic, short-term or acute. The lack of chronic toxicity data prevented OHA from developing chronic guideline values, and OHA continues to survey the literature and the work of regulatory agencies for useable chronic values. Low-dose, chronic exposure to cyanotoxins can have significant adverse health effects [1,27,28], and the absence of chronic guideline values should not imply that chronic exposure to cyanotoxins does not occur in Oregon. Many HABs in Oregon last for several weeks or months, posing the risk of prolonged or multiple intermittent exposures to a single HAB. Oregonians may frequent multiple bodies of water creating the potential for individuals to encounter multiple HABs over the course of a season and over many years. OHA does not have the resources or depth of Oregon-specific cyanotoxin concentrations over the course of a bloom or season to support a reliable or meaningful assessment of the risk to Oregonians from potential chronic exposure to cyanotoxins. Future research in this area would be extremely valuable if resources were made available.

OHA uses guideline values developed for specific structural variants of families of cyanotoxins to apply to the entire family. For example, OHA uses the guideline values developed based on microcystin-LR studies for all microcystins, and the guideline values developed for SXT-eq to apply to total saxitoxins. Many of OHA's partner agencies test for microcystin and saxitoxin using enzyme linked immunosorbent assays (ELISA), which cross-react with multiple variants within the families. Therefore, it is important for OHA to be able to use guideline values in the context of total microcystins or total saxitoxins as measured by ELISA. A limited number of studies comparing the *in vivo* toxicity of three of the more commonly detected variants (microcystins-LR, RR, YR) indicate that microcystin-LR is the most toxic of those three [28,29]. *In vitro* studies indicate that microcystins-LF and LW might be more toxic *in vitro*, perhaps because these variants are more lipophilic and enter cells more readily in an *in vitro* setting [30]. This hypothesis has not been tested *in vivo*. Overall, these studies suggest that application of the microcystin-LR-based guideline values to total microcystins is health protective. EFSA's TEF analysis [26] suggests that OHA's guideline values for saxitoxins (SXT-eq) provide a health protective approach.

Dog-specific guideline values are not used as a basis for issuing recreational HAB advisories. These values are used to communicate the significance of cyanotoxin exposures with veterinarians and pet owners to help reduce dog illnesses and death. OHA has outreach and educational materials targeted at pet owners that are available to the public and posted at monitored water bodies in Oregon.

Drinking water guideline values are not used as a basis for issuing recreational HAB advisories. These values are used by drinking water staff to determine if a cyanotoxin problem exists in raw or finished water samples taken from public drinking water facilities where a bloom has been identified in source water. These samples are taken weekly throughout the life of the bloom. Although raw water samples have tested as high as 5.24 µg/L for microcystin-LW, Oregon has not had finished drinking water samples with cyanotoxin levels above drinking water guideline values. The highest detection of any cyanotoxin in finished drinking water was 0.3 µg/L anatoxin-a.

4.2. Uncertainties and Limitations Surrounding Exposure Assumptions for Calculation of Guideline Values

When calculating cyanotoxin guideline values for Oregon, OHA selected default assumptions for inputs such as body weight and water consumption from standard government agency sources. While Oregon's guideline values are designed to be representative of the general population, it would of course be more accurate to use population-specific measurements for such inputs. Unfortunately, OHA did not have resources to develop Oregon-specific inputs for derivation of guideline values.

OHA exercised professional judgment in selecting the ages of four to six years as the youngest likely to swim for hours at a time. Of course, other ages could have been selected and different guidelines calculated for those alternate selections, but OHA considers the assumptions selected to be realistic and protective of public health.

Studies have shown that cyanotoxins, microcystins in particular, can be found in fish tissue [1,31], though at lower levels in the fillet than in lipophilic tissues. Cyanotoxins may also be found in crops irrigated with affected water [32]. Contaminated fish or crops could serve as an additional source of cyanotoxin exposure to people who consume them. This possibility could mean that an RSC other than 1 should be selected when calculating drinking water guideline values. However, exposure to cyanotoxins via food sources would be expected to constitute a more chronic exposure, and OHA's guideline values are focused on short-term, acute exposures.

4.3. Limitations and Uncertainties in Selection of Critical Toxicity Studies for TDI Derivation

4.3.1. Anatoxin-a

Very few applicable studies have been conducted with the intent to identify dose-response relationships to anatoxin-a administered orally. Therefore, OHA applied an UF for database limitations in the TDI derivation to account for possible future studies that may reveal that anatoxin-a has different toxicity than has been suggested in currently available literature.

OHA identified only two primary studies that employed oral administration of anatoxin-a: the Fawell, *et al.*, study, selected as the critical study [13,14] and an older study conducted by Astrachan, *et al.* [7,8]. Independent reviews [10,11] of the Astrachan study have derived a TDI of 0.51 µg/kg-day, a value within a factor of 5 to the TDI selected (0.1 µg/kg-day). CALOEHHA has proposed a subchronic oral reference dose (RfD) of 2.5 µg/kg-day [6], consistent with EPA's proposed RfD [20] that did not consider the death in the 500 µg/kg-day dose group to be treatment related in the critical study [13,14]. Other toxicity studies [16] have been conducted using non-oral routes of exposure (mainly intraperitoneal injection). Because human exposure to anatoxin-a in Oregon is expected to be primarily through ingestion, either in drinking water or accidental ingestion of surface water while recreating, OHA considered only those studies using oral routes of exposure.

4.3.2. Cylindrospermopsin

The EPA's 2006 toxicological review of cylindrospermopsin included a comprehensive summary of toxicological studies collected up to that time [23]. Since then a few relevant studies and reviews have been published [27,33]. However, OHA relied heavily on the EPA's 2006 review, because it is robust and comprehensive and because newer studies have not identified lower subchronic NOAELs than those described in EPA's 2006 review.

One study [27] by Sukenik, *et al.*, evaluated chronic (42-weeks) exposure in mice via drinking water and identified a LOAEL of 20 µg/kg-day based on increased hematocrit and deformed erythrocytes. This study did not include as many endpoints as the Humpage *et al.*, study [24] and exposed the same experimental groups of animals to gradually increasing doses of cylindrospermopsin, rather than treating separate groups of animals with consistent doses throughout the experiment. This dosing regimen poses difficulties in interpretation for either chronic or short-term exposure effects for the purposes of TDI development. Lower doses early in the experiment could have created tolerance in the experimental group, which could have made them resistant to higher doses later. For these reasons, OHA could not justify the use of this study in support of either a chronic TDI or chronic guideline values.

4.3.3. Microcystins

Two different critical studies have been used by different entities to develop TDIs or RfDs for microcystin-LR. The WHO used a study conducted by Fawell, *et al.* [34]. In this study, mice were dosed by oral gavage for 13 weeks. The study identified a NOAEL of 40 µg/kg-day. WHO divided this NOAEL by a total UF of 1000 to develop a TDI of 0.04 µg/kg-day. The total UF is 10 to account for interspecies variability, 10 for individual variability and 10 for limitations in the database, particularly surrounding cancer and chronic disease and reproductive health endpoints.

The second critical study was conducted and published by R. Heinze [25], which OHA used as the basis for its TDI. CALOEHHA also chose the Heinze study because "...it evaluated more endpoints, utilized a better experimental design, showed greater target organ specificity (intrahepatic hemorrhage) in the histopathological analysis, and showed a clear dose-response trend" when compared with other toxicity studies [6].

CALOEHHA applied benchmark dose (BMD) techniques to determine a BMD of 6.4 µg/kg-day [6]. They then applied an UF of 1000 to establish an acute RfD of 0.006 µg/kg-day. The total UF consisted of 10 for interspecies variability, 10 for individual variability, and 10 for limitations in the database, particularly surrounding cancer and reproductive health endpoints.

The rats of the Heinze study were also more sensitive to microcystin-LR than the mice of the Fawell study, and general toxicological practice is to use the most sensitive endpoint and species as the basis for selecting a critical study.

OHA agreed with CALOEHHA's selection of the critical study and the selection of the 50 µg/kg-day LOAEL as the basis for development of an acute TDI. However, guidance for using BMD techniques [35] recommends against using it in cases where there are fewer than three dose groups (not counting controls) and the Heinze study only had two dose groups. Instead of BMD, OHA applied an UF of 10 to achieve an estimated NOAEL of 5 µg/kg-day as is consistent with EPA guidance [36]. It is worth noting that the difference between using BMD and the UF to adjust down from the LOAEL is only 1.4 µg/kg-day and the UF is slightly more protective.

The TDI developed by WHO (0.04 µg/kg-day), based on the Fawell study [34] is very similar to the provisional acute value (0.05 µg/kg-day) proposed here. CALOEHHA's selection [6] of the Heinze study [25] also supports OHA's decision to use the same study. A chronic (18 month) mouse toxicity study of microcystin-LR in drinking water identified a NOAEL of 3 µg/kg-day [37]. This number is very similar to the estimated 5 µg/kg-day NOAEL OHA used to develop the state's provisional TDI based on the Heinze study.

4.3.4. Saxitoxins

OHA was unable to find any additional relevant studies for use in TDI development for saxitoxins. Therefore, the application of the UF for database limitations is especially important in this case.

4.4. Comparison with Guideline Values Developed by Other Nations and States

4.4.1. Anatoxin-a

The New Zealand Ministry of Health has a drinking water guideline (6 µg/L) [21] for anatoxin-a. Duy, *et al.* [11] proposed a drinking water guideline value of 2.72 µg/L for infants, 4.08 µg/L for children and 12.24 µg/L for adults. Oregon's value falls near the most protective end of this range. Codd, *et al.* [10], in an independent review of the literature, proposed supporting the 12.24 µg/L value put forward by Duy, *et al.* for adults. Ohio has a drinking water guideline of 20 µg/L [22].

CALOEHHA has also proposed a recreational water guideline value for swimmers derived using a higher TDI (2.5 µg/kg-day). However, the result (90 µg/L) [6] is similar, within a factor of 4.5 to the recreational water guideline value developed for Oregon (20 µg/L). Washington State Department of Health adopted 1 µg/L as their guidance value for recreational water [19]. Ohio has a recreational guideline value of 80 µg/L with a no contact advisory at 300 µg/L [18]. Vermont has a guideline value of 10 µg/L for anatoxin-a [18].

4.4.2. Cylindrospermopsin

New Zealand's Ministry of Health has drinking water guidelines for cylindrospermopsin equal to OHA's provisional guideline of 1 µg/L [21]. Ohio also has a drinking water guideline value of 1 µg/L [22].

OHA's provisional recreational water guideline value is similar to those proposed by other governmental bodies. CALOEHHA proposed a guideline value of 4 µg/L [6]. The Department of Health for Washington State has proposed a recreational guideline value of 4.5 µg/L [19]. Ohio has a recreational guideline value of 5 µg/L with a no-contact advisory level of 20 µg/L [18]. These values are similar to the provisional recreational water guideline value developed for Oregon (6 µg/L).

4.4.3. Microcystins

OHA's provisional drinking water guideline for microcystin-LR (1 µg/L) is identical to the drinking water guideline established by the WHO [1] and the actual calculated value of 1.5 µg/L is identical to the value finalized by Health Canada [3]. Ohio also has a drinking water guideline of 1 µg/L [22] and Minnesota has a drinking water guideline of 0.04 µg/L [18].

OHA's recreational water guideline value (10 µg/L) is the same as the upper limit of "mild and/or low probability of adverse health effects" suggested by the WHO [1]. Illinois also has a recreational guideline value of 10 µg/L [18], slightly higher than the Washington State guideline of 6 µg/L [18], which is also shared by Vermont and Virginia [18]. OHA's value is 12.5 times greater than California's recreational value of 0.8 µg/L [6]. Indiana and Kansas have tiered systems that use 4 µg/L as a threshold for recreational activities and 20 µg/L as a threshold for any water contact [18]. Ohio also has a tiered system using 6 and 20 µg/L as the guideline values [18]. Iowa, Nebraska, Oklahoma, and Texas use a 20 µg/L value [18]. Massachusetts and Rhode Island use 14 µg/L as a recreational guideline value for microcystin [18].

4.4.4. Saxitoxins

New Zealand has a recommended drinking water guideline value for STX of 3 µg/L [21]. Ohio has a drinking water guideline value of 0.2 µg/L [22]. The Ohio drinking water guideline is also based on the EFSA acute RfD, to which they applied an additional UF of 10 for individual variability. OHA did not consider this UF necessary because the study included sensitive individuals in the general population. No other states have drinking water guideline values for saxitoxin.

Washington also used EFSA's acute RfD as the basis for their recreational water guidance value of 75 µg STX-eq/L [19]. Oregon's value is different from Washington's because OHA chose to use 20 kg as the assumed body weight of a child while Washington used 15 kg. In addition, Washington did not apply the UF for database limitations to the EFSA acute RfD. Ohio uses a tiered system of 0.8 µg/L for recreational contact and 3 µg/L to avoid all contact [18].

4.5. Additional Cyanotoxins

The four cyanotoxins for which OHA has developed guideline values are a small fraction of the cyanotoxins and other metabolic products of cyanobacteria. When a person swallows water while swimming in HAB-affected surface water, they likely ingest entire cyanobacterial organisms including everything they produce and contain. When this happens, additional components of the cyanobacterial cells may increase toxicity as compared to exposure to the purified toxin alone [23,33]. How additional cyanobacterial components may increase the toxicity of known cyanotoxins has not been adequately characterized in the literature. Therefore, OHA was not able to quantitatively adjust guideline values to account for these potential increases in toxicity.

OHA focused efforts on the cyanotoxins most frequently detected in Oregon. However, there is always the risk that additional toxins could be present for which no water body managers in Oregon are currently monitoring. For example, nodularin is another hepatotoxic cyanotoxin produced by cyanobacteria of the *Nodularia* genus [1]. Nodularin has never been monitored for in Oregon, so its frequency cannot currently be determined. However, *Nodularia* organisms have never been reported above their cell-count threshold in Oregon, so this would indicate that nodularin is not currently posing significant risk to public health in the state.

All cyanobacteria produce lipopolysaccharides (LPS) as a structural component of their cell wall [1]. For allergic or sensitive individuals, dermal exposure to LPS can cause skin rashes. However, such rashes only affect a small segment of the public, are self-limiting (*i.e.*, do not require medical attention) and lack a dose-response relationship [38]. Without a dose-response relationship it is impossible to identify a threshold at which an LPS-based advisory should be issued. For this reason OHA does not base health advisories on the risk of LPS exposure alone.

Another common metabolic product of cyanobacteria is α-amino-β-methylaminoproprionic acid (BMAA). Most cyanobacteria produce this compound, which has been implicated in increased risk of neurodegenerative diseases such as amyotrophic lateral sclerosis and Parkinson's disease in human epidemiological studies [39,40]. Increasing evidence indicates that BMAA can cause these illnesses following chronic exposure, by mimicking the amino acid L-serine, causing misfolded proteins in brain cells [41]. Clear dose-response relationships have not yet been established. In the absence of definitive data on dose-response relationships, OHA is unable to create guideline values for BMAA, and as a result may be underestimating the public health risk from cyanobacterial blooms in Oregon.

For all of the reasons above, monitoring programs that exclusively focus on cyanotoxins could underestimate risk to public health. However, the overall weight of evidence suggests that most of the risk for illness and disease associated with cyanobacteria can be averted by avoiding contact with the dominant cyanotoxins that have been identified.

4.6. Benefits of Toxin Based Monitoring

Toxin based monitoring benefits Oregonians in multiple ways. Expenditure of public health resources can be focused on those blooms with greatest risk to the population. Toxin data allow OHA to communicate with the public about actual risks, as opposed to the potential risk represented by cell count data alone. Toxin data give greater credibility to health advisories when they are issued and decrease the likelihood that an advisory would be issued unnecessarily.

Our results indicate that TBM decreases the likelihood that an advisory will be issued. This allows Oregonians to enjoy more outdoor recreation, increasing physical activity and strengthening social networks without the frustration of cancelling plans or losing deposits related to unexpected HABs advisories. Decreased advisories also reduce the risk of "advisory fatigue" wherein people stop heeding advisories because they are so frequent that they do not notice them anymore.

Although OHA does not close lakes when recreational advisories are in effect, reports from partner agencies that manage these waterbodies indicate that many fewer Oregonians visit during advisories. This anecdotal evidence is supported by national studies from various waterbody types around the country that suggest significant economic burdens on tourism industries when HABs-related health advisories are in effect [42–45]. If accurate, this decrease in visitors is an economic hardship on businesses that depend on the water tourism industry. Therefore, using TBM approaches may also reduce the economic burden of HABs by focusing advisories on those water bodies that need them and avoiding them where they are not needed.

5. Conclusions

Cyanotoxins have the potential to harm public health and they are present in Oregon's fresh waters. Health-based guideline values for cyanotoxins are necessary to evaluate risks posed from cyanobacterial blooms. To address this need, Oregon established guideline values for anatoxin-a, cylindrospermopsin, microcystins, and saxitoxins. Guideline values include acute tolerable daily intakes (TDI), human drinking and recreational water and dog-specific guideline values.

Application of guideline values allowed for meaningful TBM of HABs-affected waterbodies in Oregon. TBM reduced the number of advisories, which benefited public health and the local tourism-based economy.

Acknowledgments

Much of the work represented in this paper was funded by the Centers for Disease Control and Prevention (CDC) through a five year cooperative agreement for a Harmful Algae Bloom Surveillance Program (Enhanced Surveillance of Public Health Risks from Harmful Algae Blooms in Oregon, 5U38EH000336). Additional work was funded by OHA's Drinking Water Services section. OHA also thanks those individuals who served on an informal and voluntary science advisory committee for review and approval of OHA's cyanotoxin guideline values. These individuals were David Stone (Oregon State University, Corvallis, OR, USA); Wayne Carmichael (Wright State University, Dayton, OH, USA); Al Johnson (U.S. Forest Service, Westfir, OR, USA); Jacob Kann (Aquatic Ecosystem Sciences, LLC, Ashland, OR, USA); Theo Dreher (Oregon State University); and Kurt Carpenter (U.S. Geological Survey, Portland, OR, USA). OHA also acknowledges contributions by Casey Lyon with the Oregon Drinking Water Services section, who provided information about cyanotoxins measured in raw and finished drinking water samples.

Author Contributions

David Farrer developed the cyanotoxin guideline values, organized and staffed the voluntary and informal science advisory committee for HABs, developed toxin-based monitoring guidance for partners, and drafted the majority of the paper. Rebecca Hillwig and Marina Counter provided statistics and Figures 1–3 related to recreational HABs advisories in Oregon. Curtis Cude was the program manager on the CDC Harmful Algae Bloom Surveillance cooperative agreement grant that funded much of the work and the Principal Investigator of the Oregon Environmental Public Health Tracking program which continues to support collection and reporting of HABs data and contributed substantive scientific and editorial direction on the paper.

Abbreviations

ATSDR—Agency for Toxic Substances and Disease Registry
BMAA—α-amino-β-methylaminoproprionic acid
BMD—Benchmark Dose
BW—Body weight
BWIR—Body weight normalized intake rate
C—C-toxins
CALOEHHA—California EPA's Office of Environmental Health Hazard Assessment
dcSTXs—11-hydroxy-STX and decarbamoylsaxitoxins
EFSA—European Food Safety Authority
ELISA—enzyme linked immunosorbent assay
EPA—U.S. Environmental Protection Agency
GTX—Gonyautoxins
HAB—Harmful algae bloom
IR—Intake rate
LOAEL—Lowest observable adverse effect level

LPS—Lipopolysaccharide
neoSTX—Neosaxitoxin
NOAEL—No observable adverse effect level
OHA—Oregon Health Authority
POD—Point of departure
RfD—Oral reference dose
RSC—Relative source contribution
STX—Saxitoxin
STX-eq—Saxitoxin equivalent
TBM—Toxin based monitoring
TEF—Toxic equivalency factor
TDI—Tolerable daily intake
UF—Uncertainty factor
WHO—World Health Organization

Conflicts of Interest

The authors declare no conflict of interest.

References

1. Chorus, I.; Bartram, J. *Toxic Cyanobacteria in Water: A Guide to Their Public Health Consequences, Monitoring, and Management*; World Health Organization: London, UK, 1999.
2. Meriluoto, J.A.O.; Spoof, L.E.M. Cyanotoxins: Sampling, sample processing and toxin uptake. *Adv. Exp. Med. Biol.* **2008**, *619*, 483–499.
3. ARCHIVED: Cyanobacterial Toxins-Microcystin-LR [Technical document-Chemical/Physical Parameters]. Available online: http://www.hc-sc.gc.ca/ewh-semt/pubs/water-eau/cyanobacterial_toxins/index-eng.php (accessed on 11 November 2014).
4. United States Environmental Protection Agency. *Exposure Factors Handbook*; National Center for Environment Assessment Office of Research and Development: Washington, DC, USA, 2011; Document EPA/600/R-090/052F.
5. Agency for Toxic Substances and Disease Registry. *Public Health Assessment Guidance Manual*; US Department of Health and Human Services: Atlanta, GA, USA, 2005.
6. California Environmental Protection Agency (CalEPA). *Toxicological Summary and Suggested Action Levels to Reduce Potential Adverse Health Effects of Six Cyanotoxins*; CalEPA: Sacramento, CA, USA, 2012.
7. Astrachan, N.B.; Archer, B.G. Simplified monitoring of anatoxin-a by reverse-phase high performance liquid chromatography and the sub-acute effects of anatoxin-a in rats. In *The Water Environment: Algal Toxins and Health*; Carmichael, W.W., Ed.; Plenum Press: New York, NY, USA, 1981; pp. 437–446.
8. Astrachan, N.B.; Archer, B.G.; Hilbelink, D.R. Evaluation of the subacute toxicity and teratogenicity of anatoxin-a. *Toxicon. Off. J. Int. Soc. Toxinol.* **1980**, *18*, 684–688.

9. Burch, M.D. Effective doses, guidelines & regulations. *Adv. Exp. Med. Biol.* **2008**, *619*, 831–853.

10. Codd, G.A.; Morrison, L.F.; Metcalf, J.S. Cyanobacterial toxins: Risk management for health protection. *Toxicol. Appl. Pharmacol.* **2005**, *203*, 264–272.

11. Duy, T.N.; Lam, P.K.; Shaw, G.R.; Connell, D.W. Toxicology and risk assessment of freshwater cyanobacterial (blue-green algal) toxins in water. *Rev. Environ. Contam. Toxicol.* **2000**, *163*, 113–185.

12. Falconer, I.R.; Humpage, A.R. Health risk assessment of cyanobacterial (blue-green algal) toxins in drinking water. *Int. J. Environ. Res. Public Health* **2005**, *2*, 43–50.

13. Fawell, J.F.; James, H.A. *Toxins from Blue-Green Algae: Toxicological Assessment of Anatoxin-a and a Method for Its Determination in Reservoir Water*; Foundation for Water Research: Marlow, UK, 1994.

14. Fawell, J.K.; Mitchell, R.E.; Hill, R.E.; Everett, D.J. The toxicity of cyanobacterial toxins in the mouse: II anatoxin-a. *Hum. Exp. Toxicol.* **1999**, *18*, 168–173.

15. Pegram, R.A.; Nichols, T.; Etheridge, S.; Humpage, A.; LeBlanc, S.; Love, A.; Neilan, B.; Pflugmacher, S.; Runnegar, M.; Thacker, R. Cyanotoxins Workgroup report. *Adv. Exp. Med. Biol.* **2008**, *619*, 317–381.

16. Rogers, E.H.; Hunter, E.S.; Moser, V.C.; Phillips, P.M.; Herkovits, J.; Munoz, L.L.; Hall, L.; Chernoff, N. Potential developmental toxicity of anatoxin-a, a cyanobacterial toxin. *J. Appl. Toxicol.* **2005**, *25*, 527–534.

17. Van Apeldoorn, M.E.; van Egmond, H.P.; Speijers, G.J.A.; Bakker, G.J.I. Toxins of cyanobacteria. *Mol. Nutr. Food Res.* **2007**, *51*, 7–60.

18. United States Environmental Protection Agency. Policies and Guidelines. Available online: http://www2.epa.gov/nutrient-policy-data/policies-and-guidelines (accessed on 13 November 2014).

19. Washington Department of Health. *Washington State Recreational Guidance for Cylindrospermopsin (Provisional) and Saxitoxin (Provisional)*; Washington Department of Health: Olympia, WA, USA, 2011.

20. United States Environmental Protection Agency. *Toxicological Reviews of Cyanobacterial Toxins: Anatoxin-a (External Review Draft)*; US Environmental Protection Agency: Washington, DC, USA, 2006; Document NCEA-C-1743.

21. New Zealand Ministry of Health. *Drinking-Water Standards for New Zealand 2005 (Revised 2008)*; Ministry of Health: Wellington, New Zealand, 2008.

22. Ohio Environmental Protection Agency. *Public Water System Harmful Algal Bloom Response Strategy*; Ohio EPA: Columbus, OH, USA, 2014.

23. United States Environmental Protection Agency. *Toxicological Reviews of Cyanobacterial Toxins: Cylindrospermopsin*; US Environmental Protection Agency: Washington, DC, USA, 2006; Document NCEA-C-1763.

24. Humpage, A.R.; Falconer, I.R. Oral toxicity of the cyanobacterial toxin cylindrospermopsin in male swiss albino mice: Determination of no observable adverse effect level for deriving a drinking water guideline value. *Environ. Toxicol.* **2003**, *18*, 94–103.

152

25. Heinze, R. Toxicity of the cyanobacterial toxin microcystin-LR to rats after 28 days intake with the drinking water. *Environ. Toxicol.* **1999**, *14*, 57–60.

26. European Food Safety Authority. Scientific Opinion: Marine biotoxins in shellfish-Saxitoxin group. *EFSA J.* **2009**, *1019*, 1–76.

27. Sukenik, A.; Reisner, M.; Carmeli, S.; Werman, M. Oral toxicity of the cyanobacterial toxin cylindrospermopsin in mice: Long-term exposure to low doses. *Envirion. Toxicol.* **2006**, *21*, 575–582.

28. United States Environmental Protection Agency. *Toxicological Reviews of Cyanobacterial Toxins: Microcystins LR, RR, YR and LA*; US Environmental Protection Agency: Washington, DC, USA, 2006; Document NCEA-C-1765.

29. Gupta, N.; Pant, S.C.; Vijayaraghavan, R.; Lakshmana Rao, P.V. Comparative toxicity evaluation of cyanobacterial cyclic peptide toxin microcystin variants (LR, RR, YR) in Mice. *Toxicology* **2003**, *188*, 285–296.

30. Vesterkvist, P.S.M.; Misiorek, J.O.; Spoof, L.E.M.; Toivola, D.M.; Meriluoto, J.A.O. Comparative Cellular Toxicity of Hydrophilic and Hydrophobic Microcystins on Caco-2 Cells. *Toxins* **2012**, *4*, 1008–1023.

31. Berry, J.P.; Lee, E.; Walton, K.; Wilson, A.E.; Bernal-Brooks, F. Bioaccumulation of microcystins by fish associated with a persistent cyanobacterial bloom in Lago De Patzcuaro (Michoacan, Mexico). *Environ. Toxicol. Chem.* **2011**, *30*, 1621–1628.

32. Saqrane, S.; Oudra, B. CyanoHAB occurrence and water irrigation cyanotoxin contamination: ecological impacts and potential health risks. *Toxins* **2009**, *1*, 113–122.

33. De la Cruz, A.A.; Hiskia, A.; Kaloudis, T.; Chernoff, N.; Hill, D.; Antoniou, M.G.; He, X.; Loftin, K.; O'Shea, K.; Zhao, C.; *et al.* A review on cylindrospermopsin: The global occurrence, detection, toxicity, and degradation of a potent cyanotoxin. *Environ. Sci. Process. Impacts* **2013**, *13*, 49–58.

34. Fawell, J.K.; Mitchell, R.E.; Everett, D.J.; Hill, R.E. The toxicity of cyanobacterial toxins in the mouse: I microcystin-LR. *Hum. Exp. Toxicol.* **1999**, *18*, 162–167.

35. United States Environmental Protection Agency. *Benchmark Dose Technical Guidance*; US Environmental Protection Agency: Washington, DC, USA, 2012; Document EPA/100/R-12/001.

36. Reference Dose (RfD): Description and Use in Health Risk Assessments. Available online: http://www.epa.gov/iris/rfd.htm (accessed on 17 September 2012).

37. Ueno, Y.; Makita, Y.; Nagata, S.; Tsutsumi, T.; Yoshida, F.; Tamura, S.I.; Sekijima, M.; Tashiro, F.; Harada, T.; Yoshida, T. No chronic oral toxicity of a low dose of microcystin-LR, a cyanobacterial hepatotoxin, in female BALB/c mice. *Environ. Toxicol.* **1999**, *14*, 45–55.

38. Pilotto, L.; Hobson, P.; Burch, M.D.; Ranmuthugala, G.; Attewell, R.; Weightman, W. Acute skin irritant effects of cyanobacteria (Blue-Green Algae) in healthy volunteers. *Aust. N. Z. J. Public Health* **2004**, *28*, 220–224.

39. Chiu, A.S.; Gehringer, M.M.; Welch, J.H.; Neilan, B.A. Does α-Amino-β-Methylaminopropionic Acid (BMAA) play a role in neurodegeneration? *Int. J. Environ. Res. Public Health* **2011**, *8*, 3728–3746.

40. Kisby, G.E.; Spencer, P.S. Is neurodegenerative disease a long-latency response to early-life genotoxin exposure? *Int. J. Environ. Res. Public Health* **2011**, *8*, 3889–3921.

41. Dunlop, R.A.; Cox, P.A.; Banack, S.A.; Rodgers, K.J. The non-protein amino acid BMAA is misincorporated into human proteins in place of L-serine causing protein misfolding and aggregation. *PLoS One* **2013**, *8*, e75376.

42. Larkin, S.L.; Adams, C.M. Harmful algal blooms and coastal business: Economic consequences in Florida. *Soc. Nat. Resour.* **2007**, *20*, 849–859.

43. Hudnell, H.K. The state of U.S. freshwater harmful algal blooms assessments, policy and legislation. *Toxicon* **2010**, *55*, 1024–1034.

44. Hoagland, P.; Anderson, D.; Kaoru, M.Y.; White, A.W. The economic effects of harmful algal blooms in the United States: Estimates, assessment issues, and information needs. *Estuaries* **2002**, *25*, 819–837.

45. Dodds, W.K.; Bouska, W.W.; Eitzmann, J.L.; Pilger, T.J.; Pitts, K.L.; Riley, A.J.; Schloesser, J.T.; Thornbrugh, D.J. Eutrophication of U.S. freshwaters: Analysis of potential economic damages. *Environ. Sci. Technol.* **2009**, *43*, 12–19.

Chapter 4:
Monitoring Efforts in Freshwater and Marine Water Systems

Harmful Algal Bloom Characterization at Ultra-High Spatial and Temporal Resolution Using Small Unmanned Aircraft Systems

Deon Van der Merwe and Kevin P. Price

Abstract: Harmful algal blooms (HABs) degrade water quality and produce toxins. The spatial distribution of HAbs may change rapidly due to variations wind, water currents, and population dynamics. Risk assessments, based on traditional sampling methods, are hampered by the sparseness of water sample data points, and delays between sampling and the availability of results. There is a need for local risk assessment and risk management at the spatial and temporal resolution relevant to local human and animal interactions at specific sites and times. Small, unmanned aircraft systems can gather color-infrared reflectance data at appropriate spatial and temporal resolutions, with full control over data collection timing, and short intervals between data gathering and result availability. Data can be interpreted qualitatively, or by generating a blue normalized difference vegetation index (BNDVI) that is correlated with cyanobacterial biomass densities at the water surface, as estimated using a buoyant packed cell volume (BPCV). Correlations between BNDVI and BPCV follow a logarithmic model, with r^2-values under field conditions from 0.77 to 0.87. These methods provide valuable information that is complimentary to risk assessment data derived from traditional risk assessment methods, and could help to improve risk management at the local level.

Reprinted from *Toxins*. Cite as: Van der Merwe, D.; Price, K.P. Harmful Algal Bloom Characterization at Ultra-High Spatial and Temporal Resolution Using Small Unmanned Aircraft Systems. *Toxins* **2015**, *7*, 1065-1078.

1. Introduction

Cyanobacteria are photosynthesizing prokaryotic bacteria. They are found in most surface waters worldwide, and are often important primary producers in aquatic ecosystems. Under certain environmental conditions, however, they may proliferate exponentially to form harmful algal blooms (HABs). The incidence rates of HABs have increased over time, and higher incidence rates have been linked to excess nutrient influx into surface waters [1–3]. The relentless and necessary pursuit of ever-higher agricultural production to feed growing human and livestock populations inevitably results in nutrient-rich agricultural run-off, and the trend towards more frequent HABs in surface freshwaters is therefore expected to persist unless alternative, less polluting food production methods are found and implemented.

Several common genera of cyanobacteria have the ability to produce toxins, referred to as cyanotoxins, which affect people, livestock, pets, and wildlife [4,5]. The production of toxins is influenced by algal density, genetic potential, and environmental factors. Important environmental factors include nutrient concentrations, water temperature, light intensity, water pH, wind conditions, and interactions between aquatic organisms, such as predation and competition for nutrients. Toxin production is generally more common during warmer weather in summer, but can occur at any time of the year [6–9]. Animals may be exposed to cyanotoxins when drinking from, wading in, or swimming in contaminated lakes and ponds. People are most often exposed to cyanotoxins when swimming, skiing, or boating in contaminated waters. Other routes of human exposure include drinking water, contaminated foods, and nutritional supplements [10].

Traditional risk assessments depend on the interpretation of chlorophyll-a concentrations, cell density, and toxin concentration data obtained from surface water samples, usually taken at points along a lake shoreline or from a boat [11]. Results from such samples are typically available from a laboratory after a delay of a few days. The spatial and temporal sparseness of water samples taken and analyzed in the traditional manner create challenges for adequate and timely risk assessment. HABs are highly variable over space and time, and high risk of poisoning may therefore exist where traditional methods of risk assessment indicated low risk. For example, a water sample collected at the site of lethal poisoning of a dog at Milford Lake in Kansas, USA, in 2011, within one day of the exposure, indicated a safe density of *Microcystis* cells, and a safe concentration of cyanotoxins [12]. There is, therefore, a need for a more immediate, efficient, and locally relevant method of risk assessment to enable effective and appropriate local risk management. Remote sensing offers an alternative to direct water sampling for determining the presence of HABs, and can be a valuable supplement to direct water sampling in the process of risk assessment. It has been used to detect and quantify HABs based on visual identification of scums, and estimates of phycocyanin and chlorophyll-a concentrations [13–17].

The purpose of this study was to assess the use of small, unmanned aircraft systems (sUAS), and cameras modified to capture near infrared (NIR) and blue light wavelengths to produce color-infrared reflectance data, for remote sensing of cyanobacteria density in surface freshwaters at spatial and temporal resolutions needed for effective local risk assessment.

2. Results and Discussion

2.1. Results

2.1.1. HAB Density Variation over Space and Time

Repeated flights during a *Microcystis* HAB over Centralia Lake, KS, on 31 August, 14 September, and 24 September of 2012 followed by qualitative assessment of the resulting aerial images, revealed a highly complex distribution of cyanobacterial biomass at the water surface over space and time. Shorelines on different sides of the cove, where accumulation occurred, showed different cyanobacterial biomass densities on different shoreline directions, and also over short distances along the shoreline. Marked changes occurred over time (Figure 1).

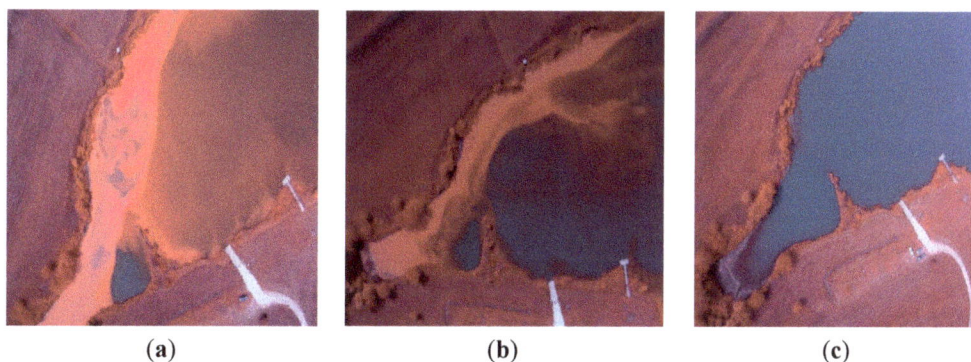

(a)   (b)   (c)

Figure 1. Color-infrared images derived from a small, unmanned aircraft system of a *Microcystis* HAB in Centralia Lake, KS, USA in 2012, on (**a**) 31 August; (**b**) 14 September; and (**c**) 24 September.

2.1.2. Buoyant Packed Cell Volume (BPCV) to Blue Normalized Difference Vegetation Index (BNDVI) Correlation

BPCV correlated strongly with blue NDVI when assessing serially diluted samples under laboratory conditions, with an r^2-value of 0.99, following a logarithmic model because blue NDVI tends to become saturated towards high BPCV levels (Figures 2–5):

$$\text{Blue NDVI} = 0.2118\ln(\text{BPCV}) + 0.0821 \tag{1}$$

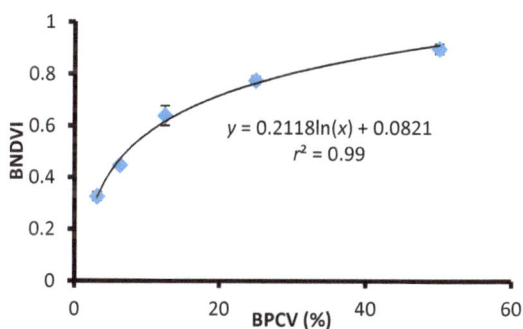

Figure 2. The correlation between Blue Normalized Difference Vegetation Index (BNDVI) and Buoyant Packed Cell Volume (BPCV) derived from a serially diluted sample of a single species of cyanobacteria in the genus *Microcystis*.

Three ponds were investigated to determine BPCV to blue NDVI correlations under field conditions. Logarithmic models provided good correlations for two ponds with pure *Microcystis* blooms (Equations (2) and (3); Figures 6 and 7), and a pond with a mixed *Microcystis* and *Aphanizomenon* bloom (Equation (4); Figure 8). Correlation between BPCV and blue NDVI remained high under field conditions, with r^2-values based on logarithmic models of 0.77, 0.79, and 0.87, respectively, for Pond 1, Pond 2, and Pond 3. The model parameters were as follows:

$$BNDVI = 0.0713\ln(BPCV) - 0.0854 \tag{2}$$

$$BNDVI = 0.0692\ln(BPCV) + 0.0938 \tag{3}$$

$$BNDVI = 0.0534\ln(BPCV) - 0.315 \tag{4}$$

Graphic depictions of results from pond 3 are represented in Figures 3–5 and 8.

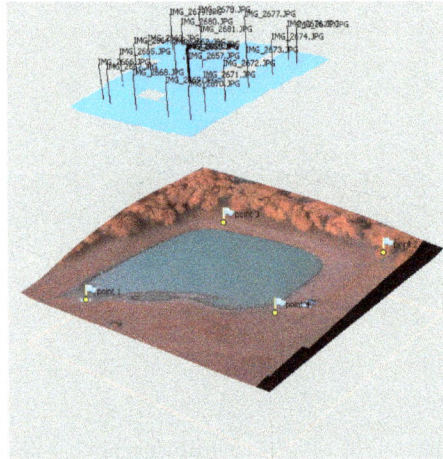

Figure 3. A texturized surface model derived from a livestock drinking water pond containing a harmful *Microcystis* algal bloom, including the calculated positions and orientations of images used to produce the surface model.

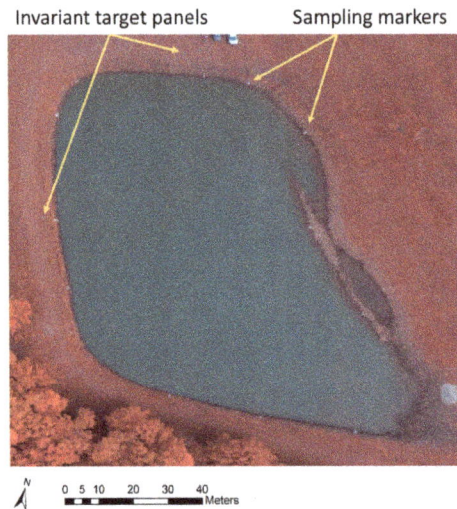

Figure 4. An averaged color-infrared orthomosaic of a livestock drinking water pond, derived from 25 aerial images captured at an altitude of 25 m, between 10:30 a.m. and 11:00 a.m. on 23 August, 2013. Average reflectance values for each point on the water surface were derived from 15–25 images.

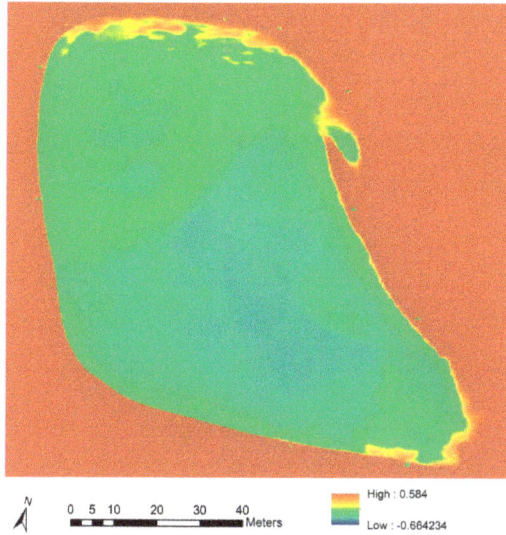

Figure 5. A colorized gradient map of blue normalized difference vegetation index values of a livestock drinking water pond, derived from averaged reflectance values from 25 color-infrared aerial images captured at an altitude of 50 m.

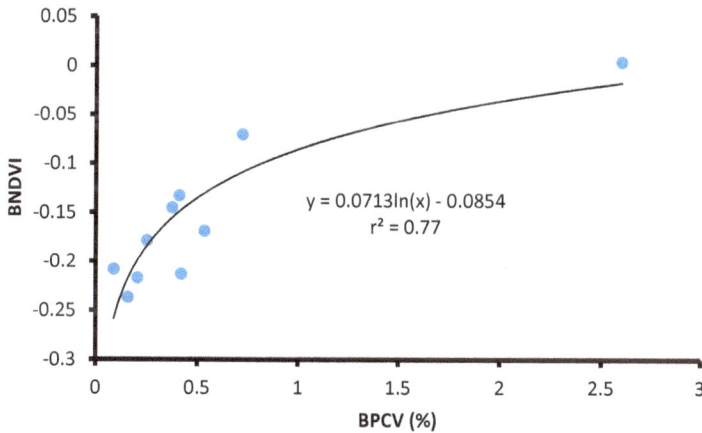

Figure 6. The correlation between Blue Normalized Difference Vegetation Index (BNDVI) and Buoyant Packed Cell Volume (BPCV) at a farm pond containing a harmful *Microcystis* algal bloom.

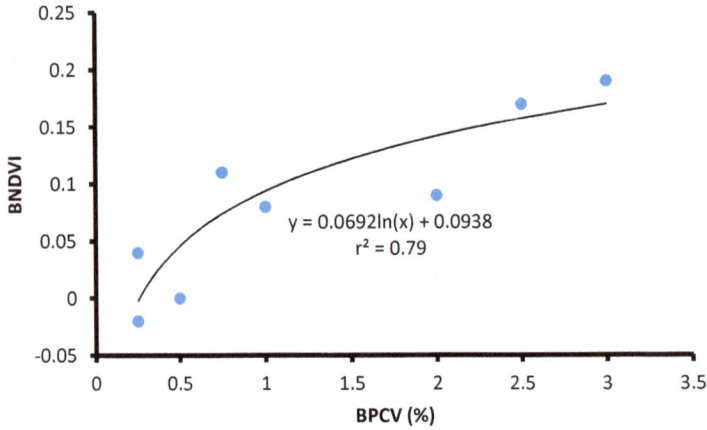

Figure 7. The correlation between Blue Normalized Difference Vegetation Index (BNDVI) and Buoyant Packed Cell Volume (BPCV) at a farm pond containing a harmful *Microcystis* algal bloom.

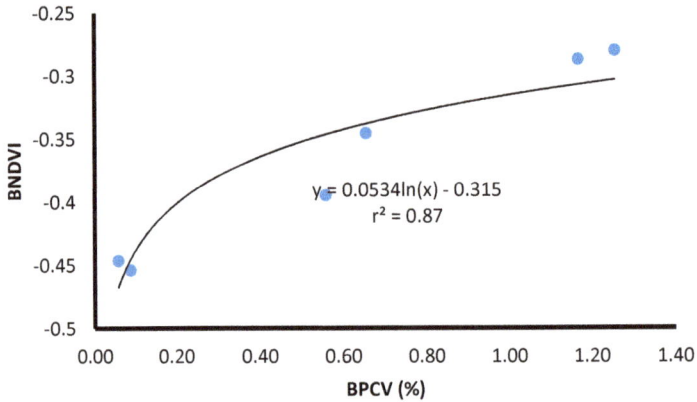

Figure 8. The correlation between Blue Normalized Difference Vegetation Index (BNDVI) and Buoyant Packed Cell Volume (BPCV) at a farm pond containing a harmful *Microcystis* algal bloom.

2.2. Discussion

The use of satellite imagery for assessment of cyanobacteria cell densities in surface waters has been well established, both for early detection and monitoring purposes, and is the preferred method for tracking blooms in oceans and large lakes [18–21]. Manned aircraft are typically able to able to carry larger and heavier payloads compared to sUAS, can stay airborne for longer, and can operate at higher altitudes. It allows manned aircraft to deploy relatively large, hyperspectral sensors that are able to differentiate relatively narrow spectral bands, over relatively large areas. The use of narrow spectral bands can be an important advantage in differentiating cyanobacteria from other photosynthetic organisms based on unique reflectance characteristics associated with pigments produced by cyanobacteria [18]. The ability to differentiate cyanobacteria from other photosynthetic organisms can be a major advantage in situations where direct water sampling and access to *in situ* data are not available. The ability of manned aircraft to cover larger areas compared to sUAS, also makes them suited for assessment of lakes that are too large for sUAS to cover effectively. It is therefore important to assess the potential role of sUAS in remote sensing in relation to traditional remote sensing approaches. Although satellite and manned aircraft remote sensing are extremely useful and are expected to continue to be important, they are limited for use in rapid, local risk assessment, particularly where there is a need for water quality information on small aquatic environments or specific areas along lake shorelines, by the cost and size of narrow band multispectral and hyperspectral sensors fitted with custom-made optics, the cost of manned aircraft and satellite operations, observation limitations imposed by cloud cover, the frequency of suitable satellite positioning over the target area, and spatial resolutions that are often inadequate for small water bodies such as livestock ponds and the detection of small pockets of cyanobacterial biomass accumulation. The different types of remote sensing therefore do not compete directly with each other, but rather provide complimentary information to the risk assessment process.

The spatial distribution of cyanobacteria over space and time is highly variable and complex, to the extent that sampling at a specific location may only be relevant to risk at that location around the time of sampling. Pockets of high biomass accumulations may be intermixed, over short distances, with areas of low biomass accumulation. Average cyanobacterial density in a lake or pond is therefore only partially related to local risk, and a large number of samples are required to produce a statistically robust estimate. These factors make it difficult to predict the local risk along a shoreline, or at specific points in a lake, based on averages derived from sparse data points generated by traditional direct sampling and analysis methods. This limitation is highly significant in the case of dogs due to their roaming and scavenging behavior, as illustrated by a case of lethal poisoning in a dog following exposure to microcystins at a lake shore site where a water sample collected within 24 hours of the exposure indicated low risk [12]. Recreational lake users such as swimmers, skiers and anglers who enter the water, livestock, and wildlife may also be at risk from localized hazards when other areas of a lake that were sampled may be safe, depending on the specific location where contact with the lake water occurs and the positioning of floating algal scums at the time. Knowledge of the specific locations of cyanobacterial biomass accumulations at the time when water contact occur are therefore critical to effective local risk management, and sUAS are likely to provide the most efficient means for generating the required data.

Two types of aircraft were used in these studies because the optimal aircraft type depends on the area that needs to be covered. Multirotor aircraft are typically limited to 25 minutes or less of flight duration with currently available battery technology. They also fly relatively slowly and are therefore limited in coverage per flight to 10s of acres. The ability to hover in place at low altitude can, however, be an advantage when specific sites need to be investigated in extremely high detail, or when suitable open areas for fixed wing aircraft takeoff and landing are not available. Fixed wing aircraft, on the other hand, are relatively efficient, fly longer and faster, and can cover larger areas of

100s of acres. Flying at an altitude of 400 feet, a fixed wing sUAS can typically cover about 600 acres within 25 to 40 minutes with a spatial resolution in the resulting images of less than 5 cm, while maintaining visual line of sight with the operator. Operations beyond visual line of sight require additional measures to ensure safe operations, and were outside the scope of this study. The costs of practical sUAS aerial photography platforms, and the complexity of their operation, have reduced dramatically in recent years. System cost and operational complexity are no longer insurmountable barriers to the use of sUAS at a local level. Airspace use regulations can be a significant barrier to sUAS use in countries where sUAS-specific regulations have not been developed, or where their use have been banned. Regulations associated with sUAS operations are, however, in flux in many parts of the world, and the trend is towards the creation of regulations that allow for the safe operation of sUAS, particularly when such operations are conducted with light-weight sUAS in rural areas, away from airports, at low altitude, and within visual line of sight.

The interpretation of data derived from sUAS can be approached in a two-tiered manner, first as qualitative assessment of single images and orthomosaics, and followed by quantitative assessment of cyanobacterial biomass concentrations based on cyanobacterial biomass density maps derived from the correlation between BNDVI and BPCV. Usefully, locally relevant risk assessment that lead to practical risk management decision can, in many cases, be based solely on qualitative assessment, particularly when the most important determination is the spatial distribution of harmful algal blooms at the time of the flight. Flights were conducted over Lake Centralia to demonstrate the utility of sUAS-based remote sensing in qualitative scouting for the presence of water surface regions with high levels of reflectance in the NIR band, which may indicate the presence of algae, and for the tracking of HAB distribution over time (Figure 1). The results indicated that sUAS-based remote sensing could be effective in this application.

Quantitative assessments are useful for tracking the density of blooms over time. It can be of value in quantitative risk assessment, and has the potential to be used in risk management decisions guided by predetermined policies regarding exposure limits. BPCV has advantages for field use because it requires relatively inexpensive, portable equipment, and very little operator training is needed to produce robust results. Although correlations between BNDVI and BPCV were strong in all three investigations, the model parameters differed. Differences could be attributed to cyanobacteria type differences, bloom stage differences, water differences, and differences in atmospheric conditions. Quantitative accuracy is therefore only possible when model calibration is performed using water samples collected at known locations at the time of the sUAS flight. The advantage of using a calibrated model in conjunction with a BNDVI map is that cyanobacterial biomass estimates can be extrapolated to the whole imaged water surface area, with a high degree of spatial resolution limited only by the resolution of the BNDVI map. Flights conducted at a low altitude using sUAS allows for very high spatial resolutions of 5 cm or less, depending on the flight altitude. It should be noted, however, that BPCV is not directly equivalent to cell density estimates derived from standard microscopy methods, and further work is needed to establish the relationship between PBCV and other cell density estimates. BPCV also does not provide information on the species composition of blooms, and traditional microscopy is still required to identify the cyanobacterial types and species composition involved in blooms.

A limitation of remote sensing methods is that they do not quantify toxin concentrations. Toxin concentrations are an essential component of risk assessment, and the sUAS-based remote sensing approach described here is therefore not suitable for risk assessment in isolation. The best use of sUAS is, arguably, as a complimentary source of data to monitor identified HABs in conjunction with other relevant data, and will be particularly useful in situations where the distribution pattern and surface density of a HAB needs to be characterized and tracked with a high level of spatial and temporal precision and accuracy after the organisms involved in the bloom have been characterized, and their potential to produce toxins have been evaluated by conventional means involving microscopy and toxin analysis on water samples.

There are environmental limitations on the use of sUAS-based remote sensing that need to be considered in the decision to deploy the technology and in the interpretation of data. Ideal atmospheric conditions are clear skies, and low wind velocity. Although data can be collected under cloudy conditions, it typically introduces variability in solar irradiance that may introduce excessive variability into the results independent of algal density. Clouds do not, however, compromise the ability to qualitatively characterize algal scum distribution patterns on the water surface or along the shoreline. Wind can be an important factor because it introduces wave-action at the water surface that degrades the consistency of reflectance values. The specific wind velocity that causes wave formation is variable and depends on the size of the water body, the wind direction, and the presence of obstacles to air movement. The presence of waves is, therefore, best evaluated locally, at the time of the intended flight. Sun angle also plays an important role in the quality and consistency of reflectance values obtained from water surfaces. Mirror-like reflections from the sun, when the sun is positioned above the sensor, causes an area of high reflectance values that are unrelated to algal density to appear on images. Flights should therefore be conducted at times when the sun angle is such that mirror-like sun reflections are not visible in images. Mid-morning and mid-afternoon are, therefore, optimal times in the day for conducting flights.

Reflectance values are influenced by the angles between the sensor, the light source, and the surface because most natural surfaces are non-Lambertian, leading to bidirectional reflectance artifacts in images [22]. Low altitude sensors using wide angle lenses are therefore associated with variations in results unrelated to algal density because the observation angle changes significantly depending on how far from the image center a surface point is. To reduce the influence of bidirectional reflectance, reflectance values were averaged for each surface point, using multiple images taken from different locations at the same altitude over the area of interest. The creation of a virtual surface model from multiple images is an essential step in data processing to enable efficient reflectance value averaging.

Atmospheric conditions, sun angles, and sun irradiance levels influence surface reflectance values, and vary over time. Sensor sensitivity may also change over time. Furthermore, internal radiometric sensor calibration as required for stable sensor sensitivity over time [23] is not feasible in converted consumer-grade sensors. Quantitative comparisons of reflectance values determined at different times therefore require that the data be normalized to a common standard. Semi-lambertian invariant target panels were deployed around livestock ponds for this purpose. The targets were not utilized for radiometric calibration in the current study because livestock ponds were not assessed over multiple time points, but it will be needed for data normalization to a common standard if comparisons over time are needed in future studies. It should be noted, however, that invariant target panels do not provide a complete solution to data normalization across time and location because panels do not account for certain sources of variation in the reflectance values of algae in water. These potential sources of error include variations in the optical properties of water depending on light absorption by organic matter and backscattering from suspended particulates [14], as well as the effects of non-Lambertian reflectance characteristics of panels that are amplified due to the use of wide angle lenses on sensors that are deployed at low altitude. These considerations support our recommendation that the sUAS approach described here is best used to compliment and expand the utility of water samples obtained at the time when flights are conducted. Aerial images processed into averaged reflectance orthomosaics can then be used to derive accurate surface algal density estimates for the entire area covered by the orthomosaic, and reduces the uncertainty associated with interpolation between sparse data points.

3. Experimental Section

Due to the presence of chlorophyll-a, light absorption and reflection patterns in cyanobacteria generally follow the patterns associated with green plants. Light in the visible spectrum is absorbed, with a relatively high absorption rate in the blue and red regions of the visible spectrum, while near infrared (NIR) light is strongly reflected. Absorption of NIR light by water provides a contrast in the NIR band between cyanobacteria at the water surface, and surrounding clear water. The contrast between clear water and cyanobacteria in color-infrared imagery can therefore be used to visually distinguish between clear water and cyanobacteria with a high degree of sensitivity, and the ratio between reflected blue light and reflected NIR can be used to quantify algal density at the water surface by creating a parameter called the blue normalized difference vegetation index (BNDVI; Equation (5)):

$$BNDVI = (NIR - blue)/(NIR + blue) \tag{5}$$

BNDVI was calculated from JPEG-format images captured by a modified digital camera (Canon Powershot S100 NDVI, LDP LLC, Carlstadt, NJ, USA). The filters on the camera sensor were modified to allow visible blue and visible green light between 400 nm and 580 nm, and the visible red edge to near infrared transition between 680 nm to 780 nm, to pass to the sensor, while blocking visible red light between 580 nm and 680 nm, and NIR light above 780 nm.

Two aircraft types, fixed wing and multirotor, were used. The fixed wing aircraft was a Zephyr sUAS. It is a flying wing with a 137 cm wingspan (RitewingRC, Phoenix, AZ, USA), controlled with an Ardupilot Mega 2.6 (3DRobotics, San Diego, CA, USA). Modifications from the standard configuration included strengthening of the leading edge of the wing to withstand landing in rough vegetation by applying laminating film of 0.254 mm thickness, and the installation of a custom camera holder constructed out of expanded polypropylene foam. The multirotor was a DJI F550 controlled with a NAZA V2 (DJI Innovations, Shenzhen, China), fitted with a camera gimbal (Gaui Crane II, TSH Gaui Hobby Corporation, New Taipei City, Taiwan), and a real-time video system (ReadymadeRC LLC, Lewis Center, OH, USA).

Flight planning for fixed wing operations was done in Mission Planner, free software under the terms of the General Public License (Free Software Foundation, Boston, MA, USA). Flights were conducted at an altitude of 122 m, with flight line intervals of 33 m, a ground speed of 15 m/s, and an image interval of 3 s, to achieve front and side overlaps of 75%. Multirotor flights were flown manually, at 25–50 m altitude, to achieve image overlap of at least 75%. Four invariant target panels of 0.37 m^2 were deployed around livestock ponds. The targets were made from particle board covered with matt acrylic latex paint (Behr Premium Plus #S-H-390, The Home Depot, Inc., Brandon, FL, USA). The targets provided semi-Lambertian surfaces with reflectance characteristics that fall within the typical reflectance value ranges of green vegetation for the bands detected by the modified digital camera used in the study.

Images were processed into averaged orthomosaics using Agisoft Photoscan Professional Version 1.0.4 build 1847 (Agisoft LLC, St. Petersburg, Russia). The image processing procedure involved the following steps: photo alignment using high accuracy and generic pair preselection, buiding a surface mesh using a high polygon count, and exporting an orthophoto in JPEG format using the average blending mode.

BNDVI maps were derived in ArcGIS Desktop 10.2.2.3552 (Esri Inc., Redlands, CA, USA), using the Raster Calculator tool in the Spatial Analyst extension. The procedure included importing NIR and blue data as separate raster layers, converting pixel values to floating-point values, and applying the BNDVI algorithm discussed above.

Surface water samples were scooped from the lake or pond water surface at the shoreline using a cup attached to a 1.8 m long handle. Locations were marked using white vinyl strips 6.5 cm wide and 90 cm long. Water samples were taken at consistent distances from the markers to facilitate identification of the sample locations on aerial images. Water samples were transferred to 50 mL polypropylene tubes (Environmental Express, Charlston, SC, USA) for storage in a cooled container, and analyzed within 48 h.

Cyanobacteria were identified to genus level based on microscopic morphology light microscopy (Olympus SZX16, Olympus Corporation, Center Valley, NJ, USA). Due to the need for a rapid quantitation method for surface cyanobacterial biomass that can be deployed under field conditions, a quantitation method was developed based on the buoyant portion of cells after using microscopy to confirm that the buoyant cells were cyanobacteria. Water samples were mixed by rapid inversion of the sample vial by hand at least 10 times, followed by immersion of one end of 75 mm capillary micro-hematocrit tubes (Cat. No. 21112, Sherwood Medical Industries, St. Louis, MO, USA) to draw water into the tubes to about 80% of the tube length, followed by sealing with clay (Seal-ease, Clay-Adams Inc., New York, NY, USA). Tubes were centrifuged for 10 minutes (International Centrifuge Model MB, International Equipment Company, Boston, MA, USA). BPCV was read as a percentage of the total sample volume using a micro-hematocrit tube reader (Critocap, Biological Research Inc., St. Louis, MO, USA). Fractions of a percent were derived from images produced using a stereo microscope (Olympus SZX16, Olympus Corporation, Center Valley, NJ, USA), and quantified by comparing the lengths of transects through the cell layer portion of the image and a 1% reference in the background.

To establish the correlation between BPCV and blue NDVI, a fresh sample of *Microcystis* algal scum derived from Centralia Lake, KS, with a BPCV of 50%, was serially diluted with tap water to 25%, 12.5%, 6.3% and 3.1%, and placed into a 96 well microplate (Cooke Microtiter, Cooke Engineering Company, Alexandria, VA, USA). Broad-spectrum light was produced with a halogen lamp source (Cole-Palmer Illuminator 41720, Cole-Palmer, Vernon Hills, IL, USA). The samples were imaged using a converted camera, followed by calculation of a blue NDVI for each sample.

4. Conclusions

sUAS-based remote sensing methods provide valuable information that is complimentary to HAB risk assessment data derived from traditional methods, and could improve risk management at the local level. It is particularly useful in situations where the distribution pattern and surface density of a HAB needs to be characterized and tracked with a high level of spatial and temporal precision and accuracy.

Acknowledgments

The authors thank Gabriel Kenne, Ali Mahdi, Huan Wang, and Gustavo de Alckmin for assistance during field investigations.

Conflicts of Interest

The authors declare no conflict of interest.

References

1. Paerl, H.W.; Fulton, R.S.; Moisander, P.H.; Dyble, J. Harmful freshwater algal blooms, with an emphasis on cyanobacteria. *Sci. World.* **2001**, *1*, 76–113.
2. De Figueiredo, D.R.; Azeiteiro, U.M.; Esteves, S.M.; Gonsalves, F.J.M.; Pereira, M.J. Microcystin-producing blooms—A serious global public health issue. *Ecotoxicol. Environ. Saf.* **2004**, *59*, 151–163.
3. Hudnell, H.K. The state of US freshwater harmful algal blooms assessments, policy and legislation. *Toxicon* **2010**, *55*, 1024–1034.
4. Briand, J.F.; Jacquet, S.; Bernard, C.; Humbert, J.F. Health hazards for terrestrial vertebrates from toxic cyanobacteria in surface water ecosystems. *Vet. Res.* **2003**, *34*, 361–377.
5. Trevino-Garrison, I.; DeMent, J.; Ahmed, F.S.; Haines-Lieber, P.; Langer, T.; Ménager, H.; Ménager, H.; Neff, J.; van der Merwe, D.; Carney, E. Human illnesses and animal deaths associated with freshwater harmful algal blooms—Kansas. *Toxins* **2015**, *7*, 353–366.
6. Dodds, W.K.; Bouska, W.; Eitzmann, J.L.; Pilger, T.J.; Pitts, K.L.; Riley, A.J.; Schloesser, J.T.; Thornbrugh, D.J. Eutrophication of US freshwaters: Analysis of potential economic damages. *Environ. Sci. Technol.* **2009**, *43*, 12–19.
7. Downing, J.A.; Watson, S.B.; McCauley, E. Predicting Cyanobacteria dominance in lakes. *Can. J. Fish. Aquat. Sci.* **2001**, *58*, 1905–1908.

8. Graham, J.L.; Jones, J.R.; Jones, S.B.; Downing, J.A.; Clevenger, T.E. Environmental factors influencing microcystin distribution and concentration in the Midwestern United States. *Water Res.* **2004**, *38*, 4395–4404.

9. Kanoshina, I.; Lips, U.; Leppanen, J. The influence of weather conditions (temperature and wind) on cyanobacterial bloom development in the Gulf of Finland (Baltic Sea). *Harmful Algae* **2003**, *2*, 29–41.

10. Azevedo, S.M.F.O.; Carmichael, W.W.; Jochimsen, E.M.; Rinehart, K.L.; Lau, S.; Shaw, G.R.; Eaglesham, G.K. Human intoxication by microcystins during renal dialysis treatment in Caruaru-Brazil. *Toxicology* **2002**, *181*, 441–446.

11. Chorus, I.; Bartram, J. *Toxic Cyanobacteria in Water: A Guide to Their Public Health Consequences, Monitoring and Management*; Spon Press: Boca Raton, FL, USA, 1999.

12. Van der Merwe, D.; Sebbag, L.; Nietfeld, J.C.; Aubel, M.T.; Foss, A.; Carney, E. Investigation of a *Microcystis aeruginosa* cyanobacterial freshwater harmful algal bloom associated with acute microcystin toxicosis in a dog. *J. Vet. Diagn. Invest.* **2012**, *24*, 679–687.

13. Lunetta, R.S.; Schaeffer, B.A.; Stumpf, R.P.; Keith, D.; Jacobs, S.A.; Murphy, M.S. Evaluation of cyanobacteria cell count detection derived from MERIS imagery across the eastern USA. *Remote Sens. Environ.* **2014**, *157*, 24–34.

14. Gitelson, A.A.; Dall'Olmo, G.; Moses, W.; Rundquist, D.C.; Barrow, T.; Fisher, T.R.; Gurlin, D.; Holz, J. A simple semi-analytical model for remote estimation of chlorophyll-*a* in turbid waters: Validation. *Remote Sens. Environ.* **2008**, *112*, 3582–3593.

15. Moses, W.J.; Gitelson, A.A.; Perk, R.L.; Gurlin, D.; Rundquist, D.C.; Leavitt, B.C.; Barrow, T.M. Estimation of chlorophyll-*a* concentration in turbid productive waters using airborne hyperspectral data. *Water Res.* **2012**, *46*, 993–1004.

16. Han, L.; Rundquist, D.C. Comparison of NIR/RED ratio and first derivative of reflectance in estimating algal-chlorophyll concentration: A case study in a turbid reservoir. *Remote Sens. Environ.* **1997**, *62*, 253–261.

17. Rundquist, D.C.; Han, L.; Schalles, J.F.; Peake, J.S. Remote measurement of algal chlorophyll in surface waters: The case for the first derivative of reflectance near 690 nm. *Photogramm. Eng. Remote Sens.* **1996**, *62*, 195–200.

18. Hunter, P.D.; Tyler, A.N.; Carvalho, L.; Codd, G.A.; Maberly, S.C. Hyperspectral remote sensing of cyanobacterial pigments as indicators for cell populations and toxins in eutrophic lakes. *Remote Sens. Environ.* **2010**, *114*, 2705–2718.

19. Keith, D.J.; Milstead, B.; Walker, H.; Snook, H.; Szykman, J.; Wusk, M.; Kagey, L.; Howell, C.; Mellanson, C.; Drueke, C. Trophic status, ecological condition, and cyanobacteria risk of New England lakes and ponds based on aircraft remote sensing. *J. Appl. Remote Sens.* **2012**, doi:10.1117/1.JRS.6.063577.

20. Wynne, T.T.; Stumpf, R.P.; Briggs, T.O. Comparing MODIS and MERIS spectral shapes for cyanobacterial bloom detection. *Int. J. Remote Sens.* **2013**, *34*, 6668–6678.

21. Gitelson, A.A.; Schalles, J.F.; Rundquist, D.C.; Schiebe, F.R.; Yacobi, Y.Z. Comparative reflectance properties of algal cultures with manipulated densities. *J. Appl. Phycol.* **1999**, *11*, 345–354.

22. Walthall, C.; Norman, J.; Welles, J.; Campbell, G.; Blad, B. Simple equation to approximate the bidirectional reflectance from vegetative canopies and bare soil surfaces. *Appl. Opt.* **1985**, *24*, 383–387.

23. Vogelmann, J.E.; Helder, D.; Morfitt, R.; Choate, M.J.; Merchant, J.W.; Bulley, H. Effects of Landsat 5 Thematic Mapper and Landsat 7 Enhanced Thematic Mapper Plus radiometric and geometric calibrations and corrections on landscape characterization. *Remote Sens. Environ.* **2001**, *78*, 55–70.

Integrative Monitoring of Marine and Freshwater Harmful Algae in Washington State for Public Health Protection

Vera L. Trainer and F. Joan Hardy

Abstract: The more frequent occurrence of both marine and freshwater toxic algal blooms and recent problems with new toxic events have increased the risk for illness and negatively impacted sustainable public access to safe shellfish and recreational waters in Washington State. Marine toxins that affect safe shellfish harvest in the state are the saxitoxins that cause paralytic shellfish poisoning (PSP), domoic acid that causes amnesic shellfish poisoning (ASP) and the first ever US closure in 2011 due to diarrhetic shellfish toxins that cause diarrhetic shellfish poisoning (DSP). Likewise, the freshwater toxins microcystins, anatoxin-a, cylindrospermopsins, and saxitoxins have been measured in state lakes, although cylindrospermopsins have not yet been measured above state regulatory guidance levels. This increased incidence of harmful algal blooms (HABs) has necessitated the partnering of state regulatory programs with citizen and user-fee sponsored monitoring efforts such as SoundToxins, the Olympic Region Harmful Algal Bloom (ORHAB) partnership and the state's freshwater harmful algal bloom passive (opportunistic) surveillance program that allow citizens to share their observations with scientists. Through such integrated programs that provide an effective interface between formalized state and federal programs and observations by the general public, county staff and trained citizen volunteers, the best possible early warning systems can be instituted for surveillance of known HABs, as well as for the reporting and diagnosis of unusual events that may impact the future health of oceans, lakes, wildlife, and humans.

Reprinted from *Toxins*. Cite as: Trainer, V.L.; Hardy, F.J. Integrative Monitoring of Marine and Freshwater Harmful Algae in Washington State for Public Health Protection. *Toxins* **2015**, *7*, 1206-1234.

1. Introduction

Both marine and freshwater toxic algal blooms are believed to be occurring more frequently in lakes, estuaries and oceans of the U.S. Recent problems with new toxic events have increased the risk for illness and negatively impacted sustainable public access to safe shellfish and recreational waters in Washington State. To address these increasing threats to public health, monitoring programs have been strengthened through collaborations that include observations and analyses performed by local, state, and federal scientists, as well as volunteer groups.

Washington State produces the highest amount of commercially harvested mussels, clams and oysters in the nation with an estimated annual production of 39 thousand metric tons that generates over $77 million in sales [2]. This commercial harvest, together with recreational shellfish harvest on Washington's public beaches by approximately 300,000 people, necessitates an effective and comprehensive monitoring program for biotoxins that can affect shellfish safety. If harmful algae producing natural toxins are present, toxins can collect in shellfish tissue and cause illness or even death in marine wildlife or people. The expansion of Washington's shellfish growing areas is evidenced by the net gain of 27,811 acres approved for commercial shellfish production from 1991 to 2010 and an increase in beaches open for recreational harvesting from 78 in 2005 to 201 in 2010 [3,4]. However, marine toxins continue to pose a severe threat to shellfish safety. Closures due to paralytic shellfish toxins are annual occurrences. For example, in 2012, 453 shellfish tissue samples had concentrations of PSP above the regulatory level of 80 μg/100 g and 50 samples had concentrations above 1000 μg/100 g, resulting in closures of numerous commercial shellfishing areas to harvesting [4]. New toxic events are also entering the scene. In 2011, Washington had a confirmed case of diarrhetic shellfish poisoning (DSP), the first known illness from this marine biotoxin-related syndrome in the United States [5].

Toxic cyanobacteria have been observed in over 132 lakes in Washington State, resulting in animal and human illnesses and animal deaths in some lakes [6–8]. Toxic cyanobacteria and blooms occur in natural lakes, manmade reservoirs, and ponds, but especially those that are influenced by watershed development and pollution. Lakes that produce toxic blooms often provide citizens with vital recreational opportunities in addition to supplying drinking water. Closures of lakes due to toxic blooms have had economic impacts in lakes from all regions of the state resulting in closure of recreational areas and restriction of fishing. With the potential for cyanotoxins to bioaccumulate in fish, public health officials are concerned about exposure through consumption [9], and freshwater toxins from lake blooms have been observed downstream in marine shellfish [10]. Furthermore, in 2014, a lake in the Puget Sound lowlands that provides drinking water to over 500 households had its first toxic bloom, provoking intense scrutiny and public concern [8]. Regional or short-term monitoring programs and opportunistic surveillance indicate that toxic blooms are becoming more frequent in the state, potentially impacting public health, regional economies, and lifestyles of citizens who use the lakes.

Here we provide an overview of marine and freshwater toxins in the region that endanger human health (Table 1) and describe the emergence of integrated, interagency monitoring programs for marine and freshwater toxins in Washington State, necessitated by increases in toxin threats to our valued shellfish and freshwater resources. First, we describe marine toxins, their algal hosts, biochemical activity, and historical trends in shellfish toxicity and illness events, followed by similar summary sections for the freshwater toxins. Finally, we provide recommendations for the future and suggestions for tools that can be used for integrative monitoring of biotoxins, marine and fresh water alike.

Table 1. Regulated marine and freshwater toxins in Washington State. [a] Relative abundance values are used by SoundToxins and ORHAB partnerships to provide rapid, early warning of shellfish toxicity in the marine environment; [b] Cell count action level is >50,000 cells/L (large *Pseudo-nitzschia*) and >1,000,000 cells/L (small *Pseudo-nitzschia*); [c] Relative abundance values. For *Dinophysis*, cell count action level is >20,000 cells/L ("common") or an increase from "present" to "common"; ELISA = enzyme-linked immunosorbent assay; LC/MS-MS = liquid chromatography tandem spectrometry; HPLC = high performance liquid chromatography; n/a = not applicable; nd = not done.

Toxins	Known causative organism(s) in WA	Regulatory Method	Action Level (Regulatory or Guidance)			Year of first known illness in WA State
			Shellfish	Water or particulate toxin	Relative cell abundance [a]	
Freshwater Toxins						
Microcystins	*Microcystis, Anabaena* / *Planktothrix* / *Aphanizomenon* / *Hapalosiphon, Nostoc* / *Anabaenopsis* / *Hapalosiphon* / *Gloeotrichia*	ELISA	n/a	6 µg/L	nd	1976
Anatoxin-a	*Anabaena* / *Aphanizomenon* / *Planktothrix* / *Oscillatoria* / *Cylindrospermopsis* / *Raphidiopsis*	LC/MS-MS	n/a	1 µg/L	nd	1989
Cylindrospermopsin	*Aphanizomenon* / *Cylindrospermopsis*	ELISA	n/a	4.5 µg/L	nd	n/a
Saxitoxin	*Anabaena* / *Aphanizomenon* / *Planktothrix* / *Cylindrospermopsin*	ELISA	n/a	75 µg/L	nd	n/a
Marine Toxins						
Saxitoxins	*Alexandrium*	Mouse bioassay	80 µg/ 100 g	~100–200 ng/L STX equiv./L [11]	present	1942
Domoic acid	*Pseudo-nitzschia*	HPLC	20 ppm	~200 ng/L [12]	common or bloom [b]	1991
Diarrhetic shellfish toxins	*Dinophysis*	LC/MS-MS	16 µg/g	~20 ng/L [13]	increase from present to common [c]	2011

2. Shellfish Monitoring for Marine Toxins

Monitoring of shellfish safety is a critical function of the Office of Shellfish and Water Protection of the Washington State Department of Health (DOH). The shellfish toxicity surveillance program was initiated by the DOH in the early 1930s as a collaboration between DOH and the George Williams Hooper Foundation for Medical Research in San Francisco [14]. Initial monitoring by DOH focused on commercial shellfish and included recreational shellfish for the first time in the early 1990s. Since the 1930s, the DOH has measured biotoxins in shellfish from hundreds of locations in western Washington waterways in order to protect consumers from shellfish poisoning. When harmful levels of biotoxins are measured, alerts are issued by DOH to shellfish growers and harvesters, local health agencies, and tribes by newspaper, television, the DOH Biotoxin Hotline (1.800.562.5632), and the internet [15]. A highly structured Sentinel Monitoring Program was established in 1990 [16] to provide early warning of the onset of biotoxin concentrations in shellfish.

Through this Sentinel Monitoring Program, caged mussels are sampled at about 40 locations in Washington's marine waters every 2 weeks throughout the year. Generally the blue mussel, *Mytilus edulis*, is sampled; however, *M. galloprovincialis* and *M. californianus* are collected at a few Puget Sound sites. Wire mesh cages are stocked with mussels and suspended from floats and docks. Caged mussels sit for at least 1 week before they are sampled and are replenished as needed. At a few sites, natural-set mussels are harvested. Seventy to 100 mussels provide the 100 grams of tissue needed for analysis. Mussels are sealed into plastic bags, chilled with frozen gel packs, and shipped to the DOH laboratory in Seattle for analysis by mouse bioassay [17] (Table 1).

When toxins are detected above the regulatory level in shellfish, the harvest area is closed. It takes two shellfish samples of the same species from same area collected 7–10 days apart with acceptable levels of toxin to reopen a closed area to harvest. When the closure is in a commercial harvest area, all licensed shellfish companies in that area are notified to stop harvesting immediately. Commercial product that came from a closed area may also be recalled from the market.

3. Marine Toxins Affecting Public Health in Washington

3.1. Saxitoxins

3.1.1. Activity and Source of Saxitoxins

Saxitoxins are among the most potent natural toxins known [18] that act by blocking sodium channels of nerves, impairing normal signal transmission [19,20]. More than 30 different saxitoxin analogues have been identified, including pure saxitoxin (STX), neosaxitoxin (neoSTX), the gonyautoxins (GTX) and decarbamoylsaxitoxin (dc-STX) of which STX, NeoSTX, GTX1 and dc-STX are the most toxic isomers. The term saxitoxin often refers to the entire suite of related neurotoxins produced by cyanobacteria and marine algae.

This suite of closely related tetrahydropurines (saxitoxins-STX) is also described as a group of carbamate alkaloid toxins that are either nonsulfated (STXs), singly sulfated (gonyautoxins, GTX), or doubly sulfated (C-toxins) [21]. Chemically, saxitoxin is stable and readily soluble in water, although it can be inactivated by treatment with a strong alkali. The half-lives for breakdown of a range of different saxitoxins in natural water have been shown to vary from 9 to 28 days, and gonyautoxins may persist in the environment for more than 3 months [22]. The toxicological database for STX-group toxins is limited and is comprised primarily of studies on acute toxicity following intraperitoneal (i.p.) administration. For monitoring purposes, toxicity equivalency factors (TEFs) have been applied to express the detected analogues (using high performance liquid chromatography, HPLC) in freshwater systems and the mouse bioassay for shellfish in marine systems) as STX equivalents (STX-equiv.). The Scientific Panel on Contaminants in the Food Chain (EFSA 2009) proposes the following TEFs based on acute intraperitoneal toxicity in mice: $STX = 1$, $NeoSTX = 1$, $GTX1 = 1$, $GTX2 = 0.4$, $GTX3 = 0.6$, $GTX4 = 0.7$, $GTX5 = 0.1$, $GTX6 = 0.1$, $C2 = 0.1$, $C4 = 0.1$, $dc\text{-}STX = 1$, $dc\text{-}NeoSTX = 0.4$, $dc\ GTX2 = 0.2$, $GTX3 = 0.4$, and $11\text{-hydroxy-}STX = 0.3$.

The dinoflagellate *Alexandrium catenella* (Balech), previously described as belonging to the genus *Gonyaulax* (Whedon and Kofoid) or *Protogonyaulax* (Taylor), has been identified as the primary causative species of paralytic shellfish poisoning on the west coast of North America [23]. However, the name *A. fundyense* [24,25] has recently been proposed to replace all Group I strains of the *A. tamarense* species complex which includes the Washington *Alexandrium* isolates.

3.1.2. Illness and Symptoms

Saxitoxins are toxic by ingestion and by inhalation, with inhalation leading to rapid respiratory collapse and death. Intoxication with saxitoxin can be a severe, life-threatening illness requiring immediate medical care. Most information on saxitoxin symptoms comes from exposure through consumption of shellfish. Within minutes of eating toxic shellfish, a person would initially develop tingling of the lips and tongue. However, it can take up to an hour or two to develop tingling, depending on the dose and individual tolerance, followed by numbness and weakness with loss of control of arms and legs, developing into difficulty in breathing. Some people feel nauseated or experience a sense of floating after saxitoxin exposure. If a person consumes enough saxitoxin, muscles of the chest and abdomen become paralyzed, including muscles used for breathing, and the victim can suffocate. Terminal stages of saxitoxin poisoning can occur 2–12 h after exposure, and death from PSP has occurred in less than 30 min [26].

Diagnosis of saxitoxin poisoning is confirmed by detection of toxin in the food, water, stomach contents, or environmental samples. Artificial respiration is used to support breathing; when such support is applied within 12 h of exposure, recovery usually is complete with no lasting side effects [27–29]. Stomach evacuation can be conducted if exposure is through ingestion. No antidote against saxitoxin exposure has been developed for human use.

3.1.3. Washington Occurrences

Closures of recreational shellfish harvesting due to paralytic shellfish toxins (PSTs) have been imposed in Washington State since 1942 when three Native American fatalities occurred in the town of Sekiu on the Strait of Juan de Fuca [13]. At that time, the Washington Department of Fisheries imposed annual closures for all shellfish harvest except razor clams from 1 April to 31 October in the area west of Dungeness Spit (near Port Angeles, WA, Figure 1) including the Pacific coast to the

Columbia River [30]. The shellfish surveillance program for PSTs was temporarily stopped in 1946 when it was believed that the seasonal blanket closure was adequately protecting public health. However, an outbreak of PSP on eastern Vancouver Island in 1957 [31] resulted in a mandatory monitoring program for PSTs in all commercial shellfish in Washington. Illnesses due to PSP were not reported in Puget Sound prior to 1978, but widespread toxicity occurred that year throughout much of the central basin [30]. High numbers of illnesses include 14 in 1978, nine in 2000, and 7 in 2012, all in Puget Sound [32–34] (Table 2). Toxins causing PSP are now found in most areas of Puget Sound after a massive event in 1978 that caused spreading into the main basin, then further migration into the southernmost reaches of the Sound in the 1980s and 1990s. Multiple closures due to PSTs occur annually at many locations throughout Puget Sound.

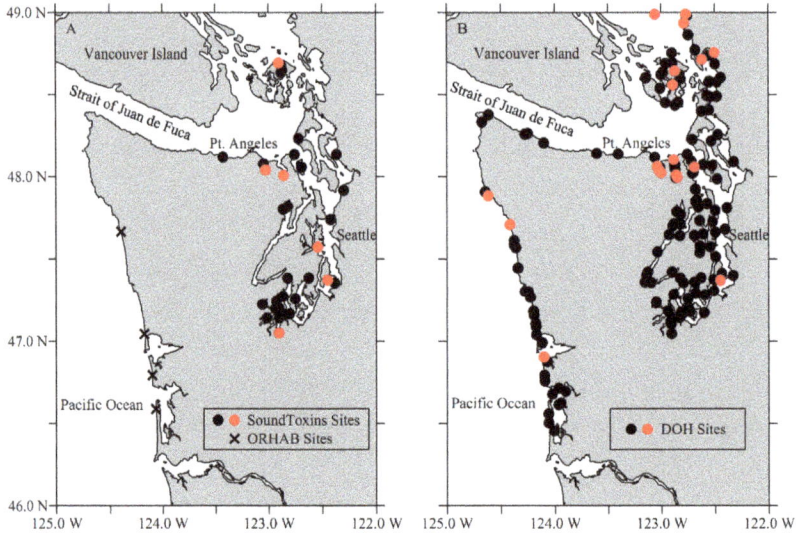

Figure 1. Phytoplankton monitoring locations and DOH shellfish biotoxin management sites in 2014. A. SoundToxins monitoring sites (black circles), including locations where *Dinophysis* was quantified as common or greater (red circles), B. DOH shellfish biotoxin monitoring sites (black circles) include locations where diarrhetic shellfish toxins were at or above the regulatory level of 16 µg/kg (red circles). Routinely monitored, core ORHAB sites are marked with X.

3.2. Domoic Acid

3.2.1. Activity and Source of Domoic Acid

Several species of pennate, chain-forming diatoms in the genus *Pseudo-nitzschia* are known to produce domoic acid (DA), a toxin that bioaccumulates through the food chain to shellfish and planktivorous fish, then to vertebrates such as birds, marine mammals, and humans. The toxin, DA, acts at the same nerve receptor as glutamate, the major excitatory neurotransmitter in the mammalian central nervous system that is responsible for many of the functions within the brain, including learning and memory. Several comprehensive recent reviews are available for more information on *Pseudo-nitzschia* and DA [35–39].

Table 2. Marine biotoxin-related illnesses, 1942–2014. [a] Includes 3 deaths; [b] Probable illnesses with only one illness confirmed; [c] Domoic acid concentration in ppm. Source: DOH.

Year	Month	Illnesses	Shellfish	Toxin Concentration (µg/100 g)
1942	May	6 PSP [a]	Mussels, Clams	3500
1978	August	4 PSP	Scallops	2597
1978	September	10 PSP	Mussels	1415
1979	July	3 PSP	Clams	2597
1985	September	2 PSP	Scallops	1107
1985	November	1 PSP	Scallops	338
1988	May	2 PSP	Clams	1200
1988	September	5 PSP	Oysters	2171
1991	October	25 ASP [b]	Razor Clams	26 ppm [c]
1998	October	5 PSP	Mussels	10,928
2000	August	9 PSP	Mussels	13,769
2007	April	1 PSP	Clams	709
2011	June	3 DSP	Mussels	160
2012	August	1 PSP	Mussels	1621
2012	September	1 PSP	Mussels	10,304
2012	September	7 PSP	Mussels	6250

3.2.2. Illness and Symptoms

Domoic acid poisoning is formally known as amnesic shellfish poisoning in humans. Gastrointestinal symptoms can appear 24 h after ingestion of shellfish containing DA and may include vomiting, nausea, diarrhea, abdominal cramps and bleeding in the gastrointestinal system. Neurological symptoms in more severe cases can take hours to three days to appear and include headaches, hallucinations, confusion and impairment of short-term memory, unstable blood pressure, cardiac arrhythmia and coma [40]. People poisoned with very high doses of the toxin or those who display risk factors such as old age or renal failure can die after exposure.

3.2.3. Washington Occurrences

The razor clam and Dungeness crab fisheries on the outer coast of Washington have been plagued by DA closures since 1991 [41–43]. Commercial, recreational and subsistence razor clam fisheries suffered total coastwide closures in 1991, 1998 and 2002. However, due to enhanced information about specific locations of *Pseudo-nitzschia* species attributable to the monitoring efforts of the ORHAB partnership, formed in 2000, selective closures were possible in 2001 and 2003–2005. Because razor clams can retain DA for periods of up to a year due to the presence of a high affinity glutamate binding protein [44], closures on the outer coast lasting for up to a year caused serious economic hardship to the tribal communities which rely on this subsistence fishery.

DA closures occurred in Puget Sound in 2003 and 2005, causing great concern to shellfish managers. To date, concentrations of DA below the regulatory level of 20 ppm have been detected in Puget Sound blue mussel (*Mytilus edulis*), littleneck clam (*Protothaca staminea*), geoduck clam (*Panopea abrupta*), manila clam (*Tapes philippinarum*), Pacific oyster (*Crassostrea gigas*), and Dungeness crab (*Cancer magister*) [45]. If future DA concentrations are found at levels in excess of the regulatory level in more areas of Puget Sound, resulting economic losses could be severe.

3.3. Diarrhetic Shellfish Toxins

3.3.1. Activity of Diarrhetic Shellfish Toxins

These lipophilic toxins that are often found in combination in shellfish can be divided into four groups with different chemical structures and relative toxicities in humans: Okadaic acid (OA and its derivatives, the DTXs; the pectenotoxins (PTXs); the yessotoxins (YTXs); and the azaspiracids (AZAs). Both OA and the DTXs are lipid polyethers with inhibitory effects on protein phosphatases [46,47] and are the only toxins of the DSP group that can cause diarrhea in mammals [48]. The PTXs and YTXs are toxic in animal studies [49] but have not yet been associated with human poisonings [50]. The AZAs were first described after several people became ill after consuming contaminated mussels in Ireland [51] and have recently been measured in shellfish from Washington State at low concentrations [5].

3.3.2. Illness and Symptoms

Diarrhetic shellfish poisoning (DSP) is a human syndrome caused by consumption of shellfish contaminated by toxins produced by *Dinophysis* and benthic species of *Prorocentrum* [52–54]. However, no DSP outbreaks associated with *Prorocentrum* have been described in Washington. DSP symptoms are gastrointestinal and include diarrhea, nausea, vomiting, and abdominal distress starting a few minutes to hours after ingestion of the toxic shellfish. Recovery occurs within three days [55].

3.3.3. Washington Occurrences

The first clinical report of DSP in the in the Pacific Northwest and in the U.S. with coincident high concentrations of diarrhetic shellfish toxins was due to the consumption of toxin-laced mussels collected from a pier at Sequim Bay State Park in northwest Washington in June 2011. Nine mussel samples collected immediately after the illnesses were reported, contained toxins at 2–10 times above the regulatory level. Coincidently, about 60 DSP illnesses associated with the ingestion of mussels occurred on Salt Spring Island, British Columbia, the first reports of DSP in western Canada [56], resulting in the recall of almost 14,000 kg of shellfish. Sites with shellfish testing positive for diarrhetic shellfish toxins above the regulatory level of 16 µg/g in 2014 are shown in Figure 1.

4. Integrative Monitoring of Marine Toxins in Washington

In most coastal regions of the world, shellfish harvesting closures based on monitoring for toxins are primarily reactionary. These systems have succeeded in protecting human health but often have led to conservative, blanket closures of shellfish harvesting operations, thereby negatively impacting the economy of the shellfish industry. The recent appearance of new toxins in Washington challenges the capacity and effectiveness of monitoring programs that are based solely on assessment of shellfish toxicity. The National Shellfish Sanitation Program (NSSP) recommends phytoplankton monitoring as an early warning for the control of shellfish safety to provide the assurance that states are taking adequate measures to prevent harvesting, shipping, and consumption of toxic shellfish. The plan encourages communication with other states, researchers and other environmental professionals [57–59]. Washington is one of the US states that has successfully integrated phytoplankton and shellfish monitoring through collaboration of DOH with two phytoplankton monitoring programs, the ORHAB partnership on the Pacific coast of Washington [12] and the SoundToxins program in Puget Sound [60].

The ORHAB partnership was established in 1999 and uses a combination of analytical techniques, including weekly quantification of total numbers of harmful algae using microscopes and determination of DA concentration in seawater and razor clams, to give an effective early warning of shellfish toxin events (see Figure 1 for primary ORHAB sites denoted with X). Because razor clams are the main recreationally-harvested shellfish on the outer coast of Washington and accumulate and retain more DA than any other shellfish [44], the ORHAB early warning system is focused solely on DA testing in these shellfish using enzyme-linked immunosorbent assay (ELISA). The efficacy and accuracy of ELISA for diarrhetic shellfish toxin screening are currently being tested for eventual use by the State's phytoplankton monitoring programs [61].

Using ORHAB as a model, SoundToxins was established in 2006 and has grown from four partner sites in 2006 to >30 monitoring locations today (Figure 1). Seawater samples are collected weekly by the participants at ORHAB sites on the outer coast and SoundToxins sites throughout Puget Sound and are analyzed for salinity, temperature, nutrients, chlorophyll, and particulate toxins, including paralytic shellfish toxins, DA, and diarrhetic shellfish toxins. Phytoplankton relative abundance focuses on four target genera *Pseudo-nitzschia*, *Alexandrium*, *Dinophysis* species, and *Heterosigma akashiwo*. In addition, SoundToxins participants recently have assisted with the identification of *Azadinium* species in Puget Sound.

Through its weekly monitoring of phytoplankton at sites around Puget Sound, the SoundToxins partnership has allowed the state to target monitoring for diarrhetic shellfish toxins to those sites that have the greatest risk of toxicity due to increases in relative abundance of *Dinophysis* spp. from present to common or greater (Figure 1, see definitions in Table 1). SoundToxins participants, including environmental learning centers, Native Tribes, shellfish growers, state and federal researchers and private citizens enter weekly phytoplankton relative abundances into a web-based system [60], allowing rapid visualization of data and decision making by DOH officials. Future improvements will include closer pairing of SoundToxins phytoplankton monitoring sites with shellfish harvesting areas (Figure 1) and rapid toxin testing at the sites of shellfish harvest by volunteers to provide a swift assessment of toxin risk for managers.

5. Monitoring for Freshwater Cyanobacteria and Their Toxins

Cyanobacteria blooms are common in numerous Washington lakes. Cyanobacteria (also known as blue-green algae) can create toxins collectively called cyanotoxins. A documented public health concern, cyanotoxins include the liver toxins microcystins and cylindrospermopsins and the nerve toxins anatoxin-a and saxitoxins. Historically, many animals have become ill or have died after exposure to cyanotoxins in state lakes. To address this issue, the DOH and Washington State Department of Ecology (Ecology) have conducted surveillance of blooms and human and animal illnesses related to cyanotoxin exposure for several years.

Freshwater algae and cyanobacteria produce blooms that may be non-toxic one day but may become toxic the next day or later in the growing season. The only way to know whether a cyanobacterial bloom is toxic is to test for the presence of toxins. Due in part to citizens' mounting concerns over potential health impacts from exposure to rapidly appearing freshwater cyanotoxins, the state legislature created and funded a Freshwater Algae Control Program in 2005. This Ecology program provides funds to conduct toxicity testing by King County Environmental Laboratory (KCEL) on samples collected by local health jurisdictions, lake managers, other agencies or lake residents from lakes with blooms. Originally, analysis was done on samples collected under the passive surveillance program only for microcystins, but KCEL later developed the capacity to test for anatoxin-a, cylindrospermopsins, and saxitoxins.

During initial development of the Freshwater Algae Control Program, stakeholders requested that state guidelines be developed to help with interpretation of toxicity results. In the absence of recreational guidance (based on actual toxicity levels and not cell concentrations) from the United States or the World Health Organization (WHO) for microcystins and anatoxin-a, DOH developed provisional guidance values (health-based recommendations that are not formal regulatory values) for both cyanotoxins based on a review of toxicology literature and standard risk assessment methods [62]. Later, DOH developed provisional recreational guidance for saxitoxins and cylindrospermopsins [63]. As part of the effort to provide assistance to local health jurisdictions and lake managers, DOH also developed a lake protocol that incorporated these guidance values as a reference for use by managers, agencies, and local health jurisdictions (LHJs) (Table 1). While the most likely exposure pathways to freshwater cyanotoxins are through recreational contact or contaminated drinking water, long-term chronic ingestion via drinking water and exposure through consumption of fish and shellfish were not considered in development of recreational guidance. Recreational exposure includes activities such as swimming, wind surfing, jet skiing, and water skiing. The calculations used to determine these provisional recreational guidance values are described below.

DOH incorporated the approach used by Oregon and Vermont in initial derivation of recreational guidance for microcystins [64]. Oregon has recently updated its guidance values to include anatoxin-a, cylindrospermopsin, and saxitoxin and to address acute or short-term exposures for human drinking water exposure, human recreational exposure, and dog-specific exposures [65].

DOH calculations assume a default child's body weight (BW) of 15 kg and an ingestion rate (IR) of 0.1 L based on 2 h exposure by a swimmer or other lake user with an exposure lasting for two hours per day [62]. Using the WHO tolerable daily intake (TDI) of 0.04 µg/kg-day [66] and other assumptions, above, DOH recommends a provisional recreational guidance value of 6 µg/L for microcystins, calculated as follows:

$$\text{Recreational guidance value (µg/L)} = \frac{\text{TDI} \times \text{BW}}{\text{IR}} \tag{1}$$

DOH recommends a provisional recreational guidance value of 4.5 µg/L cylindrospermopsin, assuming a subchronic RfD of 0.03 µg/kg-day (EPA 2006) calculated using EPA assumptions, as above (RfD, in place of a TDI in the above equation). Similarly, for saxitoxins, DOH recommends a provisional recreational guidance value of 75 µg/L saxitoxin, calculated using an acute RfD developed by the European Food Safety Association [67] based on acute toxicity of STX-equivalent intoxications in humans (>500 individuals) [63]. For anatoxin-a, DOH recommends a provisional recreational guidance value of 1 µg/L based on a systemic toxicity study in mice exposed to anatoxin-a for 28 days [62,68]. When an acute reference dose (RfD) or estimate of daily oral exposure becomes available for anatoxin-a, DOH will reassess this interim anatoxin-a guidance value. All recommended recreational guidance values are considered "provisional" and will be reassessed when national or international guidance values become available.

In 2009, DOH and partners began a five-year cooperative agreement with the Centers for Disease Control and Prevention (CDC) to expand efforts to address HABs in Washington. Part of this project involved monitoring 30 Puget Sound lowland lakes for microcystins and anatoxin-a, and by 2010 the project added cylindrospermopsin and saxitoxin (Figure 2). Of the four cyanotoxins, microcystins were most frequently observed in the region, followed by anatoxin-a. Cylindrospermopsin and saxitoxin were each observed in only two Puget Sound lakes during the 2009 and 2010 sampling seasons of the 30-lake monitoring project.

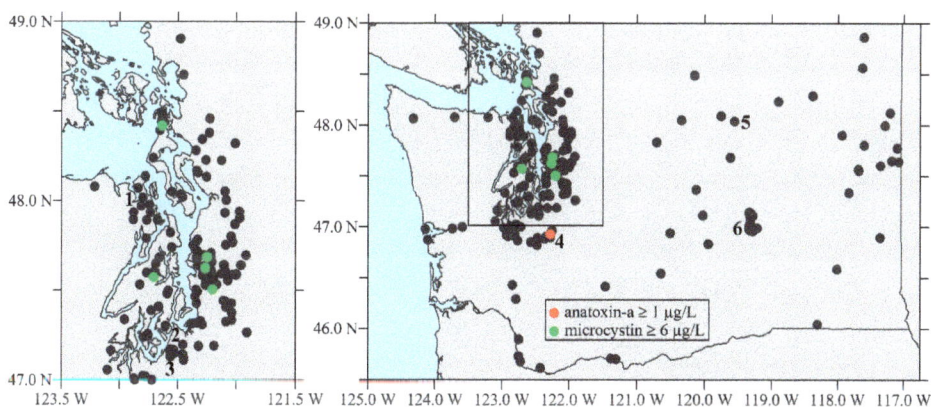

Figure 2. Washington lakes sampled for freshwater biotoxins (shown here are January 2014 data from [8]). Site names mentioned in the text are numbered: 1. Anderson Lake, 2. Waughop Lake, 3. American Lake, 4. Clear Lake, 5. Rufus Woods Lake, 6. Potholes Reservoir. Due to the size of the figure, sampled lakes are not visible.

6. Summary of Freshwater Toxins Affecting Public Health in Washington

Early in the program, DOH identified a list of cyanobacteria genera and species of concern for lakes in Washington. Toxicity testing is recommended when lake samples contain the following genera: *Microcystis, Anabaena, Aphanizomenon, Gloeotrichia, Oscillatoria/Planktothrix, Cylindrospermopsis, Lyngbya,* and/or *Nostoc.* In a summary report for the 2008–2009 state legislature, the top three toxic cyanobacteria genera in Washington lakes were identified as *Anabaena, Aphanizomenon,* and *Microcystis* [69]. *Gloeotrichia* was also included because a recent study confirmed microcystin-LR production by *Gloeotrichia echinulata* [70], and exposure to this genus has led to reports of human health impacts in Washington lakes.

Cyanotoxins are a diverse group of natural toxins that fall into three broad chemical structure groups [66,71]. These are cyclic peptides (microcystins and nodularin), alkaloids (anatoxins, saxitoxins, cylindrospermopsin, aplysiatoxins, and lyngbyatoxin), and lipopolysaccharides (irritants). Anatoxin-a(s) is a naturally-occurring organophosphate. Some genera, especially *Anabaena*, can produce both neuro- and hepatotoxins. If a toxic algal bloom contains both types of toxins, signs of neurotoxicity are usually observed first. Neurotoxic effects occur within minutes whereas effects due to liver toxins take one to a few hours to appear. Below we describe the freshwater toxins, microcystins, anatoxin-a, cylindrospermopsins and saxitoxins, which currently are monitored in Washington lakes.

6.1. Microcystins

6.1.1. Microcystins

Microcystins are the most thoroughly investigated cyanobacterial toxins [72]. At least 90 structural variants have been identified, and microcystin-LR is the variant most commonly found in cyanobacteria [73–75]. Microcystins have been identified in *Anabaena, Microcystis, Oscillatoria* (*Planktothrix*), *Nostoc* and *Anabaenopsis* species and from the terrestrial genus *Hapalosiphon* [66]. More than one microcystin may be found in a particular cyanobacteria strain. Microcystins are cyclic heptapeptides that primarily affect the liver in animals. A lethal dose of microcystins in vertebrates causes death by liver necrosis within hours or up to a few days. Microcystins block protein phosphatases 1 and 2A (important molecular switches in all eukaryotic cells) using an irreversible covalent bond [76] in [77]. Liver injury is likely to go unnoticed and results in (external) noticeable symptoms only when it is severe [77]. Other studies have shown that microcystin toxicity is cumulative [78]. Researchers suspect microcystins are liver carcinogens, which could increase cancer risk to humans following continuous, low level exposure.

6.1.2. Illness and Symptoms

Symptoms of microcystin poisoning may take 30 min to 24 h to appear, depending upon the size of the animal affected and the amount of toxic bloom consumed. Gross and histopathologic lesions caused by microcystins are quite similar among species, although species sensitivity and signs of poisoning can vary depending on the type of exposure. One of the earliest effects (15–30 min) of microcystin poisoning is increased serum concentration of bile acids, alkaline phosphatase, γ-glutamyltransferase, and aspartate aminotransferase. Microcystin symptoms in mammals and other animals may include jaundice, shock, abdominal pain and distention, weakness, nausea and vomiting, severe thirst, rapid and weak pulse, and death. It is likely that the number of incidents with low-level symptoms such as nausea, vomiting and diarrhea associated with recreational exposure to cyanobacterial toxins are underreported. Death may occur following exposure to very high concentrations within a few hours (usually within 4–24 h) or up to a few days. Death is due to intrahepatic hemorrhage and hypovolemic shock. In animals that survive more than a few hours, hyperkalemia or hypoglycemia, or both, may lead to death from liver failure within a few days [79]. Surviving animals have a good chance for recovery because the toxins have a steep dose-response curve. Activated charcoal oral slurry is likely to benefit exposed animals, even though therapies for cyanobacterial poisonings have not been investigated in detail.

6.1.3. Washington Occurrences

Microcystins are the most abundant cyanotoxins in Washington lakes. From the beginning of 2009 through the end of October 2014, 535 samples (representing 60 waterbodies) were observed with microcystin concentrations >6 µg/L (Figure 3). The number of samples above 6 µg/L each year ranged from 68 to 114 (2009–2013). The distribution of concentrations indicates that the majority of samples fell between 6 and 100 µg/L; 9 samples were above 10,000 µg/L microcystins (Figure 3). Seasonal distribution of microcystin samples with concentrations >6 µg/L illustrates that the number of samples greater than the state's recreational guidance value increases steadily from June through October (Figure 4).

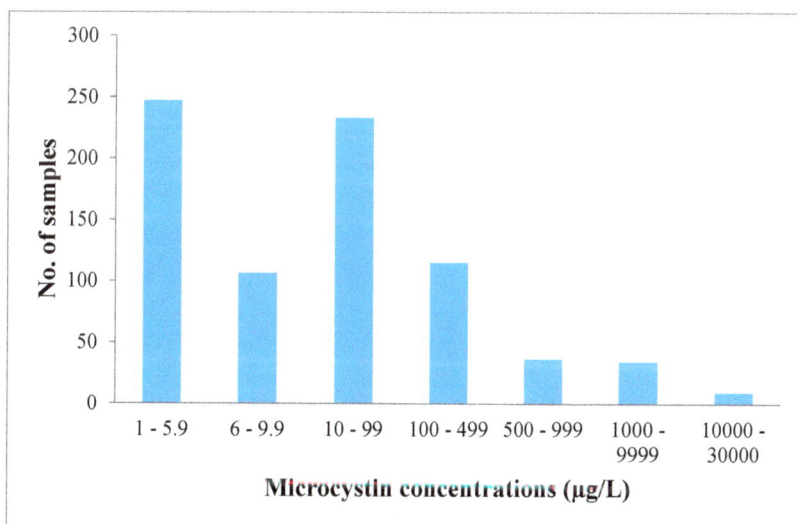

Figure 3. Distribution of the number of samples above 1 µg/L microcystin from 2009 through October 2014.

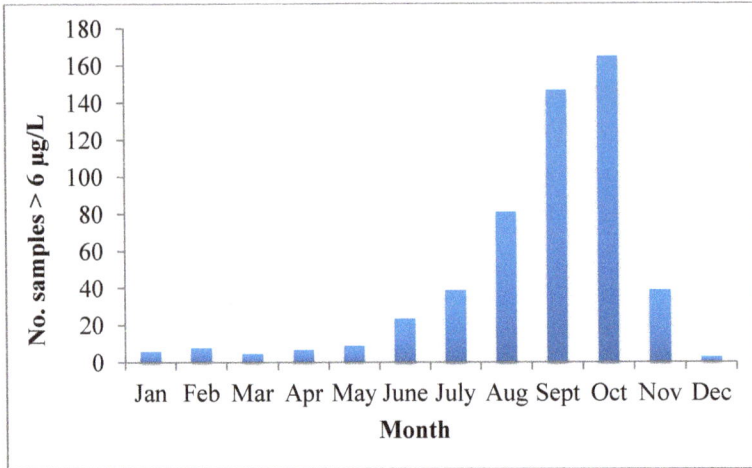

Figure 4. Monthly distribution of the sum of the number of microcystin samples above state recreational guidance value of 6 µg/L from 2009 through October 2014.

6.2. Anatoxin-a

6.2.1. Activity and Source of Anatoxin-a

Anatoxin-a is one of three neurotoxic alkaloids that have been isolated from cyanobacteria [72]. It is produced by various species of cyanobacteria including *Anabaena*, *Planktothrix* (*Oscillatoria*), *Aphanizomenon*, *Cylindrospermum* and *Microcystis* spp. Anatoxin-a was first detected in Canada in the 1960s [80]. Between 1961 and 1975, cattle and dog poisonings associated with *Anabaena flos-aquae* blooms occurred in six locations in Canada. Most anatoxin-a has been detected in Europe. Second to Europe, most reports of anatoxin-a have been in North America [74].

Anatoxin-a is a bicyclic secondary amine. It binds to the nicotinic acetylcholine receptor at the axon terminal at the neuromuscular interface [73,74]. Binding of anatoxin-a is irreversible causing the sodium channel to be locked in an open position, resulting in symptoms in humans including overstimulation, fatigue, and eventual paralysis. In the respiratory system, anatoxin-a exposure results in a lack of oxygen to the brain, subsequent convulsions and death by suffocation. Anatoxin-a is about 20 times more potent than acetylcholine, a compound involved in transmission of nerve impulses [74].

Alkaloid toxins are more likely to be present in free (non-cellular) form in water than the cyclic peptide toxins microcystins and nodularin [77]. While microcystins appear to be more common than freshwater neurotoxins, the latter have caused severe animal poisonings in North America, Europe and Australia [77]. Anatoxin-a degrades readily to nontoxic products upon exposure to sunlight and at a high pH [74]. In natural blooms in eutrophic lakes, the anatoxin-a half-life is typically less than 24 h, while its half-life in the laboratory is about five days [66]. This rapid degradation of anatoxin-a presents problems with determining accurate toxin concentrations associated with exposures. According to Botana [74], samples should be protected from light and acidified prior to storage at −20 °C in order to limit anatoxin-a degradation.

6.2.2. Illness and Symptoms

Neurotoxins are notoriously rapid acting poisons; anatoxin-a was originally called very fast death factor (VFDF) due to its potency [74]. Animal illness and death may occur within a few minutes to a few hours after exposure, depending on the size of the animal and amount of toxic bloom consumed. An animal with anatoxin-a toxicosis may exhibit staggering, paralysis, muscle twitching, gasping, convulsions, backward arching of neck (in birds), and death. Livestock that drink large amounts of contaminated water and pets that lick scum on their fur are at highest risk from anatoxin-a exposure. While anatoxin-a is largely retained within cells when conditions for growth are favorable, toxins will be liberated in the gastrointestinal tract if water containing toxic cells is consumed [66,74]. However, ingestion of a sublethal dose of these neurotoxins leaves no chronic effects and recovery appears to be complete with no ongoing injury [77]. Exposure leaves no sign of organ damage and residual toxin is rapidly degraded [74].

The first report of an animal illness in Washington due to a freshwater toxic bloom occurred in 1976 in Spokane County [7]. Four dogs died after drinking water during a toxic *Anabaena* bloom and an additional seven dogs, one horse, and one cow were reportedly sickened [81]. In the 1980s, another two hunting dogs died in eastern Washington, and five cats died during a toxic *Anabaena* bloom in American Lake, Pierce County. More recently, two dogs died after exposure to a toxic *Anabaena* bloom in Anderson Lake (2006), and two hunting dogs died in the Potholes Reservoir after exposure to a toxic bloom (2007). Each year roughly 4–5 reports of animal illness (including cats, dogs, cows, elk, and horses) are investigated, with approximately 2 probable or confirmed cases per year. Outreach and education efforts such as posting signs at lakes with confirmed toxicity began in 2009 and are thought to have decreased pet exposures in lakes with blooms [82].

6.2.3. Washington Occurrences

Three state waterbodies have long-term reoccurring anatoxin-a blooms with unique seasonal patterns [8]. For example, Clear Lake, Pierce County, exhibited blooms three years in a row that became toxic in late fall and continued through the winter (maximum 1170 µg/L anatoxin-a). Testing of Anderson Lake, Jefferson County, from 2009 to 2014 showed reoccurring blooms that began in April, May, or June in most years and continued through August, September, or October (maximum 1090 µg/L anatoxin-a, June 2011; Figures 2 and 5). Rufus Woods Lake, a reservoir behind Chief Joseph Dam on the Columbia River (for locations, see Figure 2), also has reoccurring blooms producing anatoxin-a with a unique seasonal pattern: July and August 2011; July, August, September 2012; May through September in 2013; and May through July in 2014 (maximum 110 µg/L anatoxin-a, July 2012).

Seasonal distribution of anatoxin-a concentrations above 1.0 µg/L was determined for 11 other state lakes and reservoirs. Levels above the state recreational guidance value were observed during each month of the year at various sites around the state. Ten lakes produced only one to three samples with anatoxin-a above 1.0 µg/L (maximum 592 µg/L). Most short-term blooms occurred in September, October, November or December.

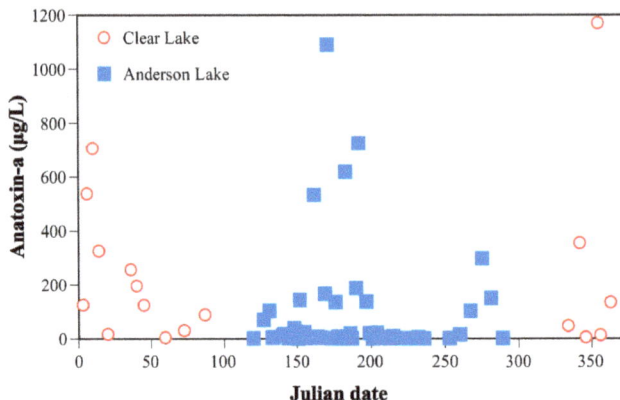

Figure 5. Seasonal distribution of anatoxin-a concentrations above 1 µg/L in Clear and Anderson Lakes.

6.3. Cylindrospermopsin

6.3.1. Activity and Source of Cylindrospermopsin

Cylindrospermopsin is comprised of a tricyclic guanidine moiety combined with a hydroxymethyl uracil. Production of the toxin is strain- not species-specific [83]. Cylindrospermopsin exhibits a completely different mechanism of toxicity than the liver toxin microcystin [84–86]. Damage to cells is caused by blockage of key protein and enzyme functions, thereby inhibiting protein synthesis. Cylindrospermopsin targets the liver and kidneys but can also injure the lung, spleen, thymus, and heart as demonstrated in mouse studies [66,72,87,88]. Animal toxicity studies also suggest that cylindrospermopsin may be carcinogenic [72,89] and may produce genotoxicity in a human lymphoblastoid cell line [90]. Laboratory studies have shown that some of the compounds produced by *Cylindrospermopsis* may be carcinogenic and genotoxic [83,90–93]

Cylindrospermopsin is found in certain strains of five genera: *Cylindrospermopsis raciborskii* (Australia, Hungary, and the U.S.), *Umezakia natans* (Japan), *Anabaena bergii* and *Raphidiopsis curvata* [94], and *Aphanizomenon ovalisporum* (Australia, Israel) [95]. It is most commonly observed in tropical and subtropical waters of Australia [83]. The first report of animal poisonings attributed to cylindrospermopsin was in drinking water in a farm pond in Queensland, Australia, where it was responsible for cattle deaths [96]. Further, *Cylindrospermopsis raciborskii* was implicated in one of the most significant cases of human poisoning from exposure to a cyanobacterial toxin in 1979 on Palm Island, northern Queensland, Australia. Generally, toxins are retained in cyanobacterial cells when conditions are favorable; however studies have shown that it is not uncommon for 70%–98% of total cylindrospermopsin produced by cells to be dissolved in the water [83,97].

6.3.2. Illness and Symptoms

Symptoms of exposure to cylindrospermopsin include nausea, vomiting, diarrhea, abdominal tenderness, pain, and acute liver failure. Clinical symptoms after exposure to cylindrospermopsin may not appear immediately but may occur several days later. Thus, it is often difficult to determine a cause-effect relationship between cylindrospermopsin exposure and symptoms.

The degree of the cyanotoxin impact for cylindrospermopsin and other cyanotoxins is influenced by animal size, species sensitivity, and individual sensitivity. According to the Merck Veterinary Manual, animals may need to ingest only a few ounces or up to several gallons to experience acute or lethal toxicity, depending on bloom densities and toxin content [79]. After removal from the contaminated water supply, affected animals should be placed in a protected area out of direct sunlight. The animal should have access to an unrestricted supply of clean water and good quality feed. Surviving animals have a good chance for recovery because both hepatotoxins and neurotoxins have a steep dose-response curve. Although no therapeutic antagonist has been found to be effective against cylindrospermopsin, activated charcoal oral slurry is likely to benefit exposed animals. An ion-exchange resin such as cholestyramine has proved useful to absorb the toxins from the gastrointestinal tract [79].

6.3.3. Washington Occurrences

The state's passive surveillance effort and monitoring results from the CDC 30-lake study show that cylindrospermopsins have been found in only six Washington lakes at very low concentrations. No results were above the state recreational guidance value of 4.5 µg/L cylindrospermopsins, with concentrations above the minimum detection level (MDL; 0.10 µg/L) ranging from 0.11 to 1.12 µg/L.

6.4. Saxitoxins

6.4.1. Source of Freshwater Saxitoxins

Saxitoxins are found in both marine and freshwater systems and have been observed in numerous lakes around the world. Their toxicity has been described in detail, above. Cyanobacteria genera that are documented as producing saxitoxin include *Aphanizomenon sp.* (U.S.); *Aphanizomenon gracile, Aphanizomenon issatschenkoi, and Aphanizomenon flos-aqua* (Europe); *Anabaena circinalis* (Australia); *Anabaena lemmermannii* (Denmark); *Lyngbya wollei* (U.S.); *Cylindrospermopsis* (Brazil); and *Planktothrix* (Italy) [21,98–100].

6.4.2. Washington Occurrences

Since 2009, saxitoxins have been detected in ten state lakes and one pond. Waughop Lake was the only waterbody with multiple samples higher than the MDL (0.020 µg/L), one of which was above the state recreational guidance value of 75 µg/L (193 µg/L, August 2009). Saxitoxin concentrations in the other lakes and pond ranged from 0.021 to 71.0 µg/L. With the exception of Waughop Lake (Figure 2), saxitoxins do not occur at levels of human health concern.

7. Washington Lakes: Three-Tiered Approach to Managing Lakes with Cyanobacterial Blooms

DOH recommends a three-tiered approach for managing toxic or potentially toxic cyanobacterial blooms. The approach applies recreational guidance values derived by DOH for managing Washington lakes (Table 1). Observers look for developing blooms and surface accumulations that can occur in any nutrient-rich water such as lakes, ponds, or river embayments. Upon notification of a potential bloom, the LHJ or other agency staff (or lake resident) will: (1) obtain a sample number from the state Freshwater Algae website [8], (2) sample the water body experiencing the bloom, then (3) send the sample to the laboratory for toxicity tests. Sampling and shipping directions are available at the website [8] or from Ecology's Freshwater Algae Control Program [101].

At present the KCEL is under contract with Ecology to test for microcystins, anatoxin-a, cylindrospermopsin, and saxitoxin. Results of toxicity analyses are incorporated into the Freshwater Algae website as they are received from the laboratory. In Washington, local jurisdictions have the authority to post advisories on water bodies within their districts (RCW 70.05.070) and actions taken such as posting or closing a lake based on toxicity results are published on the website and on Ecology's list serve.

Tier I

A sample of a visible cyanobacteria bloom or scum is sent for phytoplankton examination and toxicity testing. If the sample is dominated by potentially toxic cyanobacteria, the LHJ should post a CAUTION sign (Figures 6 and 7). Given the tremendous spatial and temporal variability in toxin concentrations, LHJs are encouraged to factor in the spatial extent of the bloom when deciding if a warning level or closed level advisory is warranted.

Tier II

When recreational guidance values for microcystin, anatoxin-a, cylindrospermopsin and/or saxitoxin are exceeded (Table 1), the LHJ posts a WARNING sign (Figures 6 and 7). The lake is sampled weekly, because toxin levels may be variable, e.g., they may be at their highest during bloom die-offs even though the water looks "normal" or may be significantly lower due to temporary changes in weather such as heavy wind and/or intense rainfall which could redistribute cyanobacteria throughout the lake and throughout the water column with little change in the total number of cyanobacteria cells. This makes assessment of bloom density quite difficult. Therefore, DOH recommends that LHJs not lift advisories unless they check the lake under weather conditions that are conducive to biomass accumulation (relatively calm or a light steady wind and little or no rainfall).

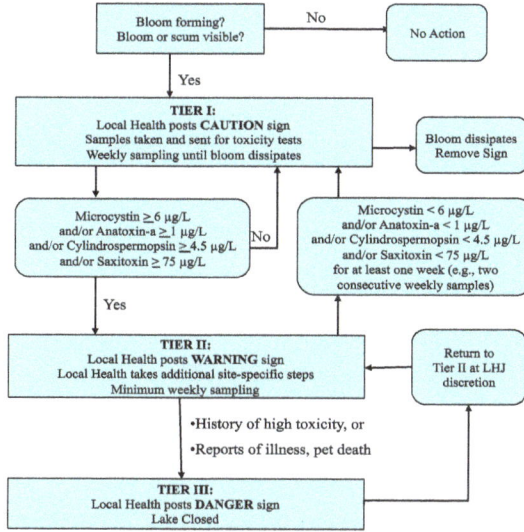

Figure 6. Three... ...periencing cyanobacterial bl

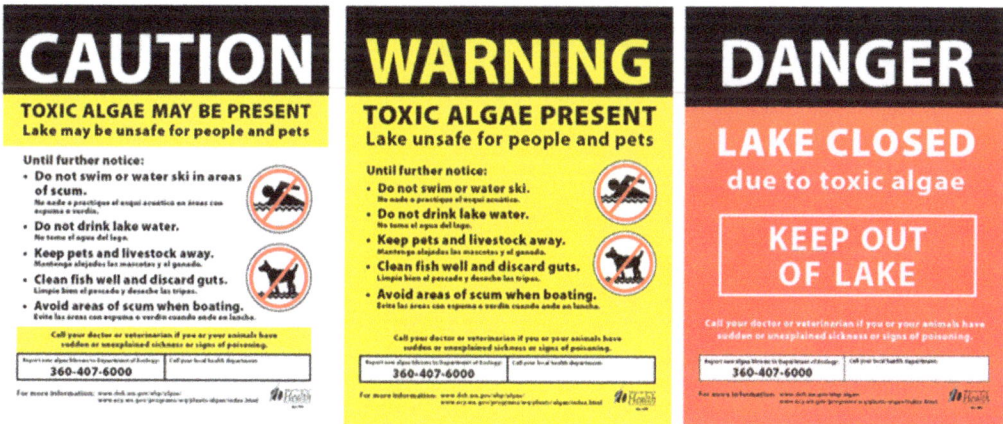

Figure 7. Advisory signs used in Washington's Freshwater Algae Control Program.

Additional steps can be taken to communicate risk (*i.e.*, press release, notification of veterinarians and fish and wildlife officials) depending on severity of the bloom, time of year, and historical use of the lake (*i.e.*, a highly used access point such as a dog park might warrant greater outreach efforts as compared with a lake not known for any recreational activity). In certain situations, some LHJs have mailed notifications to local lakefront residents after confirmation of cyanobacterial toxicity. Other possible measures that have been used to reach lakefront residents include radio messages or the internet via a list serve or "blast" email.

Tier III

Under certain circumstances, a LHJ may close a lake with unusually high microcystin, anatoxin-a, cylindrospermopsin, or saxitoxin concentrations. At the discretion of the LHJ, a water body can be posted as DANGER—Closed (Figures 6 and 7). Examples include:

- Very dense blooms covering an entire lake
- Confirmed pet illnesses or death
- Reported human illness

The LHJ will post a press release to notify the general public of a lake closure. Also, LHJs follow whatever additional methods of outreach, including those listed under Tier II, that best inform public beach users and lake front residents of the risks from cyanotoxins and how to avoid these risks. Retraction of lake closures is also at the discretion of the LHJ. DOH recommends posting a WARNING sign and following Tier II recommendations after retracting a lake closure until microcystin levels are less than the recreational guidance levels (Figure 2).

8. Human Illnesses Associated with Freshwater HABs

Human illness reports following HAB exposure are investigated; however, definitions of suspected, probable, or confirmed human illnesses have changed over time making quantitative reporting problematic. Symptoms following exposure are similar but criteria for illness reporting have changed. At present, the CDC is working on case definitions for national consistency in reporting human illnesses following HAB exposure with the realization that underreporting likely is an issue. Acknowledging these shortcomings, DOH reported 2–4 human illness investigations per year for 2010–2013, with a high of 122 human investigations in 2009, a year with unusually high temperatures during late July–early August.

The risk of illness due to exposure to toxins in freshwater will be reduced through more extensive communication and outreach. To that end, Washington has a database of freshwater toxicity data available for the public to access via the web ([8]; Supplementary Figure 1). Toxicity results can be searched and retrieved by lake, county, water resource inventory area, and toxin with defined concentrations and dates (e.g., Figure 2).

9. Future Threats, Needs and Recommendations

Although our understanding of toxic blooms in marine waters and state lakes is improving each year, many questions remain. Below is a list of suggested topics recommended for future work on freshwater and marine HABs in Washington.

- Lake and reservoir HABs in Washington pose a potential new public health threat from exposure via drinking water. In 2014, a 500 household community used untreated drinking water from a lake during a period when anatoxin-a concentrations were low but still above state recreational guidelines; no illnesses were reported. In another case, the drinking water source for Friday Harbor, an island town, had a toxic bloom that resulted in the need to import water for the community. Future efforts will be needed to improve testing in lakes used as drinking water sources and to coordinate with drinking water managers of surface water systems that may develop toxic blooms.

• The additive toxicity of co-occurring blooms in lakes and marine waters must be studied. Further, as microcystin variants become easier to identify and quantify, toxicologists will need to determine actual toxicities to improve upon the current assumption for public health guidance that all toxin variants are equally potent. In the future, our state will adopt national recreational values for freshwater cyanotoxins following EPA guideline development. CDC and the states are collaborating on an enhanced National Outbreak Reporting System that will fill the current gap at the state level for tracking animal and human health illness events.

• The impact of climate change on marine HABs and cyanobacteria is also a subject that needs to be addressed. Cyanobacteria and some marine HABs favor warm temperatures and other environmental conditions such as increased nutrient inputs from land that will be associated with climate change. If long-term climate projections for the Pacific Northwest are correct, rain events will increase, which may influence nutrient runoff from impervious surfaces, particularly as land is developed and regional populations increase.

• Washington has an effective Freshwater Algae Control Program based on passive surveillance, legislatively funded toxicity tests, and established cooperation between state agencies and local health jurisdictions. The state's 39 counties (35 local health jurisdictions) have a range of staff and resources available for water surveillance and sampling. Therefore, this program, together with the marine biotoxin monitoring program, will require continued and repeated outreach efforts to local health jurisdictions regarding blooms, toxicity testing, and toxicity postings. Thus, periodic seminars and webinars will be needed to ensure all areas of the state are aware of the program and knowledgeable about state-level technical support.

• Outreach efforts on marine and freshwater HABs have met some needs but other educational needs remain unmet. Outreach to veterinary clinics regarding differential diagnoses and distribution of posters for pet owner education has been effective in the state. Annual outreach to the public and to hunters owning dogs will need to continue. More recently, DOH has included outreach to drinking water operators about available toxicity tests, bloom identification, and options for treatment when blooms occur. However, a major outreach and education gap in the state is for physicians who treat those exposed to toxic marine and freshwater blooms.

• Standardized and consistent posting at lakes and shellfish harvesting beaches experiencing toxic blooms is essential for public health protection. Some local health jurisdictions have raised concerns about over-posting, which can lead to the public ignoring CAUTION and WARNING signs, and under-posting, which may not be protective of public health. Since blooms in lakes and marine waters are notoriously patchy, some areas of a lake may be below recreational standards while high toxicity scums in smaller areas remain a health threat. We recommend that managers, local health professionals, and state staff work together to refine outreach and offer additional posting options to reflect more complicated local conditions.

• Recommendations for future work include ongoing collaborative work investigating the link of freshwater toxins with marine bivalve bioaccumulation of toxins. Further investigation of HAB genetics may help explain why some blooms are toxic and others are not. Another recommended effort is to investigate if satellite imagery using smaller pixels can identify lakes with dominant cyanobacteria that are not under current surveillance.

10. Overall Summary and Conclusions

The integration of phytoplankton monitoring into regulatory programs to ensure shellfish safety has been promoted by European countries for many years and should be encouraged throughout the U.S., in particular in those states, such as Alaska, where regulatory monitoring of vast coastlines is challenging [102]. In some regions of the U.S., including Florida, cell counts of harmful algae are used together with satellite imagery and automated environmental observations to provide early warning of the development and movement of *Karenia brevis* blooms in the Gulf of Mexico [103]. Currently, each European state monitors marine HAB species in addition to toxins in shellfish along the Atlantic coastline. These data are interpreted and incorporated by each national monitoring program into national forecast bulletins that were developed during the program, Applied Simulations and Integrated Modeling for the Understanding of Toxic and Harmful Algal Blooms (ASIMUTH) project, as a demonstration of a downstream service [104].

For freshwater HABs, each state has developed a unique approach for monitoring and regulating toxic blooms. The most extensive effort is in Florida, where the Florida Department of Health (FDOH) has developed the Harmful Algal Bloom Online Tracking Module, which allows public health professionals and environmental scientists/managers to collaborate on cyanobacteria bloom reporting through a secure web-based data management system, hosted in *Caspio.* There are currently 86 users from 18 different organizations utilizing the system. Other examples of states integrating monitoring into regulatory programs include Oregon's collaboration with the State Drinking Water Program and an effective emphasis on education and outreach; Massachusett's collection of bloom data to serve as guidance for local health officials; New York's collaboration with the Citizen Statewide Lake Assessment Program; Wisconsin's interactive website for incident reporting by citizens and local health departments and strong partnerships with WI Department of Natural Resources and poison control centers; Maryland, Virginia, and South Carolina's integration of freshwater and marine HAB monitoring and tracking of blooms; and Iowa's effective partnership between health and natural resource departments. Such programs provide an effective interface between formalized state and federal programs while observations by trained citizen volunteers offer the best possible early warning systems for surveillance of known HABs as well as for the reporting and diagnosis of unusual events that may impact the future health of oceans, lakes and humans.

The vision for the future includes interfacing current monitoring and management programs with efforts in basic research and model development to develop forecasting systems for marine and freshwater HABs. Early warning networks will monitor changes in the abundance and location of toxic blooms using an integrated suite of sensors on satellites and stationary sensor platforms that together can measure ocean water properties including temperature, current speed and direction, chlorophyll, cell species and abundance, and toxins. Data will be telemetered and incorporated with real-time shore-based monitoring. An example of a remote sensing technology is the automated molecular detection and quantification of cells and toxins, using the environmental sample platform (ESP; e.g., [105–108]), which recently has been funded for deployment in the Pacific Northwest as part of the Integrated Ocean Observing System [109]. Rapidly-accessed data from remote platforms will be used to calibrate and fine-tune physical and biological models and HAB forecasts. One such forecasting bulletin for the Washington State coast is in its pilot stage [110]. These models and forecasts will allow shellfish managers and early warning programs to take preventive actions (such as increasing monitoring efforts, closing targeted shellfish beds, and warning at-risk communities) to safeguard public health, local economies and fisheries. In addition, some proactive management will be facilitated, e.g., early opening of the shellfish harvesting seasons or early posting of toxin threats to recreational users of lakes. A combination of technologies, from volunteer-based phytoplankton monitoring programs, to state and federal regulatory analysis of toxins in shellfish and drinking water, to the newest remote sensing technologies, will provide the most comprehensive system for the protection of public health from documented marine and freshwater HABs as well as new and emerging biotoxins in Washington State.

Supplementary Materials

Supplementary materials can be accessed at: http://www.mdpi.com/2072-6651/7/4/1206/s1.

Acknowledgments

We thank Nick Adams, NOAA Northwest Fisheries Science Center for assistance with the figures, and Jerry Borchert, DOH, Office of Shellfish and Water Protection for help with Table 2. We also thank Kathy Hamel and Lizbeth Seebacher, Washington State Department of Ecology for their ongoing support.

Author Contributions

Both authors contributed equally in the writing of this paper.

Conflict of Interest

The authors declare no conflict of interest.

Disclaimer

The contents of this article are solely the responsibility of the authors and do not necessarily represent the official views or policies of the Washington State Department of Health.

References

1. Puget Sound Action Team. *Puget Sound Water Quality Work Plan*; Puget Sound Water Quality Action Team: Olympia, WA, USA, 2003.
2. Jacobs, J. *Shellfish Safety Report*; Washington State Department of Health: Olympia, WA, USA, 2002.
3. Borchert, J. (Washington State Department of Health, Olympia, WA). Personal communication; 28 January 2015.

4. Trainer, V.L.; Moore, L.; Bill, B.D.; Adams, N.G.; Harrington, N.; Borchert, J.; da Silva, D.A.M.; Eberhart, B.-T.L. Diarrhetic Shellfish toxins and other lipophilic toxins of human health concern in Washington State. *Mar. Drugs* **2013**, *11*, 1815–1835.

5. Hilborn, E.D.; Roberts, V.A.; Backer, L.; DeConno, E.; Egan, J.S.; Hyde, J.B.; Nicholas, D.C.; Wiegert, E.J.; Billing, L.M.; DiOrio, M.; *et al.* Algal bloom-associated disease outbreaks among users of freshwater lakes—United States, 2009–2010. *Morb. Mortal. Wkly. Rep.* **2014**, *63*, 11–15.

6. Backer, L.C.; Landsberg, J.H.; Miller, M.; Keel, K.; Taylor, T.K. Canine cyanotoxin poisonings in the United States (1920s–2012): Review of suspected and confirmed cases from three data sources. *Toxins* **2013**, *5*, 1597–1628.

7. Washington State Toxic Algae, Freshwater Algae Bloom Monitoring Program. Available online: http://www.NWToxicalgae.org (accessed on 9 February 2015).

8. Johnson, A.; Friese, M.; Coots, R. *Microcystins and Other Blue-Green Algae Toxins Analyzed in Fish and Sediment from Washington Lakes*; Washington State Department of Ecology: Olympia, WA, USA, 2013.

9. Preece, E.; Moore, B.; Hardy, F.J.; Deobold, L. First detection of microcystin in Puget Sound, Washington, mussels (*Mytlilus trossulus*). *Lake Reserv. Manag.* **2015**, *31*, 50–54.

10. Lefebvre, K.A.; Bill, B.D.; Erickson, A.; Baugh, K.A.; O'Rourke, L.; Costa, P.R.; Nance, S.; Trainer, V.L. Characterization of intracellular and extracellular saxitoxin levels in both field and cultured *Alexandrium* spp. samples from Sequim Bay, Washington. *Mar. Drugs* **2008**, *6*, 103–116.

11. Trainer, V.L.; Suddleson, M. Approaches for early warning of domoic acid events in Washington State. *Oceanography* **2005**, *18*, 228–237.

12. Trainer, V.L.; Moore, L.; Bill, B.D.; Adams, N.G.; Harrington, N.; Borchert, J.; da Silva, D.A.M.; Eberhart, B.-T. Diarrhetic shellfish toxins and other lipophilic toxins of human health concern in Washington State. *Mar. Drugs* **2013**, *11*, 1815–1835.

13. Lilja, J. *Shellfish Control Program*; Food and Housing Section, Health Services Division, Department of Social and Health Services: Olympia, WA, USA, 1978.

14. Marine Biotoxin Bulletin. Available online: http://www.doh.wa.gov/ehp/sf/biotoxin.htm (accessed on 29 December 2014).

15. Nishitani, L. *Suggestions for the Washington PSP Monitoring Program and PSP Research*; DOH Office of Shellfish Programs: Olympia, WA, USA, 1990; p. 12.

16. American Public Health Association (APHA). *Laboratory Procedures for the Examination of Seawater and Shellfish*; APHA: Washington, DC, USA, 1984.

17. Araoz, R.; Molgo, J.; Tandeau de Marsac, N. Neurotoxic cyanobacterial toxins. *Toxicon* **2010**, *56*, 813–828.

18. Kao, C. Tetrodotoxin, saxitoxin and their significance in the study of excitation phenomena. *Pharmacol. Rev.* **1966**, *18*, 997–1049.

19. Narahashi, T.; Moore, J.W. Neuroactive agents and nerve membrane conductances. *J. Gen. Physiol.* **1968**, *51*, 93–101.

20. Van Apeldoorn, M.E.; van Egmond, H.P.; Speijers, G.J.A.; Bakker, G.J.I. Toxins of cyanobacteria. *Mol. Nutr. Food Res.* **2007**, *51*, 7–60.

21. Jones, G.J.; Negri, A.P. Persistence and degradation of cyanobacterial paralytic shellfish poisons (PSPs) in freshwaters. *Water Res.* **1997**, *31*, 525–533.

22. Horner, R.A.; Garrison, D.L.; Plumley, F.G. Harmful algal blooms and red tide problems on the U.S. west coast. *Limnol. Oceanogr.* **1997**, *42*, 1076–1088.

23. John, U.; Litaker, R.W.; Montresor, M.; Murray, S.; Brosnahan, M.; Anderson, D.M. Proposal to reject the name *Gonyaulax* (*Alexandrium catenella*) (Dinphyceae). *Taxon* **2014**, *63*, 932–933.

24. Wang, J.; Zhuang, Y.; Zhang, H.; Lin, X.; Lin, S. DNA barcoding species in *Alexandrium tamarense* complex using ITS and proposing designation of five species. *Harmful Algae* **2014**, *31*, 100–113.

25. Centers for Disease Control and Prevention. Available online: http://www.bt.cdc.gov/ agent/saxitoxin/casedef.asp (accessed on 9 February 2015).

26. Fleming, L.E. Paralytic Shellfish Poisoning. Available online: http://www.whoi.edu/science/B/ redtide/illness/psp.html (accessed on 17 March 2015).

27. Halstead, B. *Poisonous and Venomous Marine Animals of the World*; Darwin Press: Princeton, NJ, USA, 1988.

28. Kao, C. Paralytic shellfish posioning. In *Algal Toxins in Seafood and Drinking Water*; Falconer, I.R., Ed.; Academic Press: London, UK, 1993; pp. 75–86.

29. Nishitani, L.; Chew, K. PSP toxins in the Pacific coast states: Monitoring programs and effects on bivalve industries. *J. Shellfish Res.* **1988**, *7*, 653–669.

30. Waldichuk, M. Shellfish toxicity and the weather in the Strait of Georgia during 1957. *Fish Res. Board. Can.* **1958**, *112*, 10–14.

31. Erickson, G.; Nishitani, L. The possible relationship of El Niño/southern oscillation events to interannual variation in *Gonyaulax* populations as shown by records of shellfish toxicity. In *Seattle: El Niño North*; Wooster, W., Fluharty, D., Eds.; Washington Sea Grant Program: Seattle, WA, USA, 1985; pp. 283–289.

32. Trainer, V.L.; Eberhart, B.T.L.; Wekell, J.C.; Adams, N.G.; Hanson, L.; Cox, F.; Dowell, J. Paralytic shellfish toxins in Puget Sound, Washington State. *J. Shellfish Res.* **2003**, *22*, 213–223.

33. Moore, S.K.; Mantua, N.J.; Hickey, B.M.; Trainer, V.L. Recent trends in paralytic shellfish toxins in Puget Sound, relationships to climate, and capacity for prediction of toxic events. *Harmful Algae* **2009**, *8*, 463–477.

34. Bates, S.S.; Trainer, V.L. The ecology of harmful diatoms. In *Ecology of Harmful Algae*; Graneli, E., Turner, J.W., Eds.; Springer Verlag: Heidelberg, Germany, 2006; pp. 81–93.

35. Bejarano, A.C.; VanDola, F.M.; Gulland, F.M.; Rowles, T.K.; Schwacke, L.H. Production and toxicity of the marine biotoxin domoic acid and its effects on wildlife: A review. *Hum. Ecol. Risk Assess.* **2008**, *14*, 544–567.

36. Trainer, V.L.; Hickey, B.M.; Bates, S.S. Toxic diatoms. In *Oceans and Human Health: Risks and Remedies from the Sea*; Walsh, P., Smith, S., Fleming, L.E., Solo-Gabriele, H., Gerwick, W., Eds.; Elsevier Science: New York, NY, USA, 2008; pp. 219–237.

37. Trainer, V.L.; Bates, S.S.; Lundholm, N.; Thessen, A.E.; Cochlan, W.P.; Adams, N.G.; Trick, C.G. *Pseudo-nitzschia* physiological ecology, phylogeny, toxicity, monitoring and impacts on ecosystem health. *Harmful Algae* **2012**, *14*, 271–300.

38. Lelong, A.; Hégaret, H.; Soudant, P.; Bates, S.S. *Pseudo-nitzschia* (Bacillariophyceae) species, domoic acid and amnesic shellfish poisoning: Revisiting previous paradigms. *Phycologia* **2012**, *51*, 168–216.

39. Perl, T.M.; BÈdard, L.; Kosatsky, T.; Hockin, J.C.; Todd, E.C.; Remis, R.S. An outbreak of toxic encephalopathy caused by eating mussels contaminated with domoic acid. *N. Engl. J. Med.* **1990**, *322*, 1775–1780.

40. Horner, R.A.; Kusske, M.B.; Moynihan, B.P.; Skinner, R.N.; Wekell, J.C. Retention of domoic acid by Pacific razor clams, *Siliqua patula* (Dixon, 1789): Preliminary study. *J. Shellfish Res.* **1993**, *12*, 451–456.

41. Horner, R.A.; Postel, J.R. Toxic diatoms in western Washington waters (US west coast). *Hydrobiologia* **1993**, *269*, 197–205.

42. Wekell, J.C.; Gauglitz, E., Jr.; Barnett, H.J.; Hatfield, C.L.; Simons, D.; Ayres, D. Occurrence of domoic acid in Washington State razor clams (*Siliqua patula*) during 1991–1993. *Nat. Toxins* **1994**, *2*, 197–205.

43. Trainer, V.L.; Bill, B.D. Characterization of a domoic acid binding site from Pacific razor clam. *Aquat. Toxicol.* **2004**, *69*, 125–132.

44. Bill, B.D.; Cox, F.H.; Horner, R.A.; Borchert, J.A.; Trainer, V.L. The first closure of shellfish harvesting due to domoic acid in Puget Sound, Washington, USA. *Afr. J. Mar. Sci.* **2006**, *28*, 435–440.

45. Takai, A.; Bialojan, C.; Troschka, M.; Ruegg, J.C. Smooth-muscle myosin phosphate inhibition and force enhancement by black sponge toxin. *FEBS Lett.* **1987**, *217*, 81–84.

46. Fujiki, H.; Suganuma, M. Tumor promotion by inhibitors of protein phosphatase-1 and phosphatase-2A—The okadaic acid class of compounds. *Adv. Cancer Res.* **1993**, *61*, 143–194.

47. Burgess, V.; Shaw, G. Pectenotoxins—An issue for public health—A review of their comparative toxicology and metabolism. *Environ. Int.* **2001**, *27*, 275–283.

48. Tereo, K.; Ito, E.; Yasumoto, T.; Yamaguchi, K. *Hepatotoxic and Immunotoxic Effects of Dinoflagellate Toxins on Mice*; Elsevier Science Publishing Co., Inc: New York, NY, USA, 1990.

49. Draisci, R.; Lucentini, L.; Mascioni, A. Pectenotoxins and yessotoxins: Chemistry, toxicology, pharmacology, and analysis. In *Seafood and Freshwater Toxins: Pharmacology, Physiology, and Detection*; Botana, L., Ed.; Marcel Dekker, Inc.: New York, NY, USA, 2000; pp. 289–324.

50. Satake, M.; Ofuji, K.; James, K.J.; Furey, A.; Yasumoto, T. New toxic event caused by Irish mussels. In *Harmful Algae*; Reguera, B., Blanco, J., Fernandez, M.L., Wyatt, T., Eds.; Xunta de Galicia and Intergovernmental Oceanographic Commission of UNESCO: Santiago de Compostela, Spain, 1998; pp. 468–469.

51. Van Egmond, H.P.; van Apeldoorn, M.E.; Speijers, G.J.A. *Marine Biotoxins*; Food and Nutrition Paper 80; FAO: Rome, Italy, 2004; pp. 53–96.

52. Heymann, D.L. *Control of Communicable Diseases Manual*; 19th ed.; American Public Health Association Press: Washington, DC, USA, 2008.

53. Cembella, A.D. Occurrence of okadaic acid, a major diarrhetic shellfish toxin, in natural populations of *Dinophysis* spp. from the eastern coast of North America. *J. Appl. Phycol.* **1989**, *1*, 307–310.

54. Barceloux, D.G. Diarrhetic shellfish poisoning and okadaic acid. In *Medical Toxicology of Natural Substances: Foods, Fungi, Medicinal Herbs, Plants, and Venomous Animals*; John Wiley & Sons: Hoboken, NJ, USA, 2008; pp. 222–226.

55. Taylor, M.; McIntyre, L.; Ritson, M.; Stone, J.; Bronson, R.; Bitzikos, O.; Rourke, W.; Galanis, E.; Outbreak Investigation, T. Outbreak of diarrhetic shellfish poisoning associated with mussels, British Columbia, Canada. *Mar. Drugs* **2013**, *11*, 1669–1676.

56. Felsing, W., Jr. *Proceedings of a Joint Seminar on North Pacific Clams*; US Public Health Service: Washington, DC, USA, 1966.

57. Quayle, D. Paralytic shellfish poisoning in British Columbia. In *Fish Res Bd Canada Bull*; Fisheries Research Board of Canada: Ottawa, ON, Canada, 1969; p. 168.

58. Prakash, A.; Medcof, J.C.; Tennant, A.D. *Paralytic Shellfish Poisoning in Eastern Canada*; Fisheries Research Board of Canada: Ottawa, ON, Canada, 1971; p. 98.

59. SoundToxins.org. Available online: http://www.soundtoxins.org (accessed on 7 April 2015).

60. Eberhart, B.-T.L.; Moore, L.K.; Harrington, N.; Adams, N.G.; Borchert, J.; Trainer, V.L. Screening tests for the rapid detection of diarrhetic shellfish toxins in Washington State. *Mar. Drugs* **2013**, *11*, 3718–3734.

61. Department of Health. *Washington State Recreational Guidance for Microcystins (Provisional) and Anatoxin-a (Interim/Provisional)*; Department of Health: Olympia, WA, USA, 2008; p. 19.

62. Department of Health. *Washington State Provisional Recreational Guidance for Cylindrospermopsin and Saxitoxin*; Department of Health: Olympia, WA, USA, 2011; p. 36.

63. Stone, D.; Bress, W. Addressing public health risks for cyanobacteria in recreational freshwaters: The Oregon and Vermont framework. *Integr. Environ. Assess. Manag.* **2007**, *3*, 137–143.

64. Farrer, D.; Counter, M.; Hillwig, R.; Cude, C. Health-based cyanotoxin guideline values allow for cyanotoxin-based monitoring and efficient public health response to cyanobacterial blooms. *Toxins* **2015**, *7*, 457–477.

65. WHO. *Toxic Cyanobacteria in Water: A Guide to their Public Health Consequences, Monitoring and Management*; Taylor and Francis: New York, NY, USA, 1999; Volume I, p. 416.

66. EFSA. Scientific opinion of the panel on contaminants in the food chain on a request from the european commission on marine biotoxins in shellfish—Domoic acid. *Eur. Food Saf. Auth. J.* **2009**, *1181*, 1–61.

67. Fawell, J.; Mitchell, R.; Hill, R.; Everett, D. The toxicity of cyanobacterial toxins in the mouse: II Anatoxin-a. *Hum. Exp. Toxicol.* **1999**, *18*, 168–173.

68. Department of Ecology. *Freshwater Algae Control Program*; Report to the Washington State Legislature (2008–2009); Department of Ecology: Olymnia, WA, USA, 2009.

69. Carey, C.C.; Haney, J.F.; Cottingham, K.L. First report of microcystin-LR in the cyanobacterium *Gloeotrichia echinulata*. *Environ. Toxicol.* **2007**, *22*, 337–339.

70. Graham, J.; Loftin, K.; Ziegler, A.; Meyer, M. *Guidelines for Design and Sampling for Cyanobacterial Toxins and Taste-and-Odor Studies in Lakes and Reservoirs*; U.S. Department of the Interior U.S. Geological Survey: Reston, VI, USA, 2008.

71. Falconer, I.R. *Cyanobacterial Toxins of Drinking Water Supplies: Cylindrospermopsins and Microcystins*; CRC Press: Boca Raton, FL, USA, 2005.

72. Huisman, J.; Matthijs, H.; Visser, P. *Harmful Cyanobacteria*; Springer: Dordrecht, The Netherlands, 2005; p. 241.

73. Botana, L. *Phycotoxins: Chemistry and Biology*; Blackwell Publishing: Hoboken, NJ, USA, 2007; p. 345.

74. Welker, M.; von Dohren, H. Cyanobacterial peptides—Nature's own combinatorial biosynthesis. *FEMS Microbiol. Rev.* **2006**, *30*, 530–563.

75. Mackintosh, C.; Beattie, K.A.; Klumpp, S.; Cohen, P.; Codd, G.A. Cyanobacterial microcystin-LR is a potent and specific inhibitor of protein phosphatases i and 2a from both mammals and higher plants. *Fed. Eur. Biochem. Soc. Lett.* **1990**, *264*, 187–192.

76. World Health Organization (WHO). *Guidelines for Safe Recreational Water Environments*; WHO: Geneva, Switzerland, 2003; Volume 1, p. 219.

77. Fitzgeorge, R.; Clark, S.; Keevil, C. Routes of intoxication. In *Detection Methods for Cyanobacterial Toxins*; Codd, G.A., Jefferies, T., Keevil, C., Potter, P., Eds.; Royal Society of Chemistry: Cambridge, UK, 1994; pp. 69–74.

78. *Merck Veterinary Manual*; Merck Manual: Whitehouse Station, NJ, USA, 2008.

79. Gorham, P. Toxic algae. In *Algae and Man*; Jackson, D., Ed.; Plenum Press: New York, NY, USA, 1964; pp. 307–336.

80. Edmondson, W. *Uses of Ecology: Lake Washington and Beyond*; University of Washington Press: Seattle, WA, USA, 1996.

81. KCDNR. *Harmful Algae Bloom-Related Illness Surveillance System (HABISS)*; Science Technical Support Section; King County Department of Natural Resources and Parks: King County, WA, USA, 2013; p.34.

82. National Institute of Environmental Health Sciences. *Cylindrospermopsin [CASRN 143545-90-8] Review of Toxciological Literature*; NIEHS: Research Triangle Park, NC, USA, 2000.

83. Hawkins, P.R.; Runnegar, M.T.C.; Jackson, A.R.B.; Falconer, I.R. Severe hepatotoxicity caused by the tropical cyanobacterium (blue-green alga) *Cylindrospermopsis raciborskii* (Woloszynska) Seenaya and Subba Raju isolated from a domestic water supply reservoir. *Appl. Environ. Microbiol.* **1985**, *50*, 1292–1295.

84. Metcalf, J.S.; Codd, G.A. *Cyanobacterial Toxins in the Water Environment*; Foundation for Water Research: Marlow, UK, 2004; p. 36.

85. Griffiths, D.J.; Saker, M.L. The Palm Island mystery disease 20 years on: A review of research on the cyanotoxin cylindrospermopsin. *Environ. Toxicol.* **2003**, *18*, 78–93.

86. Froscio, S.; Humpage, A.; Burcham, P.; Falconer, I.R. Cylindrospermopsin-induced protein synthesis inhibition and its dissociation from acute toxicity in mouse hepatocytes. *Environ. Toxicol.* **2003**, *18*, 243–251.

87. Terao, K.; Ohmori, S.; Igarashi, K.; Ohtani, I.; Watanabe, M.F.; Harada, K.I.; Ito, E.; Watanabe, M. Electron microcopic studies on experimental poisoning in mice induced by cylindrospermopsin isolated from blue-green alga *Umezakia natans. Toxicon* **1994**, *32*, 833–843.

88. Falconer, I.R.; Humpage, A. Preliminary evidence for *in vivo* tumour initiation by oral administration of extracts of the blue-green *Cylindrospermopsis raciborskii* containing the toxin cylindrospermopsin. *Environ. Toxicol.* **2001**, *16*, 192–195.

89. Humpage, A.R.; Fenech, M.; Thomas, P.; Falconer, I.R. Micronucleus induction and chromosome loss in transformed human white cells indicate clastogenic and aneugenic action of the cyanobacterial toxin, cylindrospermopsin. *Mutat. Res.* **2000**, *472*, 155–161.

90. Shen, X.Y.; Lam, P.K.S.; Shaw, G.R.; Wickramasinghe, W. Genotoxicity investigation of a cyanobacterial toxin, cylindrospermopsin. *Toxicon* **2002**, *40*, 1499–1501.

91. Humpage, A.R.; Fontaine, F.; Froscio, S.; Burcham, P.; Falconer, I.R. Cylindrospermopsin genotoxicity and cytotoxicity: Role of cytochrome P-450 and oxidative stress. *J. Toxicol. Environ. Health. A Curr. Issues* **2005**, *68*, 739–753.

92. USEPA. *Toxicological Review of Cyanobacterial Toxins: Cylindrospermopsin*; U.S. Environmental Protection Agency: Washington, DC, USA, 2006.

93. Fastner, J.; Heinze, R.; Humpage, A.; Mischke, U.; Eaglesham, G.; Chorus, I. Cylindrospermopsin occurrence in two German lakes and preliminary assessment of toxicity and toxin production of *Cylindrospermopsis raciborskii* (cyanobateria) isolates. *Toxicon* **2003**, *42*, 313–321.

94. Banker, R.; Teltsch, B.; Sukenik, A.; Carmeli, S. 7-Epicylindrospermopsin, a toxic minor metabolite of the cyanobacterium *Aphanizomenon ovalisporum* from Lake Kinneret, Israel. *J. Nat. Prod.* **2000**, *63*, 387–389.

95. Saker, M.L.; Thomas, A.D.; Norton, J.H. Cattle mortality attributed to the toxic cyanobacterium *Cylindrospermopsis raciborskii* in an outback region of North Queensland. *Environ. Toxicol.* **1999**, *14*, 179–182.

96. Chiswell, R.K.; Shaw, G.R.; Eaglesham, G.; Smith, M.J.; Norris, R.L.; Seawright, A.A.; Moore, M.R. Stability of cylindrospermopsin, the toxin from the cyanobacterium, *Cylindrospermopsis raciborskii:* Effect of pH, temperature, and sunlight on decomposition. *Environ. Toxicol.* **1999**, *14*, 155–161.

97. Lagos, N.; Onodera, H.; Zagatto, P.A.; Andrinolo, D.; Azevedo, S.; Oshima, Y. The first evidence of paralytic shellfish toxins in the freshwater cyanobacterium *Cylindrospermopsis raciborskii*, isolated from Brazil. *Toxicon* **1999**, *37*, 1359–1373.

98. Pomati, F.; Sacchi, S.; Rossetti, C.; Giovannardi, S.; Onodera, H.; Oshima, Y.; Neilan, B.A. The freshwater cyanobacterium *Planktothrix* sp FP1: Molecular identification and detection of paralytic shellfish poisoning toxins. *J. Phycol.* **2000**, *36*, 553–562.

99. Castro, D.; Vera, D.; Lagos, N.; Garcia, C.; Vasquez, M. The effect of temperature on growth and production of paralytic shellfish poisoning toxins by the cyanobacterium *Cylindrospermopsis raciborskii* C10. *Toxicon* **2004**, *44*, 483–489.

100. Department of Ecology, State of Washington, Freshwater Algae Control Program. Available online: http://www.ecy.wa.gov/programs/wq/plants/algae/monitoring/index.html (accessed on 9 February 2015).

101. Trainer, V.L.; Sullivan, K.; Le Eberhart, B.-T.; Shuler, A.; Hignutt, E., Jr.; Kiser, J.; Eckert, G.L.; Shumway, S.E.; Morton, S.L. Enhancing shellfish safety in Alaska through monitoring of harmful agae and their toxins. *J. Shellfish Res.* **2014**, *33*, 531–539.

102. Stumpf, R.P.; Culver, M.E.; Tester, P.A.; Tomlinson, M.; Kirkpatrick, G.J.; Pederson, B.A.; Truby, E.; Ransibrahmanakul, V.; Soracco, M. Monitoring *Karenia brevis* blooms in the Gulf of Mexico using satellite ocean color imagery and other data. *Harmful Algae* **2003**, *2*, 147–160.

103. ASIMUTH: Applied Simulatiions and Integrated Modelling for the Understanding of Toxic Algal Blooms. Available online: http://www.sams.ac.uk/keith-davidson/asimuth (accessed on 9 February 2015).

104. Scholin, C.A.; Marin, R.; Miller, P.E.; Doucette, G.J.; Powell, C.L.; Haydock, P.; Howard, J.; Ray, J. DNA probes and a receptor-binding assay for detection of *Pseudo-nitzschia* (Bacillariophyceae) species and domoic acid activity in cultured and natural samples. *J. Phycol.* **1999**, *35*, 1356–1367.

105. Greenfield, D.I.; Marin, R., III; Jensen, S.; Massion, E.; Roman, B.; Feldman, J.; Scholin, C.A. Application of environmental sample processor (ESP) methodology for quantifying *Pseudo-nitzschia australis* using ribosomal RNA-targeted probes in sandwich and fluorescent *in situ* hybridization formats. *Limnol. Oceanogr. Methods* **2006**, *4*, 426–435.

106. Greenfield, D.I.; Marin, R., III; Doucette, G.J.; Mikulski, C.; Jones, K.; Jensen, S.; Roman, B.; Alvarado, N.; Feldman, J.; Scholin, C. Field applications of the second-generation Environmental Sample Processor (ESP) for remote detection of harmful algae: 2006–2007. *Limnol. Oceanogr. Methods* **2008**, *6*, 667–679.

107. Doucette, G.J.; Mikulski, C.M.; Jones, K.L.; King, K.L.; Greenfield, D.I.; Marin, R., III; Jensen, S.; Roman, B.; Elliott, C.T.; Scholin, C.A. Remote, subsurface detection of the algal toxin domoic acid onboard the Environmental Sample Processor: Assay development and field trials. *Harmful Algae* **2009**, *8*, 880–888.

108. Integrated Ocean Observing System, Detecting Harmful Algal Blooms in the Pacific Northwest. Available online: http://www.ioos.noaa.gov/marine_sensors/habs_pnw.html (accessed on 9 February 2015).

109. Pacific Northwest Harmful Algal Blooms Bulletin. Available online: http://pnwhabs.org/pnwhabbulletin/100908/pnw_hab_bulletin_100908.pdf (accessed on 18 February 2015).

Spatial and Temporal Patterns in the Seasonal Distribution of Toxic Cyanobacteria in Western Lake Erie from 2002–2014

Timothy T. Wynne and Richard P. Stumpf

Abstract: Lake Erie, the world's tenth largest freshwater lake by area, has had recurring blooms of toxic cyanobacteria for the past two decades. These blooms pose potential health risks for recreation, and impact the treatment of drinking water. Understanding the timing and distribution of the blooms may aid in planning by local communities and resources managers. Satellite data provides a means of examining spatial patterns of the blooms. Data sets from MERIS (2002–2012) and MODIS (2012–2014) were analyzed to evaluate bloom patterns and frequencies. The blooms were identified using previously published algorithms to detect cyanobacteria (~25,000 cells mL^{-1}), as well as a variation of these algorithms to account for the saturation of the MODIS ocean color bands. Images were binned into 10-day composites to reduce cloud and mixing artifacts. The 13 years of composites were used to determine frequency of presence of both detectable cyanobacteria and high risk (>100,000 cells mL^{-1}) blooms. The bloom season according to the satellite observations falls within June 1 and October 31. Maps show the pattern of development and areas most commonly impacted during all years (with minor and severe blooms). Frequencies during years with just severe blooms (minor bloom years were not included in the analysis) were examined in the same fashion. With the annual forecasts of bloom severity, these frequency maps can provide public water suppliers and health departments with guidance on the timing of potential risk.

Reprinted from *Toxins*. Cite as: Wynne, T.T.; Stumpf, R.P. Spatial and Temporal Patterns in the Seasonal Distribution of Toxic Cyanobacteria in Western Lake Erie from 2002–2014. *Toxins* **2015**, *7*, 1649-1663.

1. Introduction

Lake Erie (Figure 1) has experienced a recurrence of blooms with potentially toxic cyanobacteria this century [1], with six of the last seven years having significant blooms [2]. The dominant species of cyanobacteria in Lake Erie is *Microcystis aeruginosa* (henceforth referred to as *Microcystis*). *Microcystis* typically forms dense monospecific (single species) blooms, although *Anabaena*, *Planktothrix*, and other genuses of cyanobacteria may sometimes appear. These blooms have a variety of detrimental impacts, such as: taste and odor issues in municipal water supplies, potential human health issues, mortalities in domestic and wild animal populations, and adverse economic impacts in local communities [3,4]. Contamination of drinking water is a potential hazard, given the number of intakes around the western lake. In September, 2013, Carroll Township, Ohio (Station C on Figure 2), which supplies water to several thousand people, shut down its municipal water supplies for two days [5] owing to microcystin—the toxin found in *Microcystis*—concentrations greater than the World Health Organization guideline of 1 μg L^{-1} [6]. In August, 2014 microcystin concentrations reached the same risk level in the processed water of the city of Toledo, resulting in a two-day "do not drink" statement from its municipal water suppliers (station T on Figure 2) to approximately half a million customers [7].

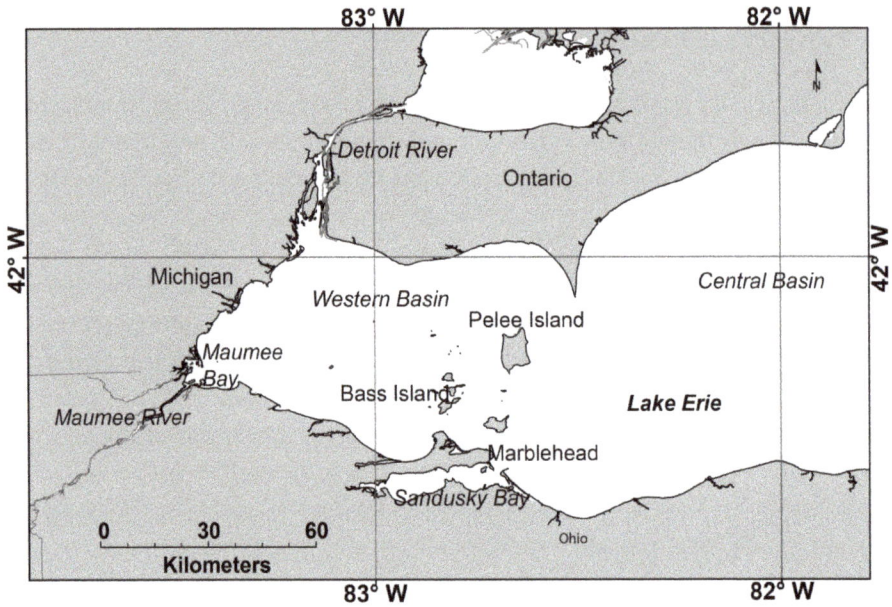

Figure 1. Study area and geographic features described in the text.

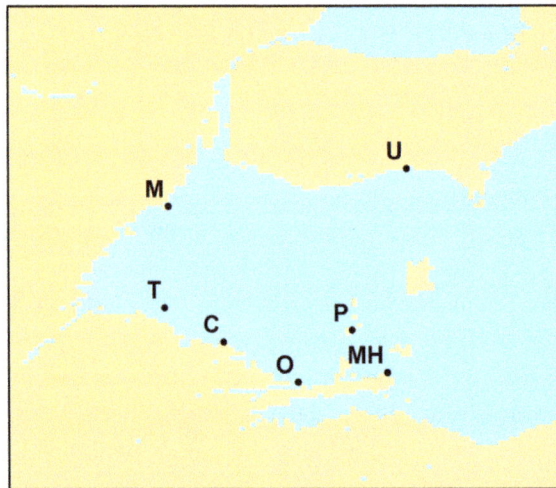

Figure 2. Location of Lake Erie municipal water intakes lettered as following: T = Toledo PWS; M = Monroe; C = Carroll Water and Sewer; O = Ottawa County Regional; P = Put-In-Bay Village PWS; MH = Marblehead Village PWS; U = Union.

NOAA has routinely issued short-term (<1 week) forecasts in Lake Erie since 2009 [2,8]. The demand for these forecasts has been high. The subscriber list for the Lake Erie forecast has experienced an annual growth rate of approximately 250% from its inception in 2009. More recently, NCCOS has started issuing seasonal forecasts [9–11] of cyanobacteria based on models previously presented [1]. A determination of the frequency of blooms over the 13 years of satellite data will provide a better understanding of timing and distributions of these potentially toxic blooms.

These frequencies may allow for spatial-temporal forecasts, which may be beneficial in both a micro and macroeconomic scale. The results could support planning by managers of public water suppliers and parks. They may also ultimately aid the public in avoiding contact with potentially toxic (and unaesthetic) cyanobacteria.

2. Results

2.1. Frequency Maps

The mean concentration of the cyanobacteria Index (CI) over the 13 years (Figure 3) shows the pattern of high concentration through the season. (The color scale is logarithmic, so the orange-red colors have 10-fold greater concentration than cyan colors.) Sandusky Bay has the highest consistent concentration, with little change through the season. This is typically a bloom from the cyanobacterium, *Planktothrix* [12]. The Maumee Bay and southwestern area of the western Lake Erie basin (WLEB) have the next highest mean concentration, with rapid increase between July 21 and August 09. In contrast, the northwest area, in the plume of the Detroit River, does not have a detectable concentration. Away from the Detroit River, low concentration may be present along the Ontario coast in early season, increasing somewhat into September.

The central basin shows two events; presence of cyanobacteria in July (July 01–10) and in early October. The July mean was produced by blooms that occurred in 2012 and 2013. The October mean owes to the severe bloom of 2011 (see the frequency discussion below).

Accumulating the biomass across lake, including Sandusky Bay (Figure 4), provides a measure of the timing of the bloom development. The minimum value on June 1 reflects the presence of a bloom in Sandusky Bay, which persists through the season. The variability above this value captures the average bloom growth in the lake proper. Early July shows the short-lived bloom in the central basin. In the WLEB, development starts by July 22 on average, and peaks in area and biomass between August 30 and September 18. Overall, the peak lasts for 40 days (*i.e.*, four 10-day periods) before decreasing rapidly in October.

The frequency distribution maps (Figures 5–8) capture key aspects of bloom development. A persistent cyanobacteria bloom is present in Sandusky Bay which is typically of the genus *Planktothrix*. Generally, the western basin blooms start in Maumee Bay, with high frequencies in the southwest corner of the WLEB at the beginning of July. The frequency is greatest in the west, with high frequency expanding eastward over the season. The greatest extent of cyanobacteria presence is from August 30 to September 18. The cyanobacteria then become slightly less prevalent during the next 30 day period, before experiencing a relatively sharp decline in abundance during the 19 September–28 September period. Cyanobacteria are no longer present over the western basin of Lake Erie after 18 October.

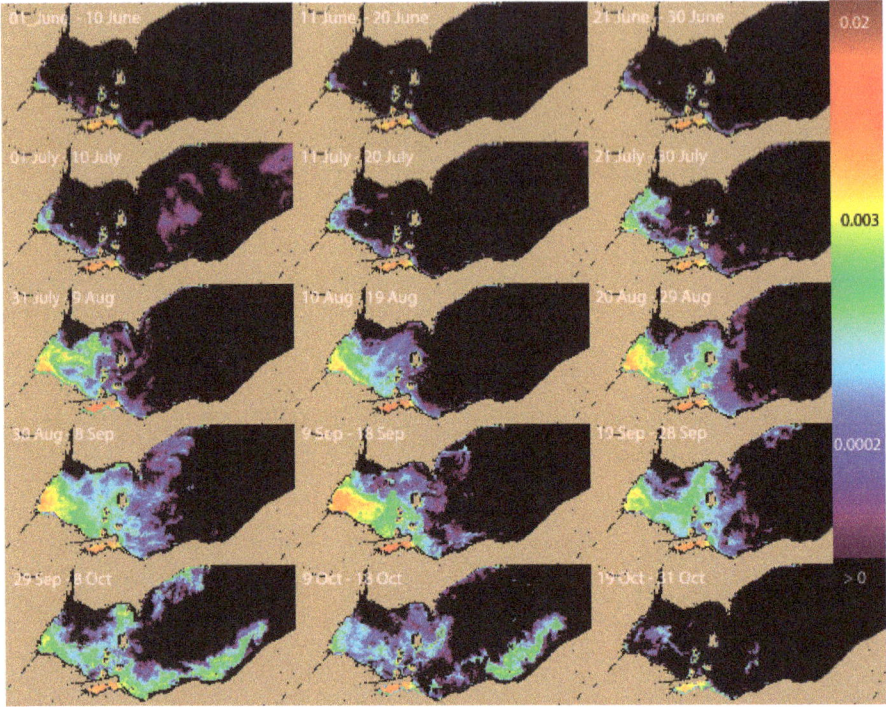

Figure 3. The average Cyanobacterial Index concentration of the 13 years (log scaled) for each 10-day period. Cell concentration can be estimated from the CI by Cells (mL^{-1}) = $10^8 \times CI$ [1]. CI > 0.001 exceeds the WHO [6] threshold of 10^5 cells mL^{-1}.

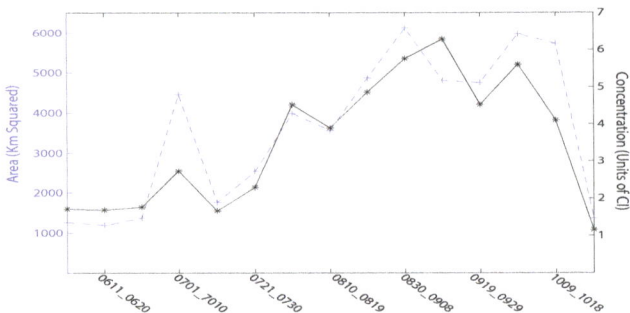

Figure 4

Figure 4. The 13-year average of the area and biomass in Lake Erie flagged by the satellite imagery for each 10-day period (0611 is June 11, *etc.*). Area is shown in blue, accumulated biomass is shown in black. The biomass is the accumulated biomass across the entire lake following previously published methods [1]. 1 CI is nominally 10^{20} cells. This is integrated spatially, thereby corresponding to biomass.

In detail, the bloom is most common first along both the west (Michigan) and south (Ohio) shorelines. However, on the Michigan coast, blooms do not occur north of Monroe (Station M on Figure 2). This area is under the influence of the Detroit River, the large volume of water keeps the bloom back near the Maumee River (discharge of the Detroit River is ~35 times that of the Maumee River [13]).

Eastward movement is not uniform. Detectable concentrations occur relatively early along the Ohio coast to Marblehead (early July). Later in the season, the pattern changes and the greatest frequency of detectable or intense blooms is near the islands in September. Ottawa County (Figure 5 station O) has about half the frequency of blooms as do the islands. Generally, the chances of encountering cyanobacteria are less than 50% until August for the island region, while the peak frequency occurs between 9 September and 18 September for the western islands (*i.e.*, Bass), and between 19 September and 28 September for the. Pelee Island region.

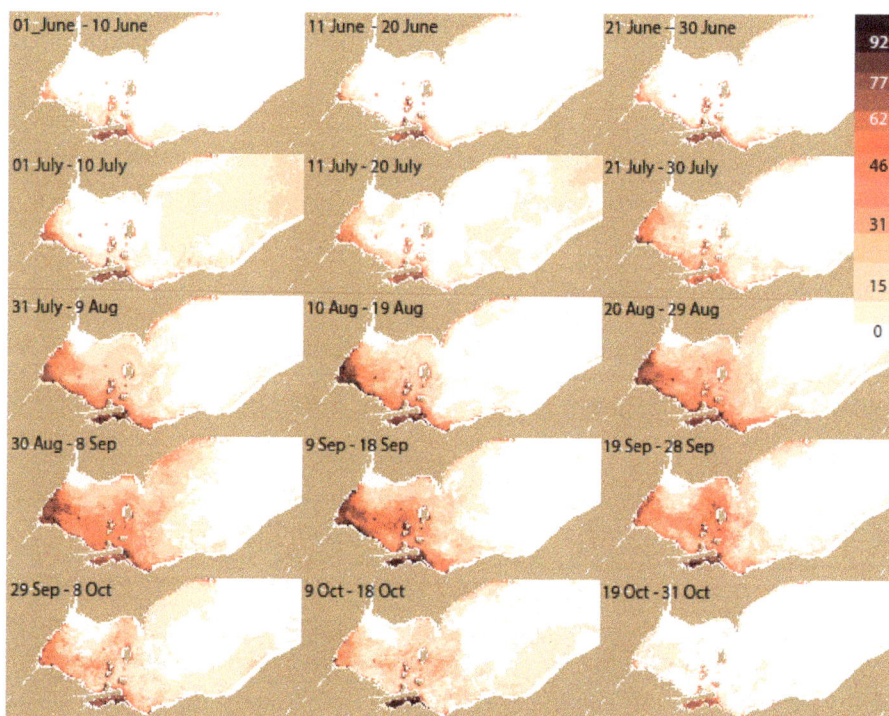

Figure 5. The spatial pattern (by pixel) of percentage frequency of detectable cyanobacteria. Analysis for each 10-day period during all years from 2002–2014.

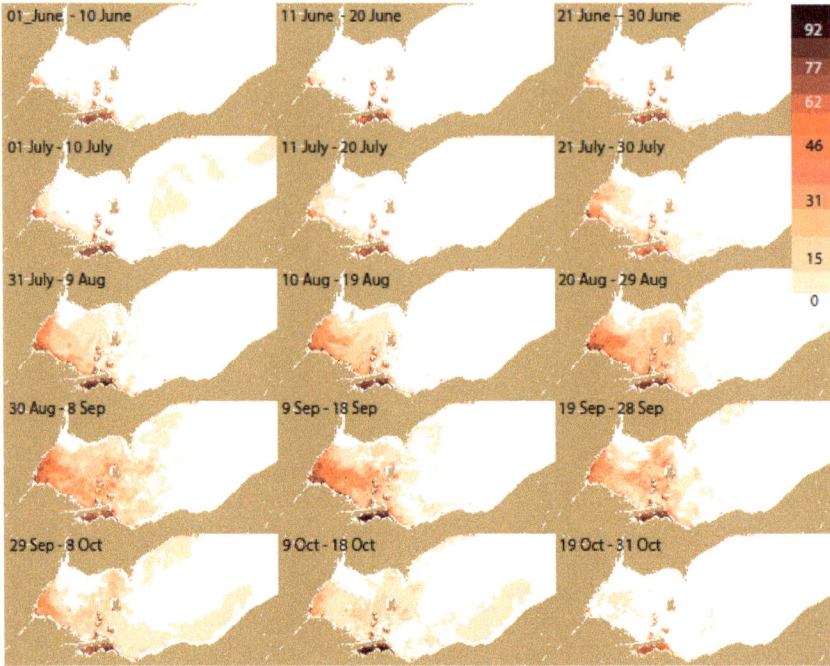

Figure 6. The spatial pattern of percentage frequency of severe cyanobacteria ($>10^5$ cells mL^{-1}, CI > 0.001) for each 10-day period during all years from 2002–2014.

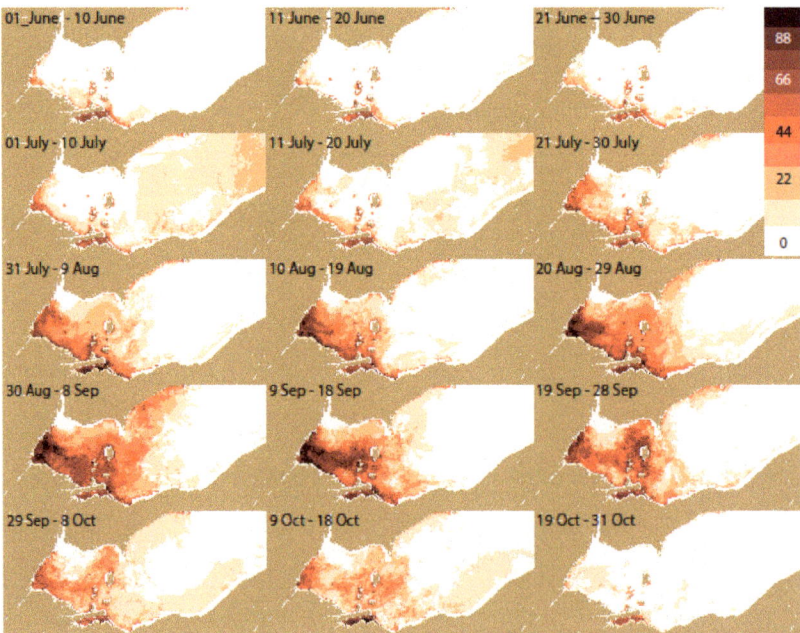

Figure 7. Same as Figure 5 for only years with blooms (percentage frequency of detectable cyanobacteria).

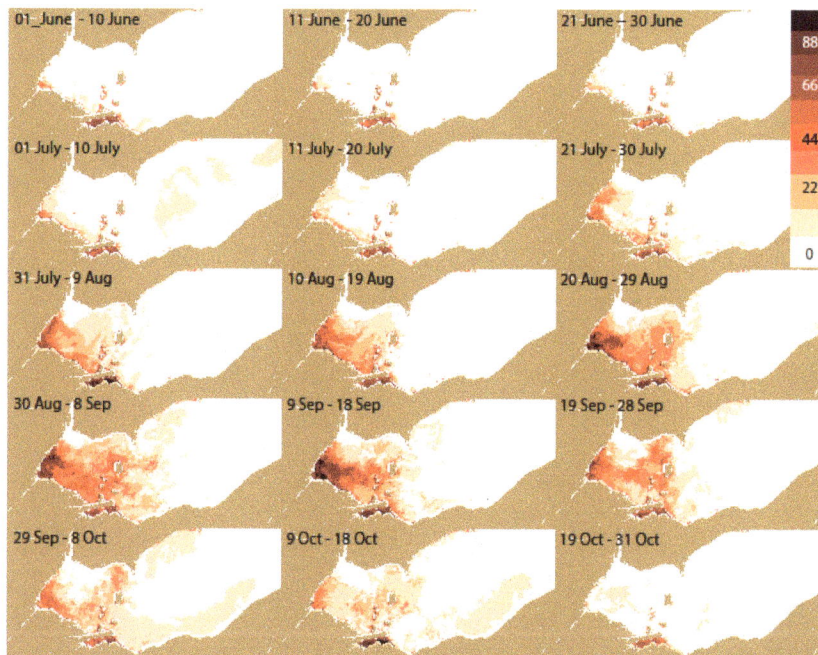

Figure 8. Same as Figure 6 for only years with blooms (percentage frequency of severe cyanobacteria).

2.2. Ontario Shoreline

The northern shoreline (Ontario) as a general rule is much less impacted relative to the southern shore (Ohio). The area east of Pelee Point is generally unaffected by cyanobacteria, with the only incident in the area occurring in 2011, the largest bloom in presented in the dataset show here [14]. The area between Pelee Point and the Detroit River Plume is more regularly affected and, like the Ohio shoreline, blooms are more likely to be encountered from 20 August though 28 September.

2.3. Drinking Water Supplies

As most intakes are within one km of the shore, we examined the frequency patterns of CI > 0.001 at three km offshore near several intakes. These water intake facilities covered a relatively large disparate area of western Lake Erie, with one station in Ontario, one in Michigan, and the remaining five in Ohio. The timing of risk for water suppliers varies (Figure 9). Toledo has the highest frequency, with 70 days having 5–6 years of intense blooms. Monroe, in Michigan, is on the edge of the influence of the Detroit River plume, and has significantly less bloom activity most years relative to Toledo. Moving eastward, there is a difference with the mainland when compared to the islands. Carroll and Ottawa County have early blooms, while Put-in Bay (Bass Island) has less frequent blooms in early August, with a short peak of high frequency at the end of August. It should be noted that the CI can only be used as a proxy for cyanobacteria biomass and not the toxin concentration. The biomass and the toxin concentration may covary, but do not necessarily do so.

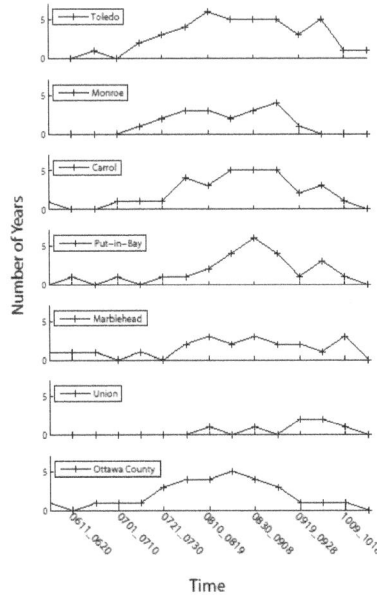

Figure 9. Frequency of severe blooms during the 2002–2014 record at the approximate location of selected water treatment intakes from Figure 2. Except for Toledo station (station 1), the data from the other stations were taken 2 pixels (~2 km) into the center of the lake to obtain valid data without land contamination or masking.

3. Discussion

Creating two frequency maps based on bloom years and all years is based on the value of the seasonal predictions issued by NOAA [9–11]. In these seasonal predictions, NOAA predicts whether a bloom of cyanobacteria is to be expected in Lake Erie based on a statistical model using discharge of total phosphorus concentration from the Maumee River as outlined previously [1]. If a bloom is to be expected, the frequency map using just the bloom years would be more likely to be an accurate assessment of the probability map of the bloom relative to the frequency map using all years.

Distinguishing between bloom and non-bloom years allows for application of the annual forecasts [9–11]. A detailed method to calculate summer peak *Microcystis* biomass using spring discharge from the Maumee River has been presented elsewhere and is appropriate to use for this application [1]. This has been used as the basis of a forecast issued annually by NOAA since 2012. The previous year's forecast is validated prior to the new forecast being issued. Thus far the accuracy of the forecast has been well received by users [15], and the forecast will continue to be issued.

The maps can assist natural resource managers as they plan on mitigation for the blooms. The municipalities that use Lake Erie for drinking water can make plans to avoid intake issues during times when blooms are likely to be present, or to plan for supplies to treat water to mitigate the risk to drinking water. Sampling of parks and public beaches for toxins can be made more strategically, as well. Even the public can use the maps to plan recreational activities to gain maximum use of the lake, while reducing risk. This could have positive impacts to the local economy as it would encourage repeat visitors if negative experiences can be avoided. Furthermore, actual mitigation of blooms may become possible if it is known when and where they will occur.

The distribution has provided insight into the patterns of the blooms. The contrast between the area near the Maumee River and the Detroit River is striking. It has been shown that the phosphorus load from the Maumee River drives the blooms to a large extent [1]. The results here show that the plumes are located in most years in the area of the Maumee River. In contrast, the blooms do not occur near the Detroit River. The pattern in the center of the WLEB, which has relatively high frequency of blooms, likely results from the transport of the bloom around the Detroit River plume. The blooms do not make landfall on the northern Ontario coast until far east of the Detroit River. The large difference in nutrient concentration between the Detroit River and Maumee River explains this difference; the Detroit River has less than 1/20 of the mean concentration of phosphorus of the Maumee River [13]. The disparity of the hydrodynamics is not necessarily an issue as the Detroit River discharge is ~35 times higher than the Maumee River discharge [13,16].

The forecast could also be useful for educational purposes by informing the public when and where blooms may occur and what causes them. The blooms have a tendency to congregate in harbors and on beaches where they are more likely to be encountered by the public [16]. These areas would be easier for short term mitigation of the blooms relative to the large open areas of the Lake. Mitigating the inshore areas affected by blooms would partially alleviate the local economic impacts from the blooms. The public also perceives the Lake as being polluted when it encounters blooms of cyanobacteria, and by applying short term mitigation techniques it may be possible to raise the public perception of the lake ecosystem.

Ecologically speaking, these frequency maps serve another purpose. Cyanobacteria blooms are common in western Lake Erie. The analysis in Figure 4 shows that the maximum intensity (biomass) of the blooms occurs between 9 September and 18 September. These maps give a spatiotemporal timeframe on the initiation and senescence of the blooms, which was not previously available. Furthermore, it gives a likelihood of where the bloom will likely next spread once it is underway. For instance, it seems highly probable that the blooms start in Maumee Bay, and will spread from there. In nearly all years, the bloom was essentially gone by 31 October, with the exception of Sandusky Bay.

4. Methods

The delineation and detection of these blooms has been well-documented with satellite ocean color data [1,2,8,17–20]. The Medium Resolution Imaging Spectrometer (MERIS) on board the Envisat-1 satellite provided data for the summers from 2002–2011. On April 8, 2012 Envisat failed, resulting in a cessation of MERIS data. The Moderate Resolution Imaging Spectroradiometer (MODIS) was used for 2012–2014. MERIS level 2 reflectance (R; with sr^{-1} units) data sets from the second reprocessing were obtained from the European Space Agency (ESA). MODIS was obtained as level 0 data from the National Aeronautics and Space Administration (NASA) and processed to Rayleigh corrected bi-directional reflectance (ρ_s; which is dimensionless) using NASA's SeaDAS package, with the "rhos_s" option in SeaDAS l2gen. Products were processed in equal area Sinusoidal projection, with 1.1 km pixel scale through 2013, and were processed to Albers 1.1 km equal area projection in 2014. All sinusoidal images were reprojected to the Albers equal area projection for all analysis (as all future analyses in our group will use the Albers projection).

Both data sets were then processed with equivalent spectral shape (second derivative) algorithms, based around 680 nm [17,20]. With MERIS bands the equation is:

$$S_{2d}(681) = R(681) - R(665) - \{R(709) - R(665)\}\frac{(681-665)}{(709-665)} \tag{1}$$

where R is the reflectance and the values are the band centers. For MODIS, the MERIS algorithm was adjusted to the MODIS Aqua sensor [20] to yield:

$$S_{2d}(678) = \rho_s(678) - \rho_s(667) - \{\rho_s(748) - \rho_s(667)\}\frac{(678-667)}{(748-667)} \tag{2}$$

where ρ_s is Rayleigh corrected bi-directional reflectance.

For MERIS, the cyanobacterial index (CI) is found from [17]:

$$CI = -S_{2d}(681) \tag{3}$$

and for MODIS the conversion to match MERIS [20] is:

$$CI = -S_{2d}(678) \times 1.3 \tag{4}$$

where the CI has units of sr^{-1}.

The time series shown here extends from 2002–2014. The portion of the time series covering 2002–2011 used MERIS imagery, and the portion covering 2012–2014 used MODIS imagery. MERIS produced superior results with less noise than MODIS and no saturation. MODIS saturates for bright pixels, which can result from glint, haze, and turbid water [21–23]. These conditions can occur during severe algal blooms during the summer [20], resulting in failure of the CI calculation expressed in Equation (4). While the time-series from 2012 showed a bloom, the imagery was not overly turbid and the MODIS bands used in Equation (2) did not saturate in bloom areas, so the MODIS saturation was not an issue. However, the 2013 and 2014 blooms were more intense and highly reflective, resulting in some saturation. A mechanism was needed to quantify the biomass under saturation. The "land" bands in MODIS are calibrated in such a way that they will not saturate even under the most turbid water conditions, and have been recommended for use when the nine bands commonly used for ocean color from MODIS (covering 412–869 nm) have saturated [21]. Cyanobacterial blooms are detectable as bright water, which can provide an estimate of presence and quantity of biomass [24,25]. The near-infrared (NIR) bands on the MODIS Aqua sensor were used to calculate a reflectance proxy for the CI for MODIS.

$$CI_{sat} = 0.5 * [\rho_w(859)]^{0.5} \tag{5}$$

with

$$\rho_w(859) = \rho_s(859) - \rho_s(1240) \tag{6}$$

where the 1240 band is used as a nominal atmospheric correction [23]. The derivation of Equation (5) was empirically tuned with a simple root relationship to overlap the retrieved CI values around saturated pixels. Slight errors in the tuning of Equation (5) are not important to the study, as they would apply when conditions are well above the "severe bloom" threshold discussed below. While scum or algae floating on the surface can produce saturation in the MODIS bands, saturation also occurs in areas without surface scums. As a result, using other metrics like the "floating algae index" [26] would still require yet another algorithm (like Equation (5)) to provide coverage of all saturated areas.

When saturation did not occur, the standard CI solution (Equation (4)) was used; for the conditions when saturation occurred within a bloom, the CI_{sat} from Equation (5) was applied. A tuning of reflectivity to biomass would probably vary between years, depending on the bloom characteristics, like cellular chlorophyll content. Resuspended sediment is uncommon during the summer in Lake Erie, and only the saturated pixels contained within blooms (areas of CI) were used. In 2014, the scattering appeared slightly milder, so the correction of Equation (6) was reduced proportionately.

CI varies linearly with biomass, with a value of 10^{-3} sr^{-1} corresponding to 10^5 cells mL^{-1} [1], which is the World Health Organization's (WHO) threshold of significantly increased risk for human health [6]. The minimum detection of the CI is still being assessed; however, a CI of 2×10^{-4} sr^{-1} produces consistent retrievals of the bloom edge over multiple images for both sensors, indicating that the minimum detection is less than 20,000 cells mL^{-1}, which is also the recommended threshold for avoiding irritative effects [6].

Clouds were masked and 10-day composites were made for each year during the bloom period using the maximum value of the CI at each pixel. There are several advantages to utilizing maximum value composites. The first advantage is that the composite reduces cloud interference, reducing the data to a systematic set of generally cloud-free images. The second key advantage is to estimate areal biomass. When winds are strong (>7.7 m s^{-1}, or stress of 0.1 Pa), the bloom is mixed through the water column, diluting the surface concentration [18,27]. Under calm winds, however, *Microcystis* floats upward with dense accumulations visible on the lake [28]. The surface concentration (CI) estimated from satellite during calm conditions then represents the *Microcystis* that is present in the water column [18], however, the concentration detected during high winds underestimates true biomass. Typically, during any 10-day period in the summer, there is a period of calm clear weather [8], allowing this estimate. The cells return to the surface within 24–48 hours after a wind event. The bands used for the algorithm quantify concentration within one meter of the surface in the clearest water [29], less as turbidity increases (usually because of the bloom). Finally, using a 10-day composite makes biological sense as the doubling time for *Microcystis* is as low as 10 days in the Great Lake region [30].

Blooms in Lake Erie generally occur in the summer when water temperatures exceed 15 °C, although blooms can persist in cooler waters once established [8]. As a result, the bloom season considered here is defined as 1 June through 31 October following conventions published elsewhere [1]. Fifteen separate 10-day composites covering the bloom year (1 June to 31 October) were constructed from methods detailed in elsewhere [1]. The final 10-day composite actually consists of 13 days to complete October (to October 31; See Table 1).

Table 1. Shown here are the start and end dates of each of the 15 10-day composites discussed in the text.

Composite number	Start date	End date
1	01 June	10 June
2	11 June	20 June
3	21 June	30 June
4	1 July	10 July
5	11 July	20 July
6	21 July	30 July
7	31 July	9 August
8	10 August	19 August
9	20 August	29 August
10	30 August	8 September
11	9 September	18 September
12	19 September	28 September
13	29 September	8 October
14	9 October	19 October
15	19 October	31 October

With the 10-day composites in hand, several climatological data sets were generated. The means for each of the 15 separate 10-day composites were made from the averages of all the years.

Frequency maps were made across two sets of conditions: (1) all years or bloom years, and (2) all detectable (measurable CI) and CI > 0.001. As noted previously, CI = 0.001 corresponds to the WHO significantly increased risk threshold of 10^5 cells mL^{-1}. The lower threshold indicates presence of cyanobacteria at a level that poses some (but slight) risk. Bloom years are those that had significant blooms. Negligible blooms were detected in 2002 and 2005–2007 [1,31]. While 2012 had a small bloom [2], it was locally dense and nearly equivalent to the 2004 bloom, and is included. As a result, the frequency maps were calculated just for years containing defined blooms (2003, 2004, 2008–2014). These frequency maps were made based on all bloom types during just the bloom years.

Spurious pixels due to satellite mis-navigation, cloud edges, and mixed land-water pixels were removed from analysis. It should be noted that the two pixels adjacent to the coastline in the southern shore of Lake Erie had to be masked due to somewhat severe land interference issues. These were caused mostly by mis-navigation, although in the case of MODIS, slow sensor response as the sensor scanned from land, where it always saturated, onto water was the cause. In individual MERIS scenes that do not have these issues, the nearshore, masked, pixels appear to have similar concentrations to the offshore pixels. Still, the concentration can vary nearshore, particularly with light winds moving surface scums. The frequency data sets are available in the journal's supplementary data section.

5. Conclusions

The methods used here give an approximation of the spatiotemporal cyanobacterial quantification for western Lake Erie. The frequency maps can be updated as more years of data are available from MODIS. In 2015, the European Space Administration is planning on launching the replacement for

MERIS, the Ocean Colour Land Imager (OLCI) sensor, on board the Sentinel-3 satellite. The accumulation of data will lead to increased statistical power of the frequency maps and allow for evaluation of them as tools for predicting bloom position and timing. The frequency information can allow managers to anticipate the timing of the arrival and duration of the bloom in their area when the seasonal forecast is made. This information allows planning for sampling, supplies and resources, and strategic monitoring to protect public health.

Supplementary Materials

Supplementary materials can be accessed at: http://www.mdpi.com/2072-6651/7/5/1649/s1.

Acknowledgments

MERIS imagery was provided by the European Space Agency (Category-1 Proposal C1P.3975). The project was partially supported by NASA's Applied Science Program announcement NNH08ZDA001N under contract NNH09AL53I.

Author Contributions

T.T. Wynne and R.P. Stumpf wrote the paper, analyzed and processed the data, and conceived of the study.

Conflicts of Interest

The authors declare no conflict of interest

References

1. Stumpf, R.P.; Wynne, T.T.; Baker, D.B.; Fahnenstiel, G.L. Interannual variability of cyanobacterial blooms in Lake Erie. *PLoS One* **2012**, *7*, e42444.
2. National Oceanic and Atmospheric Administration. Available online: http://www2.nccos.noaa.gov/coast/lakeerie/bulletin/ (accessed on 16 March 2015).
3. Backer, L.C. Cyanobacterial harmful algal blooms (CyanoHABs): developing a public health response. *Lake Reserv. Manag.* **2002**, *18*, 20–31.
4. Davenport, T.; Drake, W. Grand Lake St. Marys, Ohio—The Case for Source Water Protection: Nutrients And Algae Blooms, EPA Commentary. Available online: http://water.epa.gov/polwaste/upload/lakeline_article.pdf (accessed on 4 March 2015).
5. Henry, T. Carrol Township's scare with toxin a "wake-up call". *Toledo Blade*, 15 September 2013.
6. Chorus, I.; Bartram, J. *Toxic Cyanobacteria in Water: A Guide to Their Public Health Consequences, Monitoring and Management*; World Health Organization: London, UK, 1999.
7. Fitzsimmons, E.G. Tap Water Ban for Toledo Residents. *New York Times*, 3 August 2014. Available online: http://www.nytimes.com/2014/08/04/us/toledo-faces-second-day-of-water-ban.html?_r=0 (accessed on 15 March 2015).

8. Wynne, T.T.; Stumpf, R.P.; Tomlinson, M.C.; Fahnensteil, G.L.; Schwab, D.J.; Dyble, J.; Joshi, S. Evolution of a cyanobacterial bloom forecast system in western Lake Erie: Development and initial evaluation. *J. Great Lakes Res.* **2013**, *39*, 90–99.

9. National Oceanic and Atmospheric Administration. NOAA, partners predict mild harmful algal blooms for western Lake Erie this year. Available online: http://www.noaanews.noaa.gov/stories2012/20120705_habs.html (accessed on 4 March 2015).

10. National Oceanic and Atmospheric Administration. NOAA, partners predict significant harmful algal bloom in western Lake Erie this summer. Available online: http://www.noaanews.noaa.gov/stories2013/20130702_lakeeriehabs.html (accessed on 4 March 2015).

11. National Oceanic and Atmospheric Administration. NOAA, partners predict significant harmful algal bloom in western Lake Erie this summer. Available online: http://www.noaanews.noaa.gov/stories2014/20140710_erie_hab.html (accessed on 4 March 2015).

12. Millie, D.F.; Fahnenstiel, G.L.; Dyble Bressie, J.; Pigg, R.J.; Rediske, R.R.; Klarer, D.M.; Tester, P.A.; Litaker, R.W. Influence of environmental conditions on late-summer cyanobacterial abundance in Saginaw Bay, Lake Huron. *Aquat. Ecosyst. Health Manag.* **2008**, *11*, 196–205.

13. Ohio Environmental Protection Agency. Ohio Lake Erie Phosphorus Task Force Final Report. Available online: http://epa.ohio.gov/portals/35/lakeerie/ptaskforce/Task_Force_Final_Report_April_2010.pdf (accessed on 15 April 2015).

14. Michalak, A.M.; Anderson, E.J.; Beletsky, D.; Boland, S.; Bosch, N.S.; Bridgeman, T.B.; Chaffin, J.D.; Cho, K.; Confesor, R.; Daloglu, I.; *et al.* Record setting algal bloom in Lake Erie caused by agricultural and meterological trends consistent with expected future conditions. *Proc. Natl. Acad. Sci. USA* **2013**, *110*, 6448–6452.

15. Dierkes, C. *Fact-Checking the Forecast*; Twineline: Columbus, OH, USA, 2012; Volume 34, p. 12.

16. Ibelings, B.W.; Vonk, M.; Los, H.F.J.; van der Molen, D.T.; Mooij, W.M. Fuzzy modeling of cyanobacterial surface waterblooms: Validation with NOAA-AVHRR satellite images. *Ecol. Appl.* **2003**, *13*, 1456–1472.

17. Wynne, T.T.; Stumpf, R.P.; Tomlinson, M.C.; Warner, R.A.; Tester, P.A.; Dyble, J.; Fahnenstiel, G.L. Relating spectral shape to cyanobacterial blooms in the Laurentian Great Lakes. *Int. J. Remote Sens.* **2008**, *29*, 3665–3672.

18. Wynne, T.T.; Stumpf, R.P.; Tomlinson, M.C.; Dyble, J. Characterizing a cyanobacterial bloom in western Lake Erie using satellite imagery and metrological data. *Limnol. Oceanogr.* **2010**, *55*, 2025–2036.

19. Wynne, T.T.; Stumpf, R.P.; Tomlinson, M.C.; Schwab, D.J.; Watabayashi, G.Y.; Christensen, J.D. Estimating cyanobacterial bloom transport by coupling remotely sensed imagery and a hydrodynamic model. *Ecol. Appl.* **2011**, *21*, 2709–2721.

20. Wynne, T.T.; Stumpf, R.P.; Briggs, T.O. Comparing MODIS and MERIS spectral shapes for cyanobacterial bloom detection. *Int. J. Remote Sens.* **2013**, *34*, 6668–6678.

21. Franz, B.A.; Werdell, P.J.; Meister, G.; Kwiatkowska, E.J.; Bailey, S.W.; Ahmad, Z.; McClain, C.R. MODIS land bands for ocean color remote sensing applications. In Proceedings of the Ocean Optics XVIII, Montreal, QC, Canada, 9–13 October 2006.

22. Wang, M.; Tang, J.; Shi, W. MODIS-derived ocean color products along the China east coastal region. *Geophys. Res. Lett.* **2007**, *34*, L06611.

23. Wang, M.; Shi, W. The NIR-SWIR combined atmospheric correction approach for MODIS ocean color data processing. *Opt. Express* **2007**, *15*, 15722.

24. Budd, J.W.; Beeton, A.M.; Stumpf, R.P.; Culver, D.A.; Kerfoot, W.C. Satellite observations of Microcystis blooms in Western Lake Erie. *Verh. Int. Ver. Theor. Angew. Limnol.* **2002**, *27*, 3787–3793.

25. Kahru, M. Using satellites to monitor large-scale environmental change: A case study of cyanobacteria blooms in the Baltic Sea. In *Monitoring Algal Blooms: New Techniques for Detecting Large-scale Environmental Change*; Kahru, M., Brown, C.W., Eds.; Springer-Verlag: Berlin, Germany, 1997; pp. 43–61.

26. Hu, C. A novel ocean color index to detect floating algae in the global oceans. *Remote Sens. Environ.* **2009**, *113*, 2118–2129.

27. Hunter, P.D.; Tyler, A.N.; Willby, N.J.; Gilvear, D.J. The spatial dynamics of vertical migration by Microcystis aeruginosa in a eutrophic shallow lake: A case study using high spatial resolution time-series airborne remote sensing. *Limnol. Oceanogr.* **2008**, *53*, 2391–2406.

28. Aparicio Medrano, E.; Uitenbogard, R.E.; Dionisio Pires, L.M.; van de Wiel, B.J.H.; Clercx, H.J.H. Coupling hydrodynamics and buoyancy regulation in *Microcystis aeruginosa* for its vertical distribution in lakes. *Ecol. Model.* **2013**, *248*, 41–56.

29. Pope, R.M.; Fry, E.S. Absorption spectrum (380–700 nm) of pure water. II. Integrating cavity measurements. *Appl. Opt.* **1997**, *36*, 8710–8723.

30. Fahnenstiel, G.L.; Millie, D.F.; Dyble, J.; Litaker, R.W.; Tester, P.A.; McCormick, J.; Rediske, R.; Klarer, D. Factors affecting microcystin concentration and cell quota in Saginaw Bay, Lake Huron. *Aquat. Ecosyst. Health Manag.* **2008**, *11*, 190–195.

31. Bridgeman, T.B.; Chaffin, J.D.; Filburn, J.E. A novel method for tracking western Lake Erie Microcystis blooms, 2002–2011. *J. Great Lakes Res.* **2013**, *39*, 83–89.

Chapter 5:
Treatment Techniques for Toxin Removal and
Control in Reservoirs and Drinking Water

Application of Hydrogen Peroxide to the Control of Eutrophic Lake Systems in Laboratory Assays

Letizia Bauzá, Anabella Aguilera, Ricardo Echenique, Darío Andrinolo and Leda Giannuzzi

Abstract: We exposed water samples from a recreational lake dominated by the cyanobacterium *Planktothrix agardhii* to different concentrations of hydrogen peroxide (H_2O_2). An addition of 0.33 mg·L^{-1} of H_2O_2 was the lowest effective dose for the decay of chlorophyll-a concentration to half of the original in 14 h with light and 17 h in experiments without light. With 3.33 mg·L^{-1} of H_2O_2, the values of the chemical oxygen demand (COD) decreased to half at 36 and 126 h in experiments performed with and without light, respectively. With increasing H_2O_2, there is a decrease in the total and faecal coliform, and this effect was made more pronounced by light. Total and faecal coliform were inhibited completely 48 h after addition of 3.33 mg·L^{-1} H_2O_2. Although the densities of cyanobacterial cells exposed to H_2O_2 did not decrease, transmission electron microscope observation of the trichomes showed several stages of degeneration, and the cells were collapsed after 48 h of 3.33 mg·L^{-1} of H_2O_2 addition in the presence of light. Our results demonstrate that H_2O_2 could be potentially used in hypertrophic systems because it not only collapses cyanobacterial cells and coliform bacteria but may also reduce chlorophyll-a content and chemical oxygen demand.

Reprinted from *Toxins*. Cite as: Bauzá, L.; Aguilera, A.; Echenique, R.; Andrinolo, D.; Giannuzzi, L. Application of Hydrogen Peroxide to the Control of Eutrophic Lake Systems in Laboratory Assays. *Toxins* **2014**, *6*, 2657-2675.

1. Introduction

Cyanobacteria, also known as blue-green algae, are commonly observed in nutrient-rich aquatic ecosystems. Cyanobacteria can be found all over the world and often form dense blooms. Such blooms are problematic: the landscape deterioration is accompanied by a reduction in recreational value; the processing costs for water purification increase significantly and the decrease in water quality causes serious sanitary problems such as conditions that allow the settlement of disease vectors [1]. Under favorable light and nutrient conditions, some species produce toxic secondary metabolites known as cyanotoxins [2]. Cyanotoxins constitute a health-risk for human beings worldwide via recreational and drinking water and have been linked to the deaths of wild and domestic animals all over the world [3]. Evidence suggests that toxic cyanobacterial metabolites can bioaccumulate in aquatic food-webs, which can cause the additional health concern of food-borne contaminants [4].

The changes in temperature and precipitation that accompany global warning are predicted to stimulate increased cyanobacterial growth rates. The fourth assessment report of the Intergovernmental Panel on Climate Change [5] predicted more frequent toxic blooms. For this reason, controlling cyanobacterial blooms in recreational water bodies and cyanotoxin levels in tap water is essential to assure water quality.

Many methods of controlling cyanobacterial blooms have been studied, including the reduction of nutrient inputs, the mechanical removal of cyanobacterial biomass, artificial destratification, ultrasonication, bacterial and chemical degradation [6]. Several techniques are potentially harmful to the environment and destroy only cyanobacterial cells, leaving the toxins to be released into the surrounding water following cell lysis [7]. Conventional water treatment is usually not effective in removing extracellular cyanotoxins (soluble toxins). Neither aeration nor air stripping are effective treatments for removing soluble toxins or cyanobacterial cells [8]. Advanced treatment processes, such as oxidant agents, must be implemented to remove both extracellular toxins and intact cells.

Hydrogen peroxide is a well-known agent for disinfection and water treatment with a strong oxidizing capability. Its ability to inhibit coliform bacteria and remove COD could represent an important advance in methods of pre-treatment in drinking water plants. Barrington and Gadouani [9] proposed it as a cyanobacterial inhibitor compound for aquaculture and indicated that cyanobacteria were more sensitive to it than other photoautotrophs. H_2O_2 has also been demonstrated to be an effective chemical algaecide to inhibit cyanobacteria [10]. Because H_2O_2 is a strong oxidizing agent and environmentally friendly, it can be effective for removing COD and inhibiting the coliform bacteria in reservoirs used for drinking water.

The effect of light can enhance the toxicity of relatively high H_2O_2 concentrations in aquatic plants and phytoplankton [11]. In addition, hydrogen peroxide can destroy cyanobacteria and cyanotoxins [12,13], and it is well-established as an environmentally-friendly oxidizing agent because of its rapid decomposition into oxygen and water [14].

In this work, we used laboratory assays to study the effect of H_2O_2 on the parameters of eutrophication and on phytoplankton, with a focus on cyanobacteria. In addition, faecal coliform and COD were also analyzed. We used water samples taken from a shallow lake in the Province of Buenos Aires, Argentina, which has been dominated by cyanobacteria for more than ten years. Experiments were conducted with and without light in order to evaluate the effect of light on the effectiveness of H_2O_2.

2. Results and Discussion

2.1. Physicochemical and Biological Conditions of the Shallow Lake

Los Patos, a shallow lake, is highly turbid with dense phytoplankton. Its chemical parameters were measured immediately after arrival at the laboratory (time zero) and are shown in Table 1.

Phosphorus content is one of the factors most likely to limit cyanobacteria growth in water ecosystems. Lake Los Patos showed total and dissolved phosphorus values of 0.89 and 0.20 $mg \cdot L^{-1}$ respectively. When total phosphorus exceeds 0.10 $mg \cdot L^{-1}$, the lake is usually in a turbid-water stable state dominated by phytoplankton [15]. Similar levels of total phosphorus were reported by Ruiz [16] in the San Roque Dam, a hypertrophic water body placed in Cordoba, Argentina, where total phosphorus reached 0.886 $mg \cdot L^{-1}$.

High levels of chlorophyll-a (Chl-a) (530 $\mu g \cdot L^{-1}$) were also obtained. The concentration of Chl-a in water bodies provides a reasonable estimate of algal biomass. The international guidelines for safe practices in managing recreational waters [17] has linked both short-term adverse health outcomes, e.g., skin irritation and gastrointestinal illness, and the potential for long term illness to Chl-a concentrations above 50 $\mu g \cdot L^{-1}$. The Chl-a concentration registered in Los Patos lake exceeded this value more than tenfold.

COD is commonly used to represent the amount of organic materials that can be chemically oxidized, and was identified as a very significant environmental factor for algal growth in water bodies [18]. In this work, high levels of COD (243 $mg \cdot L^{-1}$) were obtained in Los Patos lake (Table 1).

The phytoplankton assemblage was mainly composed of cyanobacteria, which accounted for 99% of the total phytoplankton cell density (average density of 2.4×10^7 cells mL^{-1}). *Planktothrix agardhii* (1.7×10^7 cells mL^{-1}) and *Aphanizomenon aphanizomenoides* (7.0×10^6 cells mL^{-1}) dominated among cyanobacteria, accounting for 70.8% and 29.1% of the total phytoplankton, respectively. Other cyanobacteria such as *Anabaenopsis aff. elenkinii*, *A. cunningtoni*, *Raphidiopsis mediterranea* and *Microcystis aeruginosa* were present in percentages less than 1% (4.0×10^3 cells mL^{-1}). Chlorophyta and Chrysophyta represented less than 1% of total phytoplankton with counts lower than 2.0×10^3 cells mL^{-1}.

According to Chapman [19], the values of total phosphorus (0.84 $mg \cdot L^{-1}$), Chl-a (530 $\mu g \cdot L^{-1}$) and total phytoplankton density (2.4×10^7 cells mL^{-1}) obtained in the Los Patos lake showed that this lake could be classified as hypertrophic, with elevated concentrations of nutrients and an associated high biomass production. Trophic State Indices (TSI-$_t$P and TSI-Ch-a) were calculated following Equations (1) and (2) (see materials and methods section). Both TSI metrics (TSI-$_t$P = 96.09, TSI-Ch-a = 93.05) indicated that the ecosystem is hypertrophic.

2.2. Effect of H_2O_2 on Total and Faecal Coliform Bacteria Counts

Both total and faecal coliforms were found in high numbers, up to 600 MPN $\times$ 100 mL^{-1} before treatment (Table 1). These values exceeded the upper limit for recreational water bodies by more than a factor of 20 (200 MPN $\times$ 100 mL^{-1} of faecal coliforms) [20].

With increasing H_2O_2, the MPN $\times$ 100 mL of total and faecal coliforms decreased, and this effect was more pronounced in light (Table 1). There was complete inhibition 48 h after 3.33 $mg \cdot L^{-1}$ H_2O_2 was added. These results indicate the effectiveness of the H_2O_2 at removing these types of bacteria.

The bactericidal efficacy of hydrogen peroxide has been demonstrated in both water and food systems [21–23], with gram negative organisms showing greater susceptibility [24,25]. This antimicrobial action stems from its ability to form reactive oxygen species such as the hydroxyl radical and singlet oxygen, which can damage DNA and membrane constituents [26].

Table 1. Physicochemical characteristics of Los Patos shallow lake at the time zero and at after of 48 h of H_2O_2 addition.

Parameters	Time Zero	Light	0	48 h after H_2O_2 addition				
				0.17 (mg L⁻¹)	0.33 (mg L⁻¹)	0.83 (mg L⁻¹)	1.67 (mg L⁻¹)	3.33 (mg L⁻¹)
Conductivity (µS cm⁻¹)	599 ± 15	Yes	618 ± 12	666 ± 12	662 ± 20	665 ± 27	630 ± 19	640 ± 18
		No	680 ± 18	667 ± 19	670 ± 21	660 ± 25	630 ± 20	645 ± 20
pH	9.47 ± 0.20	Yes	8.88 ± 0.10	9.05 ± 0.13	9.00 ± 0.12	9.06 ± 0.09	9.19 ± 0.12	9.22 ± 0.12
		No	7.87 ± 0.12	7.45 ± 0.18	7.44 ± 0.10	7.68 ± 0.15	8.06 ± 0.15	8.20 ± 0.10
Optical Density	0.37 ± 0.02	Yes	0.08 ± 0.01	0.07 ± 0.01	0.09 ± 0.02	0.09 ± 0.01	0.08 ± 0.02	0.08 ± 0.02
		No	0.08 ± 0.02	0.07 ± 0.01	0.09 ± 0.02	0.09 ± 0.01	0.08 ± 0.01	0.07 ± 0.01
Total Phosphorus (mg L⁻¹)	0.89 ± 0.10	Yes	0.87 ± 0.10	0.83 ± 0.12	0.82 ± 0.09	0.81 ± 0.12	0.87 ± 0.03	0.90 ± 0.08
		No	0.89 ± 0.09	0.79 ± 0.10	0.81 ± 0.12	0.96 ± 0.15	0.91 ± 0.06	0.94 ± 0.09
Dissolved total Phosphorus (mg L⁻¹)	0.20 ± 0.08	Yes	0.18 ± 0.08	0.40 ± 0.10	0.40 ± 0.09	0.55 ± 0.13	0.53 ± 0.09	0.55 ± 0.09
		No	0.16 ± 0.08	0.30 ± 0.12	0.31 ± 0.13	0.47 ± 0.12	0.49 ± 0.10	0.53 ± 010
Chl-a (µg L⁻¹)	530 ± 10	Yes	445 ± 12	117 ± 5	74 ± 3	77 ± 8	71 ± 9	58 ± 8
		No	420 ± 22	320 ± 9	75 ± 6	81 ± 8	117 ± 7	111 ± 5
COD (mgO₂ L⁻¹)	243 ± 12	Yes	212 ± 8	142 ± 6	129 ± 9	130 ± 9	120 ± 10	126 ± 5
		No	213 ± 10	226 ± 15	205 ± 11	200 ± 12	180 ± 9	119 ± 7
Total coliforms (MPN × 100 mL⁻¹)	4600	Yes	4600	2800	2400	150	90	<3
		No	4600	2800	2400	280	93	<3
Fecal coliforms (MPN × 100 mL⁻¹)	4600	Yes	4600	2100	2100	130	11	<3
		No	4600	2100	2100	210	14	<3

2.3. Effect of H_2O_2 on Chemical Parameters

The addition of H_2O_2 caused water discoloration, which increased with increasing H_2O_2 concentrations (Figure 1). Table 1 shows the parameters measured 48 h after H_2O_2 addition. The pH values showed no statistically significant differences between H_2O_2 treatments in samples stored with light ($p > 0.05$). At the end of treatment, the pH values ranged from 8.88 to 9.22. However, in samples treated with different concentrations of H_2O_2 and without light, the pH values decreased one and two units with respect to the initial values (9.47). The final pH ranged from 7.44 to 8.20. This is to be expected since photosynthetic activity was inhibited without light. The magnitude of the pH change is dependent on the intensity of the respiration and photosynthetic activity.

Figure 1. The effect of H_2O_2 addition on the appearance of water samples after 48 h after H_2O_2 in the presence of light.

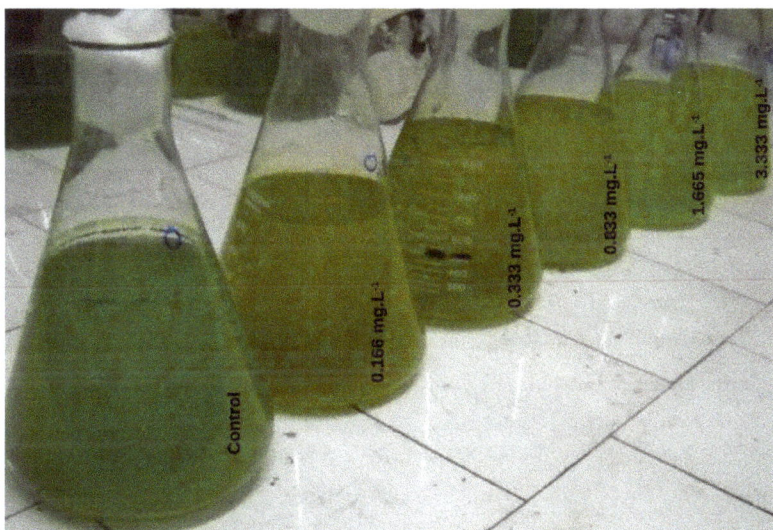

The Optical Density decreased during the assay, from 0.37 (t = 0) to values ranging from 0.08 to 0.09 at the end of the experiment (48 h) (Table 1). No statistically significant differences ($p > 0.05$) between treatments, nor with or without light, were observed.

Dissolved total phosphorus increased at the end of the experiments (Table 1) ($p < 0.05$). These increases most likely occurred as a result of the release of phosphorus during the autolysis process or bacterial lysis [27,28].

The organic matter present may react with H_2O_2 and thus degrade it [29]. In the present work, all concentrations of H_2O_2 added were rapidly degraded to below the detection limit (0.1 $mg \cdot L^{-1}$) after 48 h, both with and without light. This is in accordance with previous findings that the degradation of natural levels of H_2O_2 occurs between 6 and 24 h [30].

2.3.1. Effect of H_2O_2 and Light on Chemical Oxygen Demand (COD)

Various authors have reported that organic substances play an important role in stimulating algal blooms, and COD is the most influential factor contributing to changes in the algal blooms [18]. COD represents the loading contributed by a mixture of organic and inorganic substances, possibly including total phosphorous and total nitrogen. In this work, we evaluated the kinetics of COD degradation on addition of various H_2O_2 concentrations with and without light. Several kinetics were tested, and the pseudo-first-order kinetic was found to be the most appropriate (Equations (3) and (4) in Material and Methods Section).

The value of $(Ko)_{COD}$ was estimated through the representation of $Ln[C/Co]$ as a function of time, using a linear regression model. The proposed kinetics were successfully applied to the experimental data. Table 2 shows the findings of $(Ko)_{COD}$ values and determination coefficients.

$(Ko)_{COD}$ values were found to be greater as the H_2O_2 concentration increased and more pronounced under light, with higher $(Ko)_{COD}$ values (Table 2).

In the range of H_2O_2 studied, the times to reach half of the initial COD values were three to five times shorter in light than without light. The $(tm)_{COD}$ ranged from 142 to 36 h for different concentrations of H_2O_2 under light conditions and from 728 to 126 h in experiments performed without light; 925 h (with light) and 1050 h (without light) were obtained in the control samples (Table 2). These results indicate that H_2O_2 addition decreased COD and that the removal is dependent on light.

The greatest $(Ko)_{COD}$ was 1.90×10^{-2} h^{-1}, which corresponds to the highest concentration applied (3.33 mg·L^{-1}) with light. The $(tm)_{COD}$ values were 36 and 126 h in experiments with and without light, respectively. The degradation of hydrogen peroxide might lead to differences in the decay of the COD values as they might not follow a pseudo first order decay in this time range.

In order to take into account the effects of H_2O_2 addition on $(Ko)_{COD}$, Equation (6) was proposed. Figure 2 shows the variation of $(Ko)_{COD}$ as a function of different concentrations of H_2O_2 and presence or absence of light. $(Ko)_{COD}$ values increased when the concentration of H_2O_2 increased with a good experimental correlation ($R^2 = 0.91–0.97$) in experiments performed with and without light. $(Ko)_{COD}$ values were almost unrelated to the H_2O_2 added and light.

The parameters of Equation (6) allow us to predict the $(Ko)_{COD}$ and then use Equation (4) to estimate the COD values at times and concentrations of H_2O_2 unlike those applied in the present work in the range of H_2O_2 studied. Thus, it is possible to predict the COD values after 48 h by knowing the initial values of COD. This indicates that H_2O_2 is effective in lowering the COD and this effect is enhanced by the presence of light. Applying H_2O_2 under field conditions could reduce COD values and decrease the likelihood of blooms. COD is a synthetic indicator of water contamination representing the degree of organic pollution in water [31]. High COD levels in water are toxic and can affect the aquatic environment. Furthermore, the increase in COD can be generated by the degradation of phytoplankton blooms [32]. Thus, the application of H_2O_2 could help improve the water quality of polluted aquatic systems by reducing COD, coliforms and the algae biomass by Chl-a degradation (see Section 2.3.2).

Table 2. The parameters obtained by fitting the pseudo-first-order COD and Chl-a kinetics with experimental data. Ko: pseudo first order decay constant (h^{-1}); $(t_m)_{COD}$: time required to the concentration of COD decay to half initial values (h); $(t_m)_{Chl-a}$: time required for the concentration of Chl-a to decay to half its initial value (h). Different letters in each column indicate significant differences.

| H$_2$O$_2$ addition | Chemical oxygen demand (COD) Decay | | | | | |
| | With light | | | Without light | | |
	$(Ko)_{COD}$ (h)$^{-1}$	R^2	$(t_m)_{COD}$ (h)	$(Ko)_{COD}$ (h)$^{-1}$	R^2	$(t_m)_{COD}$ (h)
0	$7.5 \times 10^{-4} \pm 5.1 \times 10^{-4}$	0.55	925 ± 629 [a]	$6.5 \times 10^{-4} \pm 1.2 \times 10^{-4}$	0.86	1050 ± 194 [a]
0.17 mg·L^{-1}	$4.9 \times 10^{-3} \pm 1.5 \times 10^{-3}$	0.70	142 ± 43 [b]	$9.5 \times 10^{-4} \pm 3.8 \times 10^{-4}$	0.55	728 ± 291 [a]
0.33 mg·L^{-1}	$5.4 \times 10^{-3} \pm 1.0 \times 10^{-3}$	0.56	128 ± 24 [b]	$1.3 \times 10^{-3} \pm 6.3 \times 10^{-4}$	0.45	533 ± 258 [a]
0.83 mg·L^{-1}	$4.3 \times 10^{-3} \pm 9.5 \times 10^{-4}$	0.87	163 ± 36 [b]	$1.5 \times 10^{-3} \pm 1.5 \times 10^{-4}$	0.44	459 ± 46 [b]
1.67 mg·L^{-1}	$7.8 \times 10^{-3} \pm 4.9 \times 10^{-3}$	0.70	88 ± 55 [b]	$2.6 \times 10^{-3} \pm 7.5 \times 10^{-4}$	0.34	277 ± 80 [b]
3.33 mg·L^{-1}	$1.9 \times 10^{-2} \pm 9.9 \times 10^{-3}$	0.85	36 ± 18 [b]	$5.6 \times 10^{-3} \pm 2.5 \times 10^{-3}$	0.50	$126 \pm 56c$ [c]

| H$_2$O$_2$ addition | Chlorophyll-a (Chl-a) Decay | | | | | |
| | With light | | | Without light | | |
	$(Ko)_{Chl-a}$ (h)$^{-1}$	R^2	$(t_m)_{Chl-a}$ (h)	$(Ko)_{Chl-a}$ (h)$^{-1}$	R^2	$(t_m)_{Chl-a}$ (h)
0	0.010 ± 0.002	0.84	69 ± 13.8 [a]	0.011 ± 0.002	0.86	63 ± 11.4 [a]
1.67 mg·L^{-1}	0.057 ± 0.008	0.89	12 ± 1.7 [b]	0.050 ± 0.009	0.79	14 ± 2.5 [b]
0.17 mg·L^{-1}	0.042 ± 0.008	0.86	16 ± 3.1 [b]	0.025 ± 0.008	0.86	28 ± 8.8 [b]
0.33 mg·L^{-1}	0.050 ± 0.009	0.83	14 ± 2.5 [b]	0.041 ± 0.008	0.87	17 ± 3.3 [b]
0.83 mg·L^{-1}	0.050 ± 0.008	0.87	14 ± 2.2 [b]	0.045 ± 0.008	0.85	15 ± 2.6 [b]
3.33 mg·L^{-1}	0.060 ± 0.009	0.85	12 ± 1.8 [b]	0.051 ± 0.008	0.79	14 ± 2.1 [b]

Note: [a, b, c,] indicate significant differences between treatments at the 5% level of probability ($p < 0.05$).

Figure 2. The effects of H$_2$O$_2$ addition on $(Ko)_{COD}$ ● with light ■ without light. Fitting parameters of Equation (6) were a = 0.0032 ± 0.001, b = 0.005 ± 0.0007 and R^2 = 0.92 for the experiments performed with light; and a = 5.71 ± 1.63, b = 14.07 ± 1.04 and R^2 = 0.98 for experiments without light.

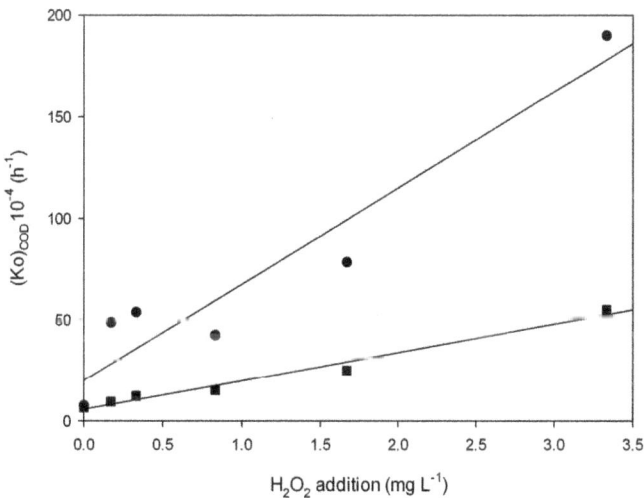

2.3.2. Effect of H_2O_2 and Light on Chl-a Degradation

We evaluated the effect of adding H_2O_2 on Chl-a degradation. Before H_2O_2 application, the Chl-a content was 530 µg·L^{-1}. In the control samples, the Chl-a contents were 446 and 420 µg·L^{-1} at 48 h of the initial experiment performed under light and without light, respectively (Table 1). The decrease in Chl-a values in the control samples could indicate that the cultures were slightly stressed (e.g., culture conditions led to a change in the diurnal rhythm as they were performed under light). In view of this, photoautotrophs could have been slightly more sensitive to the hydrogen peroxide than under optimal conditions.

After 48 h, Chl-a concentration was found to be five to ten times lower than before H_2O_2 was added, depending on the concentration of H_2O_2 added and the light conditions. In the experiments performed with light and with 0.17, 0.33, 0.83, 1.67 and 3.33 mg·L^{-1} of H_2O_2, the Chl-a content decreased by 78%, 86%, 86%, 86% and 89% respectively after 48 h. In experiments performed without light, Chl-a decreased 40%, 86%, 86%, 78% and 79%, respectively.

Our results are consistent with those of Barroin and Feuillade [33], who showed that a low concentration of hydrogen peroxide destroys Chl-a and also other cyanobacterial pigments. Randhawa [34] informed that Chl-a in cyanobacterial cultures treated with 1.6, 3.2 and 6.4 mg·L^{-1} H_2O_2 decreased more than 90% in 24 h. Qian et al. [35] found that cyanobacterial Chl-a decreased to 13.9% below the control after 48 h of 1.3 mg·L^{-1} H_2O_2 exposure under light in *Microcystis aeruginosa* cultures.

Figure 3a,b shows the natural logarithm of cyanobacterial Chl-a decay concentration obtained in the experiments as a function of time under the tested conditions. TSI values were included in the figure to visualize changes in the trophic state. It can be observed that the Chl-a decay rate increases as a function of H_2O_2 addition. We applied the pseudo-first-order kinetic in Equation (7) that was found to be the most appropriate. Table 2 shows the findings of $(Ko)_{Chl-a}$ values and coefficients of determination. $(Ko)_{Chl-a}$ values increased as the H_2O_2 concentration increased. Chl-a decay was more pronounced under light, with higher $(Ko)_{Chl-a}$ values (Table 2). Similarly, the times to reach half of the initial Chl-a concentration $(t_m)_{Chl-a}$ were calculated using $(Ko)_{Chl-a}$ values from Table 2.

The $(t_m)_{Chl-a}$ ranged between 12 and 6 h for different concentrations of H_2O_2 under light and 14–28 h in experiments performed without light. For control samples, $(t_m)_{Chl-a}$ values were 69 h (under light) and 63 h (darkness) (Table 2).

We found that 0.33 mg·L^{-1} of H_2O_2 was the lowest effective concentration to reduce the Chl-a concentration by half in 14 and 17 h under light and darkness, respectively; no statistically significant differences were found at higher concentrations of H_2O_2 (Table 2). Such concentration overlaps with the natural levels of 0.34 mg·L^{-1} observed in freshwater [35,36].

The greatest $(Ko)_{Chl-a}$ was 0.060 h^{-1}, which corresponds to the highest concentration applied (3.33 mg·L^{-1}) in experiments performed with light. In this condition, the time required for Chl-a decay to half of the initial values was 12 and 14 h under light and darkness, respectively.

Figure 3. Chlorophyll-a (Chl-a) decay upon application of different initial concentration of H_2O_2 • control; ○ 0.17 mg·L^{-1}; ▼ 0.33 mg·L^{-1}; ▲ 0.83 mg·L^{-1}; △ 1.67 mg·L^{-1}; ■ 3.33 mg·L^{-1}; (**a**) with light; (**b**) without light.

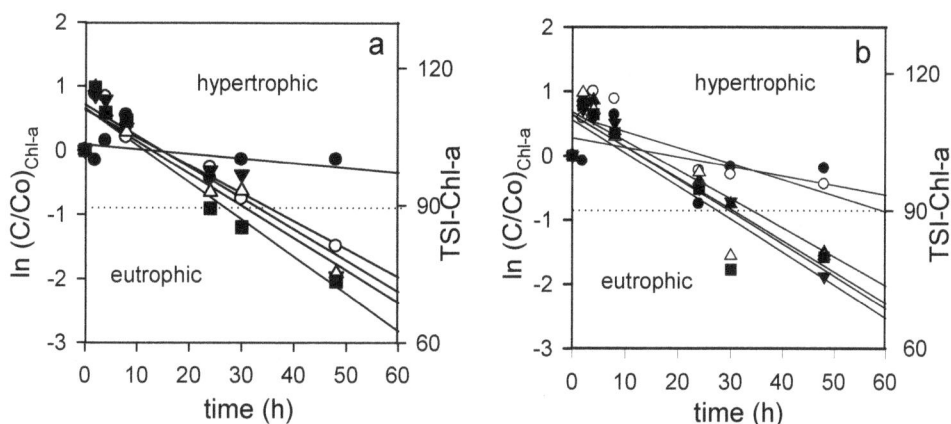

The first order rate constants for Chl-a decay $(Ko)_{Chl-a}$ exhibited a sigmoidal regression, indicating that it is likely that there is a H_2O_2 concentration below which Chl-a decay is negligible, and a concentration above which the decay rate does not increase any further.

In order to take into account the effects of H_2O_2 addition on $(Ko)_{Chl-a}$, Equation (8) was proposed. The fitting parameters were a = 0.055 ± 0.003, b = 7.93 ± 2.63 and R^2 = 0.99 and a = 0.049 ± 0.003, b = 4.54 ± 2.09 and R^2 = 0.99 in experiments performed with and without light, respectively. These parameters allow us to calculate $(Ko)_{Chl-a}$ values at H_2O_2 concentrations different from those which were applied in the present work in the range of H_2O_2 studied. Thus, it is possible to predict the Chl-a values after 48 h by knowing the initial values of Chl-a.

Figure 4 illustrates the variation in $(Ko)_{Chl-a}$ as a function of H_2O_2 concentration and the presence or absence of light, showing that $(Ko)_{Chl-a}$ values exponentially increase when the concentration of H_2O_2 rises, with a good experimental correlation (R^2 = 0.99).

These tests were conducted during a period of up to 48 h under laboratory conditions. It is possible that in aquatic environments, Chl-a levels could increase from this time due to the proliferation of phytoplankton.

2.4. The Effect of H_2O_2 and Light on Phytoplankton Counts

The effects of different concentrations of H_2O_2 on phytoplankton counts were analyzed during the experiment in both light and darkness. Before the assay, cyanobacteria predominated (2.4×10^7 cells mL^{-1}) while other phytoplankton groups remained below 1% of total phytoplankton (4.0×10^3 cells mL^{-1}). Forty-eight hours after adding H_2O_2, cyanobacteria still dominated and cell density did not change significantly in respect to the initial values ($p > 0.05$). None of the experiments showed a significant decrease in cell density after 48 h (data not show). Although the density did not change, electron microscopic observations of *Planktothrix agardhii* showed filaments and cells in several stages of degeneration, effects that were more severe under higher

H_2O_2 concentrations and longer time of exposure. Swollen cell walls and some degree of cytoplasmatic alteration were observed after 24 h of treatment with 0.83 mg·L^{-1}. After 48 h under the highest concentration (3.33 mg·L^{-1}), we observed cell wall and plasmatic membrane disruption, disorganized and degraded thylakoids and changes in the cytoplasmatic inclusions (Figure 5).

Figure 4. The effect of H_2O_2 addition on Chl-a decay (Ko)$_{Chl-a}$ ● with light ■ without light.

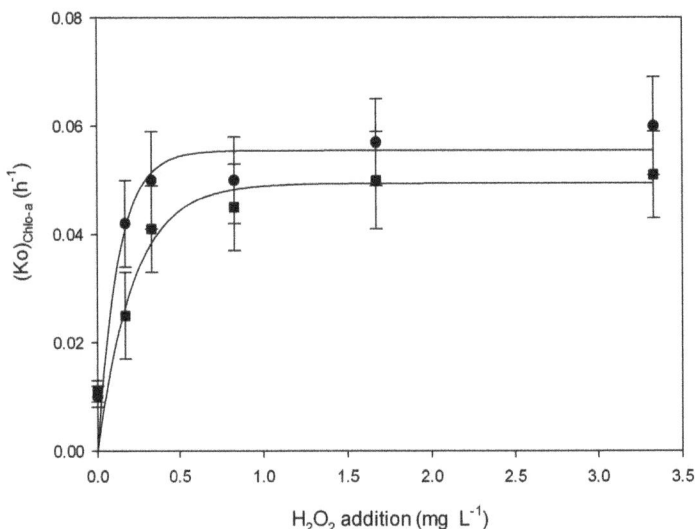

Similar results were found by Matthijs *et al.* [13], who reported a rapid decline of photosynthetic vitality in field material dominated by *Plankthotrix agardhii* after incubation with different concentrations of H_2O_2. The cyanobacterial population collapsed within a few days and stayed low for seven weeks, while the remaining plankton community appeared much less affected. Levels of 1, 2 and 4 mg·L^{-1} resulted in the suppression of the photosynthetic vitality to less than 30% of the control within 3 h.

It has been proposed that H_2O_2 may attack the cyanobacteria cells by forming hydroxyl and hydroperoxyl radicals that inhibit the photosynthesis activity by blocking photosynthetic electron transfer [9]. As in this study, Drábková *et al.* [10] reported that H_2O_2 toxicity under light condition was increased, most likely by an enhanced conversion to the hydroxyl radicals (OH*) that are known to be the strongest reactive oxygen species (ROS).

Samuilov *et al.* [37] reported that H_2O_2 inhibits photosynthetic O_2 evolution, because hydroxyl and hydroperoxyl radicals can lead to the inactivation of photosystem II, destroy pigment synthesis and the integrity of membrane, and result in cyanobacterial cell death. In the present work, no differences were found in the cells numbers of phytoplankton species to H_2O_2 addition since cyanobacteria was the predominant group in the shallow lake samples. Chlorophyta and chrysophyta represented less than 1% of total phytoplankton, quantities that did not change during the experiment. However, it is important to mention that the more sensitive parameter, TEM, showed that *Planktothrix agardhii* was damaged.

Figure 5. (A) Transverse view of the trichome of *Planktothrix agardhii* (control); **(B)** Transverse (Tv) and longitudinal (Lv) view of *P. agardhii* trichome under 3.33 mg·L^{-1} of H$_2$O$_2$, after 48 h of treatment with light.

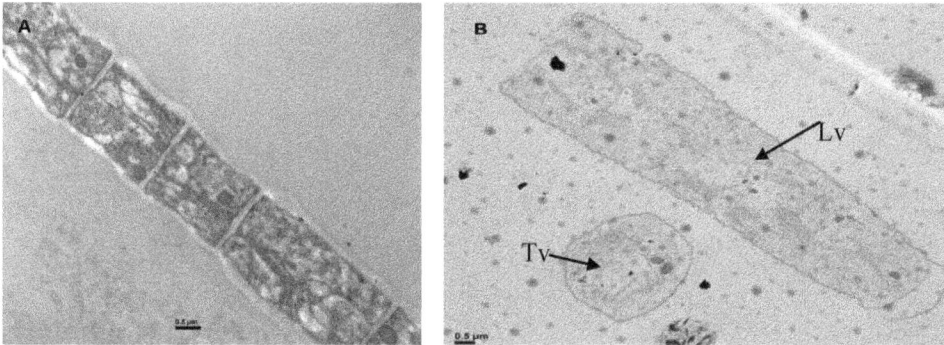

A selective effect of H$_2$O$_2$ on the phytoplankton community was reported by Drábková *et al.* [10]. Cyanobacteria was affected by H$_2$O$_2$ at 10 times lower concentrations than green alga and diatoms, and a strong light dependent toxicity enhanced the difference. Single concentrations of 0.27 mg·L^{-1} of H$_2$O$_2$ caused 50% inhibition to *M. aeruginosa* at high irradiance. The higher rate of H$_2$O$_2$ decomposition leads to stronger oxidizing and cyanobacterial effects [10]. The inhibition of photosynthesis was more severe in five tested cyanobacterial species than in three green algal species and one diatom species. Hence the inhibitory effect of H$_2$O$_2$ is especially pronounced for cyanobacteria [8], showing that hydrogen peroxide is a compound selective to cyanobacteria.

There are several reasons to justify the selectivity observed: phycobilisomes of cyanobacteria are situated on the outside of the thylakoid membranes directly exposed to the cytoplasm rather than in organised chloroplasts, and this structure makes the photosynthetic apparatus more readily susceptible to external H$_2$O$_2$ than in green alga or diatoms with photosystems enclosed in chloroplasts [6]. Furthermore, cyanobacteria have less elaborate detoxification enzymes such as catalase or catalase-peroxidase. The light inactivation of catalase [38,39] makes cyanobacteria even more susceptible to H$_2$O$_2$ in high light intensities.

The intracellular toxicity mechanisms of hydrogen peroxide in *Microcystis aeruginosa*, were studied by Mikula *et al.* [40], who reported that light is one of the critical factors affecting H$_2$O$_2$ decomposition and thus greatly influences its toxicity. Using applied flow cytometry and Chl-a fluorescence measurements, the authors suggested that hydrogen peroxide exposure elicits an immediate decline of metabolic (esterase) activity, and immediate changes in Chl-a fluorescence parameters, followed by an increase in the percentage of membrane-compromised cells.

The results of the present work show that the increase in H$_2$O$_2$ destroyed Chl-a, decreased COD, and damaged the membrane integrity of *Planktothrix agardhii* in laboratory experiments. These effects are exaggerated in the presence of light. In the same way, total and faecal coliforms were inhibited with H$_2$O$_2$ addition, and this effect was enhanced by light, suggesting that the generation of ROS could be the principal mechanism. The release of stored phosphorus during the autolysis process or bacterial lysis could explain the increase in dissolved phosphorus values. This effect was stronger in the presence of light.

Our results demonstrate that H_2O_2 could be potentially used in hypertrophic systems because it not only collapses cyanobacterial cells but may also reduce Chl-a content and chemical oxygen demand. It may also be possible to use H_2O_2 to remove cyanobacteria from shallow lakes. We propose the application of H_2O_2 when the cyanobacterial bloom starts and under higher light conditions. According to Matthijs [13], 2 mg·L^{-1} of H_2O_2 could be applied homogeneously into the entire water volume of the lake in the morning or evening to achieve more effective action. However, further investigation into the effects of H_2O_2 addition on ecosystem function must be conducted before this could be implemented. In addition, the release and increase of dissolved total phosphorus poses a problem because it can contribute to the eutrophication of the water body. The impact on elements of the ecosystem such as larval fish and macro-invertebrates and zooplankton should be assessed.

3. Experimental Methodology

3.1. Sample Collection

Sampling was carried out on December 2010 in the shallow lake of Los Patos, a small (surface area 2.5 ha, maximum depth 1 m) and hypertrophic freshwater body located in Ensenada city, 60 km south–west of the city of Buenos Aires, Argentina. Intense cyanobacterial blooms dominated by *Planktothrix agardhii* and *Raphiodiopsis mediterranea* have been frequently observed during the past decades as the result of nutrient overloading. This shallow lake contributes to the region as a valuable landscape element and is also used for recreational activities and fishing.

Water samples were taken 40 cm below the water surface at one particular point (34°50'44" S, 57°57'26" W) using a van Dorn bottle. In total, 200 mL of water were subsampled into a polyethylene bottle and preserved in Lugol's iodine solution for phytoplankton enumeration. Surface water temperature, pH and conductivity were measured *in situ* using a Sonda Sper Scientific Water Quality Meter 850081. The total orthophosphate phosphorus, dissolved total phosphorus, chemical oxygen demand (COD), Optical Density (OD), Chl-a, faecal coliforms and total coliforms were measured once samples arrived at the laboratory (see Analyzed parameters and analytical methods).

Sample collection was performed according to the GEMS/Water Operational Guide [41].

3.2. Laboratory Incubations and Experimental Design

Samples taken from Los Patos shallow lake were subdivided into 1 L aliquots that were put in 1.5 L incubation bottles.

Drábková *et al.* [10] and Matthijs *et al.* [13] showed that cyanobacteria are sensitive even to low amounts of mg·L^{-1} of H_2O_2. Accordingly, we added different volumes of a 30 g·L^{-1} (3% w/v) stock solution of H_2O_2 (Fluka), resulting in final concentrations of 0, 0.17, 0.33, 0.83, 1.67 and 3.33 mg·L^{-1}.

After adding H_2O_2, the bottles were stirred for 30 s. Bottles without H_2O_2 added were used as a control. Three replicates for each concentration were conducted.

The H_2O_2 experiments were carried out in the incubation cabinet without aeration or shaking during the incubation and stored at room temperature (24 ± 1 °C) under two experimental conditions: continuous irradiance of 50 μmol photon $m^{-2} \cdot s^{-1}$, provided by white light fluorescent tubes, and continuous darkness. Light intensity was measured in the lab using an Underwater Quantum Sensor (LI-192 US-SQS; LI-COR, Lincoln, NE, USA) and a LI-250A Light Meter (LI-COR).

Samples for Chl-a, physic-chemical parameters, faecal and total coliforms were determined at the beginning ($t = 0$) and at 2, 4, 8, 24, 30 and 48 h after 0.17, 0.33, 0.83, 1.67 and 3.33 $mg \cdot L^{-1}$ H_2O_2 addition.

At the end of the experiment (48 h) we analyzed H_2O_2 concentration by peroxide Quantofix test sticks (Machereye-Merck, Darmstadt, Germany). We were able to refine the measurements by taking photographs of each test stick and subsequent comparison to our own calibration series according to the procedure described by Matthijs et al. [13].

3.3. Analyzed Parameters and Analytical Methods

Standard analytical methods developed and/or compiled by the American Public Health Association [42] were used for each chosen parameter (the method number for each determination is provided between parentheses): pH (4500H-B), temperature (2550B), conductivity (2510A), Optical Density (OD)—measured using a Metrolab Spectrophotometer (Metrolab, Argentina) at 740 nm.

The orthophosphate phosphorus levels were determined over samples previously treated by acid hydrolysis and digested with persulphate (4500-P); dissolved total phosphorus was determined previously filtered through 0.45 μm cellulose acetate membranes (GE Osmonics).

Chemical Oxygen Demand (COD) was determined by potassium dichromate in 50% sulfuric acid solution at reflux temperature (5220D), Chl-a (10200H-spectrophotometric) with 90% buffered acetone), faecal coliforms (9221 E) and total coliforms were estimated using the multiple-tube fermentation test (9221B) and the results were expressed as Most Probable Number (MPN $\times$ 100 mL^{-1}).

Aliquots of 10 mL of the control and two H_2O_2 treatments (0.833 $mg \cdot L^{-1}$ and 3.333 $mg \cdot L^{-1}$) were preserved in Lugol's iodine solution for phytoplankton counting and immediately quenched with sodium thiosulphate. Phytoplankton was taxonomically identified using methodology described by Komàrek and Anagnostidis [43] and quantifications were done with an inverted microscope (AXIOVERT 40 C, Carl Zeiss, Jena, Germany) using the Utermöhl method [44].

Trophic State Index

The Trophic State Index (TSI) of Carlson [45] as modified by Aizaki [46] was applied to the shallow lake and calculated using the following formula:

$$TSI\text{-}_tP = 10 \times [2.46 + \frac{(6.68 + 1.15 \ln {_t}P^*)}{\ln 2.5}] \qquad (1)$$

$_tP$ = Total Phosphorus $(mg \cdot L^{-1})$

$$TSI\text{-}Chl\text{-}a = 10 \times (2.46 + \frac{\ln Chl\text{-}a^{**}}{\ln 2.5}) \tag{2}$$

Based on the values of TSI, water bodies are classified as Oligotrophic (TSI < 30), Mesotrophic (30 < TSI ≤ 60), Eutrophic (60 < TSI < 90) and Hypertrophic (TSI > 90).

3.4. Electron Microscopy Studies

Screening tests to evaluate morphological changes were studied with a JEOL JEM 1200–EX II Transmission Electron Microscope (TEM) (JEOL, Peabody, MA, USA), and images were captured using a digital camera Erlangshen ES 1000 W. We analyzed the light samples 48 h after 3.33 $mg \cdot L^{-1}$ H_2O_2 was added. For TEM preparations, cells were collected by centrifuging at 1500 rpm for 10 min. The samples were fixed in 2.0% glutaraldehyde at 4 °C for 2 h and then rinsed in phosphate buffer. Next, they were post fixed in 1% osmic acid for 2 h at 4 °C and rinsed in phosphate buffer. After that, the samples were dehydrated in increasing concentrations of alcohol (50%, 70%, 90%, and 100%, 10 min in each) and 100% acetone. The material was embedded in Epon 812 overnight at 60 °C. Using a Reichert-J Super Nova Ultracut, the Epon blocks were cut into ultrathin sections (60 nm), which were contrasted with urany acetate and lead citrate [47].

3.5. Modelling COD and Chl-a Decay

Several kinetics were tested for modelling COD decay in terms of time. The pseudo-first-order kinetic was found to be the most appropriate:

$$\frac{dC}{dt} = -(Ko)_{COD} \times C \tag{3}$$

Integrating $\int \frac{dC}{C} = -(Ko)_{COD} \cdot \int t$

$$Ln\left[\frac{C_{COD}}{C_{0COD}}\right] = -(Ko)_{COD} \times t \tag{4}$$

where $(Ko)_{COD}$ = COD pseudo first order decay constant (h^{-1}); C_{COD} = COD content at time (t) $(mg \cdot L^{-1})$; C_{0COD} = initial COD content $(mg \cdot L^{-1})$; t = time (h).

When the COD is COD/2, the time to reach half of the initial COD values $(t_m)_{COD}$ was calculated as:

$$(t_m)_{COD} = -\frac{\ln 2}{(Ko)_{COD}} \tag{5}$$

In order to take into account the effects of H_2O_2 addition on $(Ko)_{COD}$, the following Equation was proposed

$$(Ko)_{COD} = a + b \times C \tag{6}$$

where a is the interception of y axes and b is the slope and C is the concentration of H_2O_2 used.

For chlorophyll decay we applied the pseudo-first-order kinetic in Equation (7) and found it to be the most appropriate:

$$Ln\left[\frac{C_{Chl-a}}{C_{0\,Chl-a}}\right] = -(ko)_{Chl-a} \times t \tag{7}$$

where $(Ko)_{Chl-a}$ = pseudo first order Chl-a decay constant (h^{-1}); C_{Chl-a} = Chl-a concentration at time (t); C_{0Chl-a} = initial Chl-a concentration $(mg \cdot L^{-1})$; t = time (h)

The relationship between $(Ko)_{Chl-a}$ and concentration of H_2O_2 addition was modelled by

$$(Ko)_{Chl-a} = a(1 - e^{-b.c}) \tag{8}$$

where a and b are empirical constants and c is the concentration of H_2O_2 added.

3.6. Statistical Analysis

All the experiments were performed in triplicate. The Analysis of Variance (ANOVA) and the test of mean comparison according to Fisher LSD were applied with significance levels of 0.05, using a statistical package for computers (SYSTAT Inc. 2007, version 12.0, Chicago, IL, USA). The statistical requirements for the ANOVA (normal distribution, homogeneity of variance) were performed.

The parameters tested were: conductivity, pH, optical density, total and dissolved phosphorous content, phytoplankton counts, COD and Chl-a content, obtained from treated samples and the initial values.

4. Conclusions

In our laboratory assay of natural water samples from lake Los Patos, the addition of H_2O_2 reduced the Chl-a content as well as the COD by more than 90% in a few hours, depending on the experimental concentration.

Modelling COD and Chl-a decay has allowed us to calculate $(Ko)_{COD}$ and $(Ko)_{Chl-a}$ values at H_2O_2 concentrations different from those that were applied in the present work in the range of H_2O_2 studied. Thus, it is possible to predict the COD and Chl-a values after 48 h by knowing the start values of COD and Chl-a.

A concentration of $0.33 \ mg \cdot L^{-1}$ of H_2O_2 was the lowest effective concentration for half decay in Chl-a content at 14 and 17 h, with light and without light, respectively, whereas $3.33 \ mg \cdot L^{-1}$ of H_2O_2 addition reduced the COD values to half at 36 and 126 h in experiments under light and darkness, respectively. Hence, the presence of light enhanced the effects of H_2O_2 addition.

Although the densities of the dominating cyanobacterial cells did not decrease under H_2O_2, TEM observations of the trichomes of the dominating *Planktothrix agardhii* showed several stages of degeneration and cell damage 48 h after $3.33 \ mg \cdot L^{-1}$ of H_2O_2 was added in the presence of light. The relatively short period of 48 h might be the reason for missing any difference in the sensitivity of different taxa of phytoplankton, as this time was too short to cause a shift in the phytoplankton community.

In accordance with the observed cell damage (destroyed pigment and membrane integrity) in cyanobacteria, the total and faecal coliforms were also completely inhibited 48 h after adding 3.33 mg·L^{-1} of H_2O_2.

Our results indicate that H_2O_2 could be implemented to treat highly polluted systems and develop strategies for water quality management, since it can contribute to a reduction in Chl-a, coliform bacteria and COD.

Acknowledgments

The author's acknowledge the Consejo Nacional de Investigaciones Científicas y Técnicas (CONICET), Argentina, PIP 2617 and Alicia Chavez for his assistance in statistical aspects.

Author Contributions

Conceived and designed the experiments: Leda Giannuzzi, Darío Andrinolo. Performed the experiments and made the determinations: Letizia Bauzá (chemical determinations), Ricardo Echenique (species identification and phytoplankton counts). Analyzed the data: Anabella Aguilera, Letizia Bauzá, Leda Giannuzzi. Wrote the paper: Anabella Aguilera, Leda Giannuzzi.

Conflicts of Interest

The authors declare no conflict of interest.

References

1. Echenique, R.O.; Aguilera, A. Cyanobacteria toxígenas: Aspectos generales para su identificación taxonómica. In *Cianobacterias y Cianotoxinas: Identificación, Toxicología, Monitoreo y Evaluación de Riesgo*; Giannuzzi, L., Ed.; Moglia Impresiones: Buenos Aires, Argentina, 2009; pp. 37–51.

2. Environmental Protection Agency. *Cyanobacteria and Cyanotoxins: Information for Drinking Water System*; Office of Water 4304T, EPA-810F11001; Environmental Protection Agency: Washington, DC, USA, 2012.

3. Carmichael, W.W. A world overview. One-hundred-twenty-seven years of research on toxic Cyanobacteria. Where do we go from here? In *Cyanobacterial Harmful Algal Blooms: State of the Science and Research Needs*; Kenneth, H., Hudnell, H., Eds.; Springer: New York, NY, USA, 2008; pp. 105–126.

4. Berry, J. Cyanobacterial Toxins in Food-Webs: Implications for Human and Environmental Health Current Topics in Public Health. Available online: http://dx.doi.org/10.5772/55111 (accessed on 18 January 2014).

5. Intergovernmental Panel on Climate Change (IPCC). Impacts, Adaptation and Vulnerability. Contribution of Working Group II to the Fourth Assessment Report. In *Climate Change 2007*; Parry, M.L., Canziani, O.F., Palutikof, J.P., van derLinden, P.J., Hanson, C.E., Eds.; Cambridge University Press: Cambridge, UK, 2007.

6. Drábková, M. Methods for Control of the Cyanobacterial Blooms Development in Lakes. Ph.D. Thesis, Masaryk University, Faculty of Science, Research Centre for Environmental Chemistry and Ecotoxicology, Brno, Czech Republic, 2007.

7. McElhiney, J.; Lawton, L.A. Detection of the cyanobacterial hepatotoxins microcystins. *Toxicol. Appl. Pharmacol.* **2005**, *203*, 219–230.

8. Chorus, I.; Bartram, J. *Toxic Cyanobacteria in Water: A Guide to Their Public Health Consequences, Monitoring and Management*; World Health Organization, St Edmundsbury Press: Bury St Edmunds, Suffolk, London, UK, 1999.

9. Barrington, D.J.; Ghadouani, A. Application of hydrogen peroxide for the removal of toxic cyanobacteria and other phytoplankton from wastewater. *Environ. Sci. Technol.* **2008**, *42*, 8916–8921.

10. Drábková, M.; Admiraal, W.; Marsálek, B. Combined exposure to hydrogen peroxide and light: Selective effects on cyanobacteria, green algae, and diatoms. *Environ. Sci. Technol.* **2007**, *41*, 309–314.

11. Kay, S.H.; Quimby, P.C.; Ouzts, J.D. Photo-enhancement of hydrogen peroxide toxicity to submersed vascular plants and algae. *J. Aquat. Plant Manag.* **1984**, *22*, 25–34.

12. Svrcek, C.; Smith, D.W. Cyanobacteria toxins and the current state of knowledge on water treatment options: A review. *J. Environ. Eng.* **2004**, *3*, 155–185.

13. Matthijs, H.; Visser, P.; Reeze, B.; Meeuse, J.; Slot, P.; Wijn, G.; Talens, R.; Huisman, J. Selective suppression of harmful cyanobacteria in an entire lake with hydrogen peroxide. *Water Res.* **2012**, *46*, 1460–1472.

14. Antoniou, M.G.; de la Cruz, A.A.; Dionysiou, D.D. Cyanotoxins: New generation of water contaminants. *J. Environ. Eng.* **2005**, *131*, 1239–1243.

15. Wang, H.; Wang, H. Mitigation of Lake Eutrophication: Loosen nitrogen control and focus on phosphorus abatement. *Prog. Nat. Sci.* **2009**, *19*, 1445–1451.

16. Ruiz, M.; Granero, M.; Rodríguez, M.I.; Bustamante, M.A.; Ruibal, A.L. Importancia de los sedimentos como fuente interna de fósforo en el Embalse San Roque (Córdoba): Determinación de una metodología para su estudio. In Proceedings of the XX Congreso Nacional del agua y III Simposio de Recursos Hídricos del Cono Sur, Mendoza, Argentina, 9–14 May 2005.

17. World Health Organization (WHO) 1999. Available online: http://www.who.int (accessed on 25 January 2014).

18. Hou, G.; Song, L.; Liu, J.; Xiao, B.; Lui, Y. Modeling of cyanobacterial blooms in hypereutrophic Lake Dianchi, China. *J. Freshw. Ecol.* **2004**, *19*, 623–629.

19. Chapman, D. *Water Quality Assessment*; United Nations Educational, Scientific and Cultural Organization (UNESCO), World Health Organization (WHO) and UNEP Chapman and Hall: London, UK, 1992.

20. United States Environmental Protection Agency (USEPA). *Bacterial Water Quality Standards for Recreational Water (Freshwater and Marine Waters)*; EPA/823/R-98/003; USEPA: Washington, DC, USA, 2003.

21. Yoshpe-Purer, M.S.; Eylan, E. Disinfection of water by hydrogen peroxide. *Health Lab. Sci.* **1968**, *5*, 233–238.

22. Liao, C.; Sapers, G.M. Attachment and growth of *Salmonella chester* on apple fruits and *in vivo* response of attached bacteria to sanitizer treatments. *J. Food Prot.* **2000**, *63*, 876–883.

23. Forney, C.F.; Rij, R.E.; Dennis-Arrue, R.; Smilanick, J.L. Vapor phase hydrogen peroxide inhibits post-harvest decay of table grapes. *Hort. Sci.* **1991**, *26*, 1512–1514.

24. Davidson, M.P.; Branen, A.L. *Antimicrobials in Foods*, 2nd ed.; Marcel Dekker, Inc.: New York, NY, USA, 2003.

25. Lillard, H.S.; Thomson, J.E. Efficacy of hydrogen peroxide as a bactericide in poultry chiller water. *J. Food Sci.* **1983**, *48*, 125–126.

26. Juven, B.J.; Pierson, M.D. Antibacterial effects of hydrogen peroxide and methods for its detection and quantitation. *J. Food Prot.* **1996**, *59*, 1233–1241.

27. Golterman, H.L. Mineralization of algae under sterile conditions or by bacterial breakdown. *Verh. Int. Ver. Limnol.* **1964**, *15*, 544–548.

28. Fallon, R.D.; Brock, T.D. Decomposition of blue-green algal (Cyanobacterial) blooms in lake Mendota, Wisconsin. *Appl. Environ. Microbiol.* **1979**, *37*, 5820–5830.

29. Agustina, T.E.; Ang, H.M.; Vareek, V.K. A review of synergistic effect of photocatalysis and ozonation on wastewater treatment. *J. Photochem. Photobiol. C* **2005**, *6*, 264–273.

30. Cooper, W.J.; Zika, R.G. Photochemical formation of hydrogen peroxide in surface and ground waters exposed to sunlight. *Science* **1983**, *220*, 711–712.

31. Pisarevsky, A.M.; Polozova, I.P.; Hockridge, P.M. Chemical oxygen demand. *Russ. J. Appl. Chem.* **2005**, *78*, 101–107.

32. Zhang, Y.L.; van Dijk, M.A.; Liu, M.L.; Zhu, G.W.; Qin, B.Q. The contribution of phytoplankton degradation to chromophoric dissolved organic matter (CDOM) in eutrophic shallow lakes: Field and experimental evidence. *Water Res.* **2009**, *43*, 4685–4697.

33. Barroin, G.; Feuillade, G. Hydrogen peroxide as a potential algaecide for *Oscillatoria rubescens* D.C. *Water Res.* **1986**, *20*, 619–623.

34. Randhawa, V.; Thakkar, M.; Wei, L. Applicability of hydrogen peroxide in brown tide control—Culture and microcosm studies. *PLoS One* **2012**, *7*, doi:10.1371/journal.pone.0047844.

35. Qian, H.; Hu, B.; Yu, S.; Pan, X.; Wu, T.; Fu, Z. The effects of hydrogen peroxide on the circadian rhythms of *Microcystis aeruginosa*. *PLoS One* **2012**, *7*, doi:10.1371/journal.pone.0033347.

36. Skurlatov, Y.I.; Ernestova, L.S. The impact of human activities on freshwater aquatic systems. *Acta Hydrochim. Hydrobiol.* **1998**, *26*, 5–12.

37. Samuilov, V.; Timofee, K.N.; Sinitsyn, S.V.; Bezryadno, D.V. H_2O_2 induced inhibition of photosynthetic O_2 evolution by *Anabaena variabilis* cells. *Biochem. Mosc.* **2004**, *69*, 926–933.

38. Tytler, E.G.; Wong, T.; Codd, G.A. Photoinactivation *in vivo* of superoxide dismutase and catalase in the cyanobacterium *Microcystis aeruginosa*. *FEMS Microbiol. Lett.* **1984**, *23*, 239–242.

39. Tel-Or, E.; Huflejt, M.E.; Packer, L. Hydroperoxide metabolism in cyanobacteria. *Arch. Biochem. Biophys.* **1986**, *246*, 396–402.

40. Mikula, P.; Zezulka, S.; Jancula, D.; Marsalek, B. Metabolic activity and membrane integrity changes in *Microcystis aeruginosa*—New findings on hydrogen peroxide toxicity in cyanobacteria. *Eur. J. Phycol.* **2005**, *27*, 195–206.

41. World Health Organization (WHO). *GEMS/WATER Operational Guide*; WHO: Geneva, Switzerland, 1987.

42. American Public Health Association. *Standard Methods for Examination of Water and Wastewater*, 21th ed.; American Public Health Association, American Water Works Association, Water Environment Federation: Washington, DC, USA, 2005.

43. Komarek, J.; Anagnostidis, K. Modern approach to the classification system of cyanophytes. 2. Chroococcales. *Arch. Hydrobiol. Suppl.* **1986**, *73*, 157–226.

44. Utermöhl, H. Vervolkommung der quantitative phytoplankton methodik. *Mitt. Int. Ver. Theor. Angew. Limnol.* **1958**, *9*, 1–38.

45. Carlson, R.E. A trophic state index for lakes. *Limnol. Oceanogr.* **1977**, *22*, 361–369.

46. Aizaki, M.O.; Otsuki, M.; Fukushima, M.; Muraoka, H. Application of Carlson's trophic state index to Japanese lakes and relationships between the index and other parameters. *Verh. Int. Ver. Limnol.* **1981**, *21*, 675–681.

47. Reynolds, E.S. The use of lead citrate at high pH as an electron-opaque stain in electron microscopy. *J. Cell Biol.* **1963**, *17*, 208–212.

Bioreactor Study Employing Bacteria with Enhanced Activity toward Cyanobacterial Toxins Microcystins

Dariusz Dziga, Magdalena Lisznianska and Benedykt Wladyka

Abstract: An important aim of white (grey) biotechnology is bioremediation, where microbes are employed to remove unwanted chemicals. Microcystins (MCs) and other cyanobacterial toxins are not industrial or agricultural pollutants; however, their occurrence as a consequence of human activity and water reservoir eutrophication is regarded as anthropogenic. Microbial degradation of microcystins is suggested as an alternative to chemical and physical methods of their elimination. This paper describes a possible technique of the practical application of the biodegradation process. The idea relies on the utilization of bacteria with a significantly enhanced MC-degradation ability (in comparison with wild strains). The cells of an *Escherichia coli* laboratory strain expressing microcystinase (MlrA) responsible for the detoxification of MCs were immobilized in alginate beads. The degradation potency of the tested bioreactors was monitored by HPLC detection of linear microcystin LR (MC-LR) as the MlrA degradation product. An open system based on a column filled with alginate-entrapped cells was shown to operate more efficiently than a closed system (alginate beads shaken in a glass container). The maximal degradation rate calculated per one liter of carrier was 219.9 μg h^{-1} of degraded MC-LR. A comparison of the efficiency of the described system with other biological and chemo-physical proposals suggests that this new idea presents several advantages and is worth investigating in future studies.

Reprinted from *Toxins*. Cite as: Dziga, D.; Lisznianska, M.; Wladyka, B. Bioreactor Study Employing Bacteria with Enhanced Activity toward Cyanobacterial Toxins Microcystins. *Toxins* **2014**, *6*, 2379-2392.

1. Introduction

Microcystins (MCs), hepatotoxic cyclic heptapeptides, produced by several cyanobacterial species, may be transformed into non-toxic derivatives in several different ways in the natural environment. These methods include physical processes, like thermal or light-mediated decomposition, chemical oxidation or enzymatic degradation [1–3]. Furthermore, adsorption to suspended or sedimented particles and accumulation followed by transformation in aquatic organisms may occur and impact the concentration of these toxins [4–6]. However, these processes are relatively slow and do not play a crucial role in the regulation of MC concentration during and after bloom formation. Within the last few years, a notable amount of new information regarding the biodegradation of cyanotoxins has been published, and several bacteria with degradation activity against MCs were identified in the environmental samples [7]. Such discoveries should provide backing for future research to enable a general understanding of this phenomenon. Another approach is to study the possible practical application of microorganisms capable of cyanotoxin degradation. Recently, several proposals of MC biodegradation processes employed in the removal of cyanotoxins have been published. Among them, biologically-active filters (granular activated carbon and sand) have been suggested as the most attractive water treatment option [8–10]. On the other hand, the use of bacteria capable of MC degradation directly in water reservoirs was described by Ji *et al.* [11] and Sumino *et al.* [12] as an alternative to drinking water treatment. In these proposals, the introduction of bacterial strains directly into water reservoirs are suggested, and this is another option that may help in the reduction of MC occurrence below the postulated guideline value. However, such environmental manipulation should be based on local strains capable of MC degradation and requires the preparation of a large volume of bacterial culture.

Figure 1. A bioreactor employing BL21(DE3) cells modified according to *mlrA* gene expression and immobilized in alginate beads.

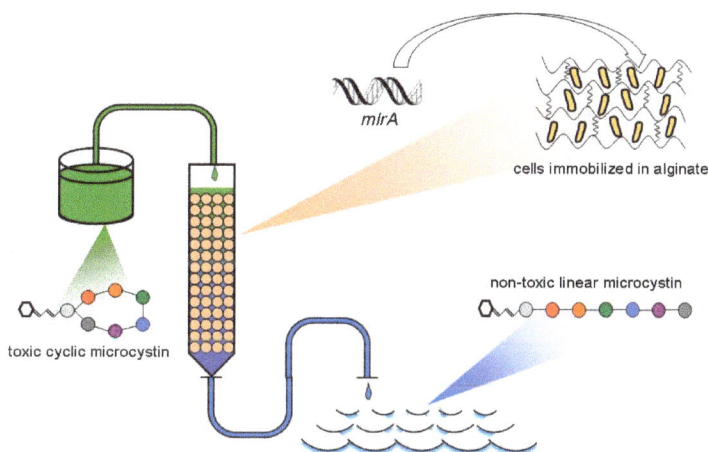

This paper presents a novel proposal based on the utilization of genetically engineered microorganisms (Figure 1). The previously investigated bioreactors employing natural microorganisms offer relatively low efficiency compared to chemical treatment, and their use in fast purification of large amounts of MC-contaminated water is questionable. Our preliminary experiments [13] indicated that bacterial cells with significantly increased biodegradation potency are still active toward MC after immobilization in alginate. In the present paper, several novel data have been provided, including: (1) the comparison of open and closed bioreactors; (2) optimizing the efficiency of MC degradation using a different length of column and different initial microcystin LR (MC-LR) concentration; and (3) assays of the long-term efficiency of columns packed with alginate bead-based MC removal at different temperatures.

2. Results

Preliminary experiments for this work were performed to confirm the hypothesis that only a part of the MlrA enzyme produced by BL21 cells is involved in MC degradation. Firstly, *E. coli* BL21-*mlrA* cells with and without induction by IPTG exhibited a similar level of activity (17.4 and 23.7 mU mL^{-1} of cell culture at stationary phase, respectively). This activity was relatively stable during long-term incubation in LB medium 100-fold diluted with freshwater. For this reason, the cultivation of BL21-*mlrA* in the further experiments described below was performed without IPTG induction. Secondly, the study on the location of MlrA in the BL21 cells (cultivated with and without IPTG) indicated that a significant amount of the enzyme is located mainly in cytosol (89.8% and 87.7% of total activity, respectively). In the periplasmic fraction, 5.5% and 5.7% of MlrA activity was noticed, whereas in membranes, 4.5% and 6.8% (induced and non-induced cells, respectively).

Different dilutions of cells were tested to optimize the maximal activity of the formed alginate beads with entrapped BL21-*mlrA* cells. The greatest potency of beads for MC degradation was found for the highest investigated cell concentration (Figure 2). On the other hand, the efficiency of immobilization (expressed as the activity of beads towards MC-LR) calculated per dilution fold was the highest for cell dilution factor 30×, and then, it decreased when the density of the culture was enhanced.

The rate and dynamics of degradation were shown to be different in a closed system when compared to beads packed in a column under continuous flow (Table 1). Independently of the column volume and applied concentration of toxin, the fast reduction of MC-LR concentration in the first minutes of the experiment was observed in a glass container with the vortexed beads, but the rate of degradation decreased during the experiment. On the other hand, in an open system, the concentration of MC-LR in the flow, as well as the rate of degradation were stable during the experiment. For example, in an open system filled with 2.23 mL of carrier (3 cm of column length), 49% of MC-LR was transformed into linear form with 1.8 min empty bed contact time (EBCT), and the rate of degradation ranged between 33.4–35.5 $\mu g\ h^{-1}\ L^{-1}$ during 3 h of continuous flow.

Figure 2. The activity of alginate-entrapped BL21-*mlrA* cells against MC-LR depending on cell concentration. The initial density (1 fold dilution) was 1.2×10^{10} cells mL^{-1}. The solid line indicates total measured activity of alginate beads, the dashed line indicates calculated efficiency of immobilization. Errors bars indicate standard deviation ($n = 4$).

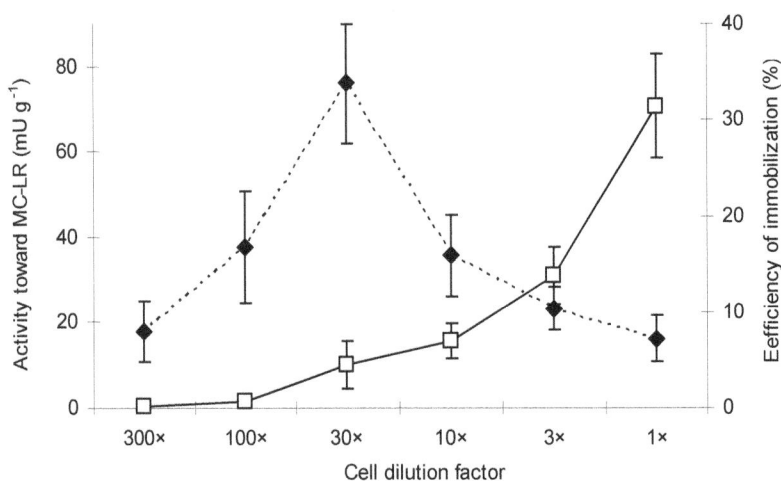

Figure 3. The collective data of MC-LR degradation efficiency depending on the column length and initial MC-LR concentration. White, gray and dark gray blocs are the response to the initial MC-LR concentration (10, 35 and 100 µg L⁻¹, respectively). Bars indicate standard deviations ($n = 9$).

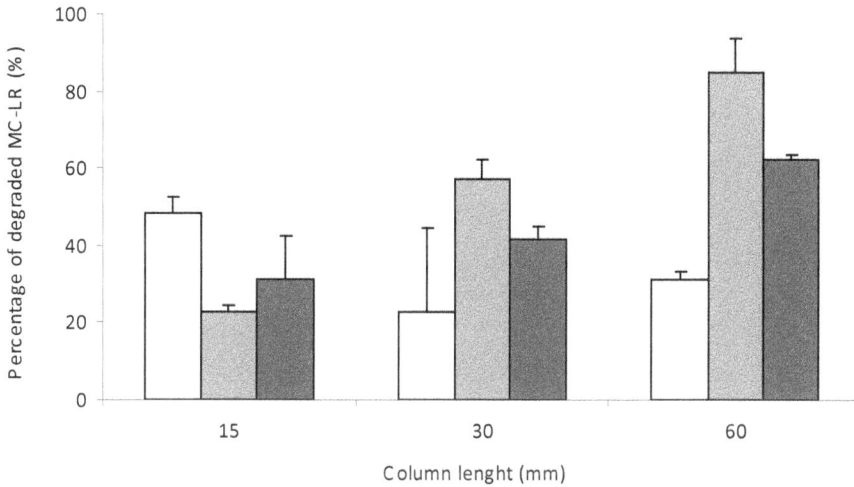

Different lengths of columns and different initial concentrations of MC-LR were tested (Figure 3) to find the optimal efficiency of MC-LR degradation in an open system. The tested MC-LR concentration ranged between 10 and 100 µg L⁻¹, which is typical during blooms [14]. As could be expected, the length of the column improved the efficiency. In a six-centimeter-column, 86.5% and 85.0% of MC-LR was degraded within a short time for a concentration of 10 and 35 µg L⁻¹, respectively; the estimated EBCT was only 3.6 min. In the case of a much higher concentration of 100 µg L⁻¹, which is extremely rare in nature, the efficiency of degradation was 62.3%. The highest documented rate of degradation in open system (calculated per 1 L of carrier) was 219.9 µg h⁻¹ of degraded MC-LR (100 µg L⁻¹ initial concentration, six-centimeter-column, 0.5 mL min⁻¹ flow rate, 20 °C).

Table 1. The efficiency of closed and open bioreactors within 3 h of operating in the different initial MC-LR concentration and volume of the carrier.

Heading	Initial MC-LR concentration ($\mu g\ L^{-1}$)	Type of system									
		Batch bioreactor (closed)					Column (open)				
time (min)		5	20	60	120	180	5	20	60	120	180
volume of carrier 2.23 mL	10										
concentration of toxin ($\mu g\ L^{-1}$)		8.77 ± 0.28	8.21 ± 0.43	4.81 ± 0.79	2.26 ± 0.44	1.16 ± 0.61	5.11 ± 0.58	4.94 ± 0.82	4.81 ± 1.07	5.10 ± 0.26	5.06 ± 0.51
total degraded toxin (μg)		0.07	0.11	0.31	0.47	0.76	0.01	0.05	0.15	0.30	0.62
rate of degradation ($\mu g\ h^{-1}\ L^{-1}$)		207.7	78.3	74.5	55.2	31.4	35.5	34.3	33.4	35.4	35.1
volume of carrier 8.46 mL	10										
concentration of toxin ($\mu g\ L^{-1}$)		7.94 ± 0.41	5.31 ± 0.38	1.29 ± 0.20	0.00	0.00	0.92 ± 0.49	1.34 ± 0.08	1.53 ± 0.25	1.29 ± 0.19	1.29 ± 0.40
total degraded toxin (μg)		0.12	0.28	0.52	0.60	0.60	0.02	0.09	0.25	0.52	1.04
rate of degradation ($\mu g\ h^{-1}\ L^{-1}$)		175.1	99.9	61.8	35.5	17.8	32.2	30.8	30.1	30.1	30.9
volume of carrier 8.46 mL	35										
concentration of toxin ($\mu g\ L^{-1}$)		20.64 ± 0.42	7.46 ± 0.38	1.43 ± 0.23	0.00	0.00	5.64 ± 0.62	7.40 ± 0.59	6.99 ± 0.37	4.40 ± 0.16	5.06 ± 0.02
total degraded toxin (μg)		0.25	0.47	0.58	0.60	0.60	0.07	0.28	0.84	1.84	3.31
rate of degradation ($\mu g\ h^{-1}\ L^{-1}$)		349.5	167.6	68.1	35.9	18.0	104.2	98.0	99.4	99.4	108.6

Previously [13], the activity of cells immobilized in alginate beads was shown to be unstable during long-term incubation (three weeks). In a subsequent experiment, the dependence of MC degradation capability on the temperature and long-term stability of the designed system was analyzed (Figure 4). The columns were under a continuous flow of freshwater (0.5 mL min^{-1}) during the experiment, and the MC-LR degradation potency was tested on the first, second, third, fifth and 28th day. The initial efficiency of the columns incubated at 20, 15 and 10 °C was 85.0% ± 3.5%, 61.6% ± 4.0% and 58.8% ± 5.5%, respectively. During two days of continuous flow, the efficiency of degradation was relatively stable, whereas in the following days, it was reduced below 35% (third day) and 12% (fifth day), which may be the result of the decreased viability of the cells.

Figure 4. The rate of MC-LR degradation (µg h^{-1} L^{-1} of carrier) in relation to the temperature in a column (6-cm length) packed with alginate-entrapped BL21-*mlrA* cells during five days of continuous flow. The initial MC-LR concentration was 35 µg L^{-1}. Solid, dashed and dotted lines show the response to the column temperatures of 20, 15 and 10 °C, respectively. Error bars indicate the standard deviation ($n = 3$).

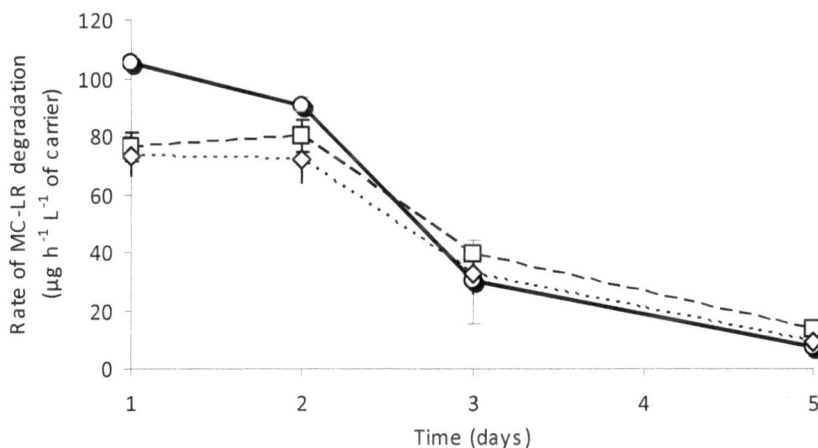

3. Discussion

3.1. Biodegradation of MCs as a Promising Alternative

The proposed biotechnological systems for the removal of cyanotoxins from drinking water indicated that biologically-active filters may be an alternative water treatment option [9,15]. Granular activated carbon (GAC) filters can be applied both for the adsorption and biodegradation, whereas the removal of MCs in sand filters has been shown to be primarily through biological degradation processes. Other materials have also been applied in the biological filtration of cyanotoxins, such as glass beads, porous ceramic materials and plastic media. So far, such proposals have assumed the use of naturally occurring bacterial strains immobilized on different carriers. However, bioreactors that employ wild strains still seem to act relatively slowly in comparison with the chemo-physical treatment of water. A possible solution to this problem may be a significant increase of the MC degradation potency of the used microorganisms. The idea of the present research is based on the utilization of genetically engineered microorganisms (GEMs).

Despite the potential risks of impacting the environment due to the persistence of undesired genes and their transfer to indigenous species, the application of GEM has been proposed as an attractive method in biological wastewater treatment and bioremediation of soil or groundwater. *Pseudomonas fluorescens* HK44, which is able to degrade polyaromatic hydrocarbons, is the first genetically engineered bacterium that has been approved by the U.S. Environmental Protection Agency for use in bioremediation of soils in the field [16]. Recently, several genetically engineered microorganisms have been successfully constructed for bioremediation purposes [17–20]; however, environmental concerns and regulatory constraints limit their application *in situ*. In this work, the construction and usage of genetically modified bacteria is assumed; however, the action of such bacteria is limited to the space of bioreactors, and no release into the environment is expected.

Within the last two years, some manuscripts documenting the heterologous expression of Mlr proteins have been published. Such an approach provides several advantages, e.g., better biochemical characterization of these important enzymes, as well as verification of their role in microcystin degradation [21–24]. Such research also provides broader perspectives for future studies and gives crucial background for original application systems for utilizing dangerous water components. The bacteria with enhanced MC-degradation capability require (in practice) the expression of only the MlrA enzyme with access to MCs, because the linear form of MCs are, in environmentally relevant concentrations, non-toxic [21].

3.2. MlrA Location

The cells of the *E. coli* BL21-*mlrA* strain tested previously [21] have indicated relatively high activity against MCs, three orders of magnitude higher than the natural degrader, the *Sphingomonas* AMC-3962 strain. Additionally, the same ratio of activity was noticed when cells of both strains were immobilized in alginate [13]. Based on the compared activity of cells and cell extracts (ratio 1:440, [21]), it was suspected that only a small portion of MlrA acts directly in the intact cells. Present data confirm such hypothesis, because an analysis of the MlrA location in BL21 cells indicated that a large portion of MlrA is located in cytosol, whereas only a few percent of MlrA activity was found in the periplasm. The possible explanation of these results may be that only a few percent of the enzyme molecules is secreted outside the inner membrane of bacteria, where the linearization of MC probably occurs. Such results suggest that the transformed BL21 cells do not use the whole potency and that a large portion of the MlrA is not employed in MC decomposition. The construction of other recombinant *mlrA* variants with a sequence delivering the enzyme into the periplasmic space may be a possible way of increasing the efficiency of MC degradation by living cells.

3.3. Efficiency of Bioreactors

In our recent report, we indicated that immobilization of MC-degrading bacteria in alginate is a promising option [13]. Among different natural polysaccharide matrices used in the immobilization technique for microorganisms, entrapment in alginate is one of the most commonly employed [25]. To mimic the natural condition, MC-LR solution was always prepared by dilution in freshwater from Dobczyckie Lake. To obtain the maximal activity of alginate beads against MC and the maximal potency of bioreactors, the highest tested value of cell condensation is preferred (Figure 2) for future experiments. However, this strategy requires a larger volume of cell culture and results in a lower immobilization efficiency. It implies a higher production cost of cells with the desired properties. In future experiments, different parameters must be tested to optimize the proportion of cells and alginate and to find more efficient immobilization conditions, as well. The choice between "closed" and "open" systems of water treatment poses another problem. In closed bioreactors, a certain volume of water with MC-LR was treated with alginate beads for different periods of time (which may be controlled), whereas in open systems, the volume of water to be purified was not limited, but the time of treatment was dependent on the flow rate. Our results indicated that the usability of the tested systems depends on the common initial concentration of MCs (Table 2). An open system is more suitable when water with a lower level of toxins ($10 \ \mu g \ L^{-1}$) is purified. In such a condition the MC-LR concentration is reduced immediately to the level close to that recommended by WHO, whereas in bath bioreactor, this value is obtained after 60 min of incubation. In the assay with $35 \ \mu g \ L^{-1}$ of MC-LR, the closed system seems to be more effective, because the recommended MC level may be reached in 60 min, whereas the column allows only partial purification of water with the MC-LR concentration significantly above the recommended level. On the other hand in both tested concentrations, the degradation rate is stable during the continuous flow of treated water, which is a big advantage in comparison with a batch bioreactor. In a closed system with a mechanical mix, the rate of degradation was very high in the first 5 min, but this parameter drastically decreased over time, and a dependence of the rate of degradation on MC-LR concentration was observed. Intensive mixing increases the probability of contact between MC molecules and the cells; however, when the MC-LR concentration is reduced (in a closed bioreactor), the interaction of MlrA with MC molecules are changed and the degradation rate decreases, as well. In an open system, continuous flow allows regular contact between the contaminant and the cells, thus, the rate of degradation may be stable for a longer period. Based on these results, an open system was analyzed in the subsequent study, as it is more suitable for continuous biodegradation of MCs. In the experiments with different column lengths and different MC-LR concentrations (tested in an open system, Figure 3), both parameters influenced the frequency of contact between MC-LR and the alginate-entrapped cells. At the initial concentration of MC-LR $10 \ \mu g \ L^{-1}$, the concentration of toxin leaking from the column was close to the WHO recommendation ($1.4 \ \mu g \ L^{-1}$). The system should be scaled-up in the future from laboratory to technical size, but we assume that in a longer column and at a relevantly faster flow rate, a similar value of MC-LR degradation efficiency may be expected.

Table 2. Compared results of selected research on different MC removal systems.

Cited work	Type of reactor	Initial MC concentration (μg L^{-1})	Calculated parameters of MC removal	
			Rate of degradation (μg h^{-1} L^{-1})	Efficiency (%)
[26]	Slow sand filter with *Sphingomonas* MJ-PV strain inoculated in column	50	1.3	80
[27]	Cells of B-9 strain immobilized on polyester pieces in closed container	200	7.5	90
[8]	Morgan WTP filter sand packed in column colonized by bacteria with *mlrA* gene	20	40	100
[28]	Photocatalytic degradation in continuous treatment system	5	225.0 [a]	85
present work	Column filled with alginate beads, BL21(DE3)-*mlrA* cells immobilized in gel	10	30.5	86
		35	105.5	85
		100	219.9	62
		35	3.8 [b]	–

Notes: [a] Rate of degradation of the whole system consisting of four 2.6 L reactors lit with four mercury vapor lamps (125 W) and treated with TiO$_2$ (250 mg L^{-1}); [b] rate of MC-LR degradation after four weeks of continuous flow.

3.4. Stability of Designed System

A crucial parameter of bioreactors is their stability in the natural environment. Our system does not provide stable operation at high intensity for a long period, and the rate of degradation decreases over time (Figure 4). This means that to obtain better efficiency, the flow rate must be relevantly reduced for longer column operation. However, even after significant efficiency decrease, the rate of MC-LR degradation observed in a bioreactor operated at 20 °C after four weeks of continuous flow is still comparable to bioreactors that employ the natural strains (Table 2).

The calculated rate of degradation documented Bourne *et al.* [26] and Tsuji *et al.* [27] was several times lower than in our system. Only the work of Ho *et al.* [8] indicated a relatively fast degradation of MC (up to 20 μg L^{-1}) in 7.5 min of empty bed contact time (Table 2). The initial rate of degradation documented in our work is also comparable with the recently published system, which assumes photocatalytic degradation of MCs [28], (Table 2). The previous proposals assumed that the bioreactors operate for several weeks or months and are able to regenerate, which is possible because the cells can proliferate inside the carrier. Additionally, the competition ability of the used natural strains is essential. However, in the cited works, the acclimation phase is required, which makes fast preparation of the system problematic. The proposal presented in this work is different. The tested stability of the system is short (a few days) and seems to be only slightly dependent on the temperature (Figure 4). However, the initial MC-LR degradation rate is very high and, after a few weeks, still similar to bioreactors proposed earlier [26,27]. This experiment indicates that despite its low stability, the proposed system may nevertheless operate better in comparison with some of the previous solutions. The application of alginate-entrapped modified cells may be different. Such a bioreactor can provide a quick reaction in sudden risk, in case of a fast bloom formation or a massive release of MCs from the cells; the documented rate of degradation depends on the initial MC concentration and is faster when the level of MCs is high. In such a situation, a high degradation rate is crucial and more important than stability. Such a column filled with carrier, which is extremely active toward MCs, may be employed in the purification of fish ponds or water reservoirs for the irrigation of fields.

4. Experimental Section

4.1. Materials

Trifluoroacetic acid (TFA) and sodium alginate were from Sigma (St. Louis, MO, USA). The RP C18 Purospher column was obtained from Merck (Darmstadt, Germany). MC-LR was extracted from a culture of Microcystis aeruginosa PCC 7813 strain obtained from the Pasteur Institute (Paris, France) and HPLC purified, as described earlier [29]. Escherichia coli BL21(DE3) (Novagen, an Affiliate of Merck KGaA, Darmstadt, Germany) with pET21a-*mlrA* used for the expression of recombinant proteins was grown at 37 °C in LB broth supplemented with ampicillin (100 µg mL^{-1}).

4.2. Expression of Recombinant MlrA

The pET21a-*mlrA* construct obtained using a procedure described earlier [21] was transformed into *E. coli* BL21(DE3), and the bacteria were plated on LB agar plates supplemented with ampicillin (100 µg mL^{-1}). Before the experiments described below, a fresh culture was prepared by incubation in LB medium supplemented with ampicillin for 24 h, until the absorbance at 600 nm (A_{600}) was in the range 1.5–2.0. In the experiments that required the induction of recombinant expression, the temperature was decreased to 30 °C when $A_{600} = 0.8$ was reached (approximately after 4 h) and IPTG (isopropyl β-D-thiogalactoside) at a final concentration of 1 mM was added; then, culturing was continued for 20 h. Subsequently, the bacteria were centrifuged (15,000× g, 10 min, 4 °C), and the pellet was further processed, as described below.

4.3. Location of MlrA Activity in Cellular Fractions

IPTG-induced and non-induced cells of 24 h-old *E. coli* BL21(DE3) cultures were centrifuged for 15 min (6,000 rpm) and washed with 100 mL of 50 mM Tris-NaCl buffer, pH 7.5. All subsequent steps were performed at 4 °C. The periplasmic fraction was isolated by suspension of pellet (1:2, w/v) in 100 mM Tris buffer (pH 7.5) with 750 mM sucrose and 1 mg mL^{-1} of lysozyme. Cells were gently shaken for 1 h. Then, EDTA was added (1 mM final concentration), and the incubation was continued for 45 min. After the addition of 5 mM MgCl$_2$ (final concentration), the pellet was centrifuged for 20 min at 6,000 rpm to obtain the periplasmic fraction. The cytosolic fraction was prepared by sonication of the pellet in 50 mM Tris buffer, pH 7.5 containing 300 mM NaCl, 1 mM PMSF and 1 mM EDTA. Subsequently, the centrifuged pellet (used to isolate the membrane fraction) was suspended in the same buffer containing 1% (v/m) of DDM (n-dodecyl β-D-maltopyranoside) and gently shaken overnight, then centrifuged at 30,000 rpm for 30 min. The

MlrA activity assays were performed for all of the fractions according to the procedure described previously [21].

4.4. Immobilization of E. coli BL21-mlrA on Alginate

The immobilization procedure was performed as described previously [13]. Forty milliliters of freshly cultured bacteria of E. coli BL21-mlrA (18 h-old culture, $OD_{600} \approx 2.0$) were centrifuged and resuspended in 2 mL of 50 mM phosphate buffer, pH 7.0. The cell suspension was mixed with 60 mg of slowly added sodium alginate. Next, it was dropped into 5% $CaCl_2$ to obtain beads of approximately 1 mm in diameter, which were then incubated in 5% $CaCl_2$ for half an hour at 5 °C. The MlrA activity of the intact E. coli BL21-mlrA cells was measured as described earlier using the HPLC method [13]. The rate of MC degradation was calculated by monitoring the level of linear MC-LR.

4.5. Activity of Alginate Beads with Entrapped E. coli BL21-mlrA

The dependence of activity of alginate beads toward MC-LR on the cells concentration was documented by the measurement of MC-LR degradation in glass vials. The beads were prepared according to the procedure described above (Section 4.4.); however, different dilutions of the cells were used (3-, 10-, 30-, 100-, 300-fold dilution; the initial density was 1.2×10^{10} cells mL^{-1}). Ten beads (0.45 g of the total mass) were placed in the glass vials filled with 1 mL of MC-LR solution (0.5 µg mL^{-1}). The level of linear MC-LR was monitored after 5, 20, 60 and 120 min of incubation at 20 °C by HPLC (20 µL injection volume). MlrA activity was expressed in mU (one unit is defined as the amount of MlrA that catalyzes the production of 1 µM of linear MC-LR per minute).

4.6. Degradation of MC-LR in the Bioreactors

In a closed bioreactor, a glass container was incubated at 20 °C and filled with 60 mL of MC-LR dissolved in filtered freshwater from Dobczyckie Lake. Alginate beads with entrapped cells were mixed on a magnetic stirrer. The open system of water treatment (Figure 1) consisted of an Econo Gradient Pump (Bio-Rad, Hercules, CA, USA), a 13.5-mm diameter glass column filled with the beads, which formed different amounts of the carrier, and a Retriever 500 autosampler (Isco, Lincoln, NE, USA). The constant flow of the MC-LR solution (10, 35 and 100 µg L^{-1}) was 0.5 mL min^{-1}, and the column was thermostated in Jetstream 2 plus column thermostat (Waters Corporation, Milford, MA, USA). In the both systems (closed and open), the level of linear MC-LR was measured after 5, 20, 40, 60, 120 and 180 min. The procedure was repeated 3 times using new, freshly prepared beads. In the 5-day experiment, three columns incubated at different temperatures (20, 15 and 10 °C) were used simultaneously.

4.7. HPLC Assays

HPLC analyses, including the MC-LR degradation rate and identification of the products, were performed using a Waters HPLC system (Waters Corporation, Milford, MA, USA) consisting of a 600E multisolvent-delivery system, a 717 plus autosampler, a 996 photodiode array detector (PDA), Millenium32 SS software and a Jetstream 2 plus column thermostat. MC-LR and its degradation product were quantified on a Purospher STAR RP-18 endcapped column, 55 mm × 4 mm, 3 μm particles (Merck, Darmstadt, Germany), as described by Meriluoto and Spoof [30]. The mobile phase consisted of a gradient of 0.05% aqueous TFA (Solvent A) and 0.05% TFA in acetonitrile (Solvent B) with the following linear gradient program: 0 min 25% B, 5 min 70% B, 6 min 70% B and 6.1 min 25% B.

5. Conclusions

The obtained results are important in assessing the benefits and obstacles associated with their applications in the removal of cyanobacterial contaminants. Further research should focus on several important parameters, of which the crucial ones are: (1) construction of bacteria with higher activity toward MCs; (2) finding the best immobilization techniques and the optimization of such a procedure; and (3) the study of the long-term stability of the designed systems in natural conditions. Such knowledge is necessary to design efficient bioreactors for MC utilization.

Acknowledgments

Grateful acknowledgement is given to Ministry of Science and Higher Education, Poland, which supported the research on biodegradation of microcystins (Grant No 4360/B/P01/2010/39). Furthermore, acknowledgement is given to Agnieszka Polit (Jagiellonian University) for the separation of cell fractions.

Author Contributions

Dariusz Dziga, Magdalena Lisznianska and Benedykt Wladyka contributed to the design and performance of the experimental work. Dariusz Dziga performed the data analysis and wrote the article, Magdalena Lisznianska and Benedykt Wladyka contributed in manuscript revision.

Conflicts of Interest

The authors declare no conflict of interest.

References

1. Welker, M.; Steinberg, C. Rates of humic substance photosensitized degradation of microcystin-LR in natural waters. *Environ. Sci. Technol.* **2000**, *34*, 3415–3419.
2. Zhang, W.H.; Fang, T.; Xu, X.Q. Study on photodegradation of cyanobacterial toxin in blooms of Dianchi Lake. *China Environ. Sci.* **2001**, *21*, 1–3.

3. Christoffersen, K.; Lyck, S.; Winding, A. Microbial activity and bacterial community structure during degradation of microcystins. *Aquat. Microb. Ecol.* **2002**, *27*, 125–136.

4. Pflugmacher, S.; Wiegand, C.; Beattie, K.A.; Codd, G.A.; Steinberg, C.E.W. Uptake of the cyanobacterial hepatotoxin microcystin-LR by aquatic macrophytes. *J. Appl. Bot.* **1998**, *72*, 228–232.

5. Tsuji, K.; Masui, H.; Uemura, H.; Mori, Y.; Harada, K.I. Analysis of microcystins in sediments using MMPB method. *Toxicon* **2001**, *39*, 687–692.

6. Holst, T.; Jorgensen, N.O.G.; Jorgensen, C.; Johansen, A. Degradation of microcystin in sediments at oxic and anoxic, denitrifying conditions. *Water Res.* **2003**, *37*, 4748–4760.

7. Dziga, D.; Wasylewski, M.; Wladyka, B.; Nybom, S.; Meriluoto, J. Microbial degradation of microcystins. *Chem. Res. Toxicol.* **2013**, *26*, 841–842.

8. Ho, L.; Meyn, T.; Keegan, A.; Hoefel, D.; Brookes, J.; Saint, C.P.; Newcombe, G. Bacterial degradation of microcystin toxins within a biologically active sand filter. *Water Res.* **2006**, *40*, 768–774.

9. Ho, L.; Newcombe, G. Evaluating the adsorption of microcystin toxins using granular activated carbon (GAC). *J. Water. Supply. Res. Technol.* **2007**, *56*, 281–291.

10. Wang, H.; Ho, L.; Lewis, D.M.; Brookes, J.D.; Newcombe, G. Discriminating and assessing adsorption and biodegradation removal mechanisms during granular activated carbon filtration of microcystin toxins. *Water Res.* **2007**, *41*, 4262–4270.

11. Ji, R.P.; Lua, X.W.; Li, X.N.; Pu, J.P. Biological degradation of algae and microcystins by microbial enrichment on artificial media. *Ecol. Eng.* **2009**, *35*, 1584–1588.

12. Sumino, T.; Ogasawara, T.; Park, H.D. Method and Equipment for Treating Microcystin-Containing Water. U.S. Patent 7.425.267, 16 September 2008.

13. Dziga, D.; Sworzen, M.; Wladyka, B.; Wasylewski, M. Genetically engineered bacteria immobilized in alginate as an option of cyanotoxins removal. *Intern. J. Environ. Sci. Develop.* **2013**, *4*, 360–364.

14. Eleuterio, L.; Batista, F.R. Biodegradation studies and sequencing of microcystin-LR degrading bacteria isolated from a drinking water biofilter and a fresh water lake. *Toxicon* **2010**, *55*, 1434–1442.

15. Ho, L.; Gaudieux, A.L.; Fanok, S.; Newcombe, G.; Humpage, A.R. Bacterial degradation of microcystin toxins in drinking water eliminates their toxicity. *Toxicon* **2007**, *50*, 438–441.

16. Sayler, G.S.; Ripp, S. Field applications of genetically engineered microorganisms for bioremediation processes. *Curr. Opin. Biotechnol.* **2000**, *11*, 286–289.

17. Dogra, Ch.; Raina, V.; Pal, R.; Suar, M.; Lal, S.; Gartemann, K.H.; Holliger, Ch.; van der Meer, J.; Lal, R. Organization of lin genes and IS6100 among different strains of hexachlorocyclohexane-degrading *Sphingomonas paucimobilis*. Evidence for horizontal gene transfer. *J. Bacteriol.* **2004**, *186*, 2225–2235.

18. Jiang, J.; Zhang, R.; Cui, Z.; He, J.; Gu, L.; Li, S. Parameters controlling the gene-targeting frequencyat the *Sphingomonas* species rrn site and expression of the methyl parathion hydrolase gene. *J. Appl. Microbiol.* **2006**, *102*, 1578–1585.

19. Jiang, J.; Zhang, R.J.; Li, R.; Gu, J.; Li, S. Simultaneous biodegradation of methyl parathion and carbofuran by a genetically engineered microorganism constructed by mini-Tn5 transposon. *Biodegradation* **2007**, *18*, 403–412.

20. Liu, Z.; Hong, Q.; Xu, J.K.; Jun, W.; Li, S.P. Construction of a genetically engineered microorganism for degrading organophosphate and carbamate pesticides. *Intern. Biodeterior. Biodegrad.* **2006**, *58*, 65–69.

21. Dziga, D.; Wladyka, B.; Zielińska, G.; Meriluoto, J.; Wasylewski, M. Heterologous expression and characterisation of microcystinase. *Toxicon* **2012**, *59*, 578–586.

22. Dziga, D.; Wasylewski, M.; Szettla, A.; Bocheńska, O.; Wladyka, B. Verification of the role of MlrC in microcystin biodegradation by studies using a heterologously expressed enzyme. *Chem. Res. Toxicol.* **2012**, *25*, 1192–1194.

23. Shimizu, K.; Maseda, H.; Okano, K.; Kurashima, T.; Kawauchi, Y.; Xue, Q.; Utsumi, M.; Zhang, Z.; Sugiura, N. Enzymatic pathway for biodegrading microcystin LR in *Sphingopyxis* sp. C-1. *J. Biosci. Bioeng.* **2012**, *114*, 630–634.

24. Yan, H.; Wang, J.; Chen, J.; Wie, W.; Wang, H.; Wang, H. Characterization of the first step involved in enzymatic pathway for microcystin-RR biodegraded by *Sphingopyxis* sp. USTB-05. *Chemosphere* **2012**, *87*, 12–18.

25. Moreno-Garrido, I. Microalgae immobilization: Current techniques and uses. *Bioresour. Technol.* **2008**, *99*, 3949–3964.

26. Bourne, D.G.; Blakeley, R.L.; Riddles, P.; Jones, G.J. Biodegradation of the cyanobacterial toxin microcystin LR in natural water and biologically active slow sand filters. *Water Res.* **2006**, *40*, 1294–1302.

27. Tsuji, K.; Asakawa, M.; Anzai, Y.; Sumino, T.; Harada, K. Degradation of microcystins using immobilized microorganism isolated in an eutrophic lake. *Chemosphere* **2006**, *65*, 117–124.

28. Jacobs, L.C.; Peralta-Zamora, P.; Campos, F.R.; Pontarolo, R. Photocatalytic degradation of microcystin-LR in aqueous solutions. *Chemosphere* **2013**, *90*, 1552–1557.

29. Gajdek, P.; Lechowski, Z.; Dziga, D.; Bialczyk, J. Detoxification of microcystin-LR using Fenton reagent. *Fresen. Environ. Bull.* **2003**, *12*, 1258–1262.

30. Meriluoto, J.; Spoof, L. Analysis of Microcystins by High Performance Liquid Chromatography with Photodiode-Array Detection. In *TOXIC: Cyanobacterial Monitoring and Cyanotoxin Analysis*; Meriluoto, J., Codd, G.A., Eds.; Åbo Akademi University Press: Turku, Finland, 2005; pp. 77–84.

Cyanobacteria and Cyanotoxins Occurrence and Removal from Five High-Risk Conventional Treatment Drinking Water Plants

David C. Szlag, James L. Sinclair, Benjamin Southwell and Judy A. Westrick

Abstract: An environmental protection agency EPA expert workshop prioritized three cyanotoxins, microcystins, anatoxin-a, and cylindrospermopsin (MAC), as being important in freshwaters of the United States. This study evaluated the prevalence of potentially toxin producing cyanobacteria cell numbers relative to the presence and quantity of the MAC toxins in the context of this framework. Total and potential toxin producing cyanobacteria cell counts were conducted on weekly raw and finished water samples from utilities located in five US states. An Enzyme-Linked Immunosorbant Assay (ELISA) was used to screen the raw and finished water samples for microcystins. High-pressure liquid chromatography with a photodiode array detector (HPLC/PDA) verified microcystin concentrations and quantified anatoxin-a and cylindrospermopsin concentrations. Four of the five utilities experienced cyanobacterial blooms in their raw water. Raw water samples from three utilities showed detectable levels of microcystins and a fourth utility had detectable levels of both microcystin and cylindrospermopsin. No utilities had detectable concentrations of anatoxin-a. These conventional plants effectively removed the cyanobacterial cells and all finished water samples showed MAC levels below the detection limit by ELISA and HPLC/PDA.

Reprinted from *Toxins*. Cite as: Szlag, D.C.; Sinclair, J.L.; Southwell, B.; Westrick, J.A. Cyanobacteria and Cyanotoxins Occurrence and Removal from Five High-Risk Conventional Treatment Drinking Water Plants. *Toxins* **2015**, *7*, 2198-2220.

1. Introduction

Cyanobacteria, also known as blue-green algae, are photosynthetic bacteria that can live in many types of water. Rapid, excessive cyanobacteria growth, often referred to as a "bloom", is linked to eutrophication and high water temperatures. Many genera of cyanobacteria are known to produce toxins. These toxins (cyanotoxins) make up a large group of chemical compounds that differ in their molecular structure and toxicological properties. They are generally grouped into major classes according to their toxicological targets: cell, liver, nervous system, skin, and tumor promotion. Microcystins are hepatotoxins commonly produced by the cyanobacteria genera *Anabaena*, *Microcystis*, *Oscillatoria*, *Planktothrix*, *Nostoc*, and *Hapalosiphon*. Cylindrospermopsin is a hepatotoxin and cytotoxin produced by the filamentous cyanobacteria *Aphanizomenon* and *Cylindrospermopsis*. Both microcystin-LR [1] and cylindrospermopsin [2] are suspected tumor promotors. Anatoxin-a is a neurotoxin produced by the cyanobacteria *Aphanizomenon*, *Anabaena*, and *Oscillatoria*. Common freshwater cyanobacteria genera like *Microcystis*, *Planktothrix*, *Aphanizomenon* and *Anabaena* contain many species and genotypes that may be both toxic and capable of forming blooms and also may cause problems not related to toxicity in water bodies used as drinking water sources [3]. A significant feature of these blooms is that their cyanotoxin production is highly variable. A single bloom may contain multiple types of cyanotoxins because a bloom may have more than one toxin-producing genus [4] and/or potentially one genus may produce more than one toxin [5]. However, occurrence of a cyanobacteria bloom does not necessarily mean there is a cyanotoxin problem. Multiple genotypes of cyanobacteria can exist in a single bloom, and some produce toxins while others do not. Even genotypes or species that can produce toxins do not always produce the toxins. Under some conditions toxic genotypes will not produce toxins at all. The environmental conditions that trigger or inhibit production of cyanotoxins remain poorly understood and remain an active area of research. Another feature common to cyanobacterial blooms is the formation of surface scums or bands of high cell concentration in the water column. Surface scums are often blown by the wind into bays and areas with poor water circulation allowing cyanobacteria and cyanotoxins to build up to very high concentrations.

There are numerous studies that have surveyed virtually all regions of the planet for the occurrence of cyanobacteria and cyanotoxins. WHO (1999) [5], and Fristachi et al. [6] provide an overview of the worldwide occurrence studies. Within the U.S. and Canada there are numerous reports from state and local health agencies that have not been published in the peer-reviewed literature but are available through websites and bulletins. The occurrence of microcystin producers and microcystins dominate these reports. Very few studies have investigated cylindrospermopsin or anatoxin-a in North America. Graham et al. [7] provides a detailed survey of cyanobacteria and cyanotoxins, including seven microcystin congeners, anatoxin-a, cylindrospermopsin, lyngbya toxin-a, and nodularin in reservoirs and lakes in the Midwestern U.S. Microcystin is the most frequently observed toxin in this study.

As of 2015, insufficient epidemiological data are available to develop a guideline value or standard for lifetime exposure to any of the cyanotoxins. High acute exposures to microcystins can cause gastroenteritis and liver damage [5]. Data and studies on chronic human exposure to microcystins are sparse. Studies that have come out of China supporting a link between elevated cancer incidence and exposure to microcystins include those by Zhou et al. (2000) [8] and works by Yu (2001) [9]. No information is available on the carcinogenicity of cylindrospermopsin in humans, and no definitive cancer studies of purified cylindrospermopsin have been conducted in animals. Falconer and Humpage (2006) observed a tenuous link between cylindrospermopsin exposure and tumor growth in a mouse study but the study lacked statistical power [10]. No studies link anatoxin-a to chronic health effects. The provisional WHO guideline value for microcystin LR is based on doses from short-term mouse studies using the no adverse effect level (NOAEL) methodology [11]. A tolerable daily intake (TDI) of 0.04 µg/kg body weight per day was derived from the 40 µg/kg NOAEL body using an uncertainty factor of 1000 (10 for intraspecies variation ×10 for interspecies variation and ×10 for less than-lifetime study). For drinking water, the WHO provisional guidance value (PGV) defines concentrations considered safe for lifetime consumption of 2 L of drinking-water per (60 kg person × day). Based on the described approach, the World Health Organization (WHO) through its updated 2011 Guidelines for Drinking-Water Quality [12] has recommended a provisional guidance value of 1 ug/L (1 ppb) total microcystin-LR in drinking water. It should be noted that this value includes free and cell-bound toxin and is for chronic exposure. Microcystins are the most widely researched group of toxins with microcystin-LR being the most frequently encountered as well as being one of the more toxic congeners. Consequently values developed for microcystin LR are generally considered to be conservative with respect to protecting public health. Some countries have used slightly different factors or included all microcystin congeners, but most worldwide guidelines range between 1.0 and 1.5 ug/L microcystin LR or LR equivalents. Some local health jurisdictions, areas of Scotland, as an example, allow short-term exposures to microcystins to exceed the WHO provisional guideline (Suggested No Adverse Effects: 24-h 12.0 ug/L and 7-day 6.0 ug/L microcystin-LR) [13]. Chorus [14] has compiled an unofficial partial list of provisional guidance values (PGVs), health alert levels (HALs) and standards from across the world. This compilation also includes values from a few countries that have set PGVs for cylindrospermopsin, anatoxin-a, and saxitoxins. PGVs for cylindrospermopsin range from 1–15 ug/L and PGVs for anatoxin-a range from 1–6 ug/L.

Currently, there are no U.S. federal regulatory guidelines or standards for cyanobacteria or their toxins in drinking water. Many states and local health authorities rely on guidelines published by the WHO or have derived their own guidelines to support public health decision-making. The Safe Drinking Water Act (SDWA) requires the U.S. Environmental Protection Agency (USEPA) to publish a list of unregulated contaminants that are present or expected to be detected in public water systems. These chemicals are on the drinking water Contaminant Candidate List (CCL). The CCL itself does not impose any requirements on public water systems. Instead, USEPA uses it to prioritize research efforts to help determine whether a contaminant has sufficient data to meet regulatory determination criteria specified in the SDWA. Freshwater cyanobacterial toxins were initially named to the drinking water Contaminant Candidate List (CCL) in 1998 by the Environmental Protection Agency (USEPA) based on insufficient data concerning toxicity, occurrence, and susceptibility to treatment (Table 2 of 63 FR 10273 [15]). In 2001 the US priority list of freshwater algal toxins included four of the more than eighty variants of microcystin (RR, LR, YR, and LA), cylindrospermopsin, and anatoxin-a. In 2012, three cyanotoxins remain listed on the CCL 3: anatoxin-a, microcystin-LR, and cylindrospermopsin. The USEPA did not implement the Unregulated Contaminant Monitoring Rule (UCMR) to more thoroughly assess the occurrence of cyanotoxins through the UCMR 3 initiated in 2012 (EPA, UCMR 3).

For the drinking water industry, the casual chain follows that when toxin producing genera are present in the source there is a risk that toxins will be present in the raw water; when toxins are present in the raw waters, there is a risk for toxins to also be present in finished drinking water. Drinking water utilities must manage this risk with appropriate responses that balance consumer safety, staff resources, economics, and the inherent variability of cyanobacteria blooms. Over the past two decades, several Risk Management Frameworks (RMFs) have been proposed by Burch [16,17], the WHO [5] and van Baalen and Du Preez [18]. All of these frameworks share a similarity in that progressive responses are based on parameters directly linked to toxic cyanobacteria such as cell numbers, chlorophyll-a, biovolume, biomass, and /or direct measurement of the cyanotoxin. In implementing any risk management plan a utility would assess its resources, treatment processes, source water(s) and geography, modify the plan for local conditions, and then implement it. In 1993 and again in 1999, the World Health Organization (WHO) presented a framework for cyanobacteria and toxin monitoring that have become the template for system specific risk management plans known as water safety plans by the WHO [5]. The original WHO risk management framework included three levels: a Vigilance Level, an Alert Level 1 and an Alert Level 2, with corresponding responses. The Vigilance Level would be achieved when cyanobacteria were detected at low concentrations. The main responses would be an increase in monitoring of the source water and monitoring of the raw water at the intakes by microscopy. Alert Level 1 would be achieved when the cyanobacterial cell concentration exceeded 2000 cyanobacteria cells/mL, or the chlorophyll-a concentration of the raw water exceeded 10 µg/L. Calculations showed that at these concentrations it was possible, but not necessarily likely, that the WHO provisional guideline, 1 ug/L, for microcystin-LR would be exceeded in the raw water. At this alert level the main responses could include increased monitoring frequency, cyanotoxin analysis, altering intake depths or locations, an assessment of the drinking water treatment barriers for cyanobacteria and cyanotoxin removal and communication with health officials and the public. Alert Level 2 would be reached when the cyanobacterial cell concentration exceeded 100,000 cells/mL, or the chlorophyll-a concentration of the raw water exceeded 50 µg/L and the cyanobacteria are shown to be toxic. The main actions during this alert level would include continued monitoring, treatment optimizations (often powdered activated carbon: PAC), consideration of alternative water supplies, and increased communication with health officials and the media. The WHO Alert Level Framework was useful, but recently the WHO has recognized limitations in a prescriptive AL risk management approach and has promoted an adaptive and holistic approach that is based on the Hazard Analysis and Critical Control Point (HACCP) approach used in the food industry. This approach recognizes that each utility is unique and that the levels and responses should be adjusted to each DWTP. Chorus [14] provides an overview of this approach and web based step by step guidance on water safety plans (WSPs).

Key information for implementation and discussion of the HAACP and water safety plan approach are the levels of cyanobacteria and cyanobacterial toxins in the raw water and finished water at each DWTP. The number of DWTP studies which measured cyanobacterial and toxins in raw and finished waters is limited. Hoeger et al. [19] provide a partial review and summary of world-wide drinking water treatment plant (DWTP) performance. Karner et al. [20] surveyed microcystin occurrence in raw and finished water from five utilities which used source water from two lakes. Bloom levels were visually noted. Lahti et al. [21] analyzed raw and finished water samples for microcystin and also determined the composition of cyanobacterial biomass by microscopy. Of particular relevance to this study are the major evaluations of North American DWTPs by Carmichael [22] and Robert et al. [23]. Carmichael [22] conducted a survey of 45 utilities across the U.S. and Canada for two years during bloom conditions when cyanobacteria reached or exceeded 2000 cells/mL. Microcystin concentrations were measured in raw and finished waters. All of these studies only investigated the occurrence of microcystin. Anatoxin-a has been rarely detected in North American drinking water sources and in general at low concentrations according to Roberts et al. [23] and Boyer et al. [24]. More recently Graham et al. [7] found that 30% of the lakes sampled in their Midwest U.S. survey contained anatoxin-a with concentrations ranging from 0.05 9.5 ug/L. The main concern with cylindrospermopsin-producing blooms, in contrast with microcystin-producing blooms, is that at different stages of a *Cylindrospermopsis* bloom, extracellular cylindrospermopsin concentrations can be substantial and range from 19 to 98% of the total amount in water [25,26].

Given the increasing presence and abundance of cylindrospermopsin and anatoxin-a-producing genera along with widespread occurrence of microcystin producers, the USEPA sought updated and expanded data for all priority toxins including the Microcystins, Anatoxin-a, and Cylindrospermopsin (MAC) [27]. Recently Zamyadi *et al.* evaluated all processes in a conventional DWTP for the removal of cyanobacteria and cyanotoxins [28]. This study intensively monitored the DWTP processes three times over 1–3 day intervals in 2008, 2009, and 2010. In 2008 and 2009 only microcystin-LR-eq were monitored. In 2010 multi-toxin LC/MS/MS method was used to identify priority microcystin congeners and cylindrospermopsin. On one occasion, traces of cylindrospermopsin were detected.

The aim of the present study was to collect concentration data regarding the MAC toxins in raw water and finished drinking water (clear well effluent) and the abundance of potential toxin producers during non-bloom and bloom conditions. Among the questions we hoped to answer from this study were:

- What is the likelihood of encountering detectable MAC toxins in different geographic areas of the U.S.?
- How do MAC concentrations from this study compare to levels found elsewhere?
- How effective are conventional DWTPs at removing MAC toxins and cyanobacterial cells?
- How do microcystin concentrations compare to the WHO provisional guideline level and to other proposed guidelines for cylindrospermopsin and anatoxin-a?
- How do measured MAC concentrations correlate with the cyanobacterial cell density alert level framework as described in Chorus and Bartram [5]?

2. Results and Discussion

A key element of a management program or water safety plan based on the WHO templates is the microscopic identification and enumeration of the cyanobacteria present in the raw water. In this study, simplified, rapid microscopic methods were used to estimate the cyanobacterial cell numbers and genus composition, at the genus level, in the raw and finished drinking water at five "high risk" DWTPs located in five states distributed across the U.S. Two graphs are presented for each DWTP. The first graph contains total algae and cyanobacteria, total cyanobacteria, and microcystin plotted on the secondary *y*-axis. Cylindrospermopsin was not plotted because it was only detected in one raw water sample. Anatoxin-a was not plotted because it was never detected. On the figures, microcystin levels below the 0.05 ug/L detection of the ELISA kit were plotted as zeros. Total algae were counted as naturally occurring colonies or cell aggregations which were referred to as units, whereas cyanobacteria were counted as individual cells or converted to individual cells. The second graph for each DWTP presents the cell concentration of the dominant potential toxin-producing cyanobacteria genera.

The goal of this study was to present a snapshot of the range of occurrence and concentration of MAC toxins and both total and potential toxin-producing cyanobacteria and to understand how conventional DWTPs performed over a 12–16 week spring-summer observation period. These five DWTPs, located in California, Texas, Oklahoma, Florida, and Vermont, were known to have potential toxin-producing cyanobacteria in their source waters and to experience a high frequency of blooms based on the author's observations, reports in the literature, or media reports. During the 12–16 week observation period, four of the five DWTPs in California, Texas, Florida (River source), and Oklahoma, total cyanobacteria cell numbers often exceeded the WHO AL 1 for cyanobacterial cells. The California DWTP raw water exceeded the WHO AL 2 on two occasions and the Texas DWTP exceeded the WHO AL 2 on one occasion. The concentrations of MAC toxins, however, were extremely low or below detection with only 1 out of the 71 (~1%) raw water samples exceeding the WHO PGV of 1 ug/L microcystin-LR.

General observations for cyanotoxins included:

- Microcystins were observed frequently in the raw water at low concentrations between 0.05 and 0.25 ug/L.
- Cylindrospermopsin was only detected in one raw water sample (Oklahoma at 0.41 ug/L in the May 2 sample).
- Anatoxin-a was not detected in any raw water sample.
- No MAC cyanotoxins were detected in any finished drinking water.
- There was no correlation between numbers of toxin-producer cyanobacteria and levels of toxins found.

The single detection of cylindrospermopsin was unexpected given the low numbers of potential cylindrospermopsin-producers present in that sample, and there were no detections of anatoxin-a in the raw water samples. It is possible that the availability and the increased sensitivity of the ELISA for microcystin compared to using only a less sensitive HPLC/PDA method for cylindrospermopsin and anatoxin-a may have skewed the frequency of detection results. Of the 43 total detections of microcystin by both ELISA and HPLC, 88% were below the detection limit for HPLC/PDA of 0.25 ug/L.

2.1. Individual Sites

2.1.1. California Plant

The greatest number of cyanobacteria found in any raw water occurred at the California DWTP (Figure 1). More than 300,000 *Microcystis* cells/mL were found on 9 May 2005 and 16 May 2005, which greatly exceeded the WHO AL 1 and WHO AL 2 monitoring framework thresholds of 2000 cells/mL and 100,000 cells/mL respectively. On two other occasions AL 1 was exceeded. On these dates, small colonies of *Microcystis* (Figure 2) accounted for almost all of the total cyanobacteria in these samples. Mid-summer samples from the California site showed that both total cyanobacteria and toxin-producing cyanobacteria declined to less than 1000 cells/mL. Figure 2 shows that through most of the sample period potential microcystin-producers outnumbered potential producers of cylindrospermopsin or anatoxin-a at the California site. No algal/cyanobacteria cells were found in any finished drinking water sample except for 1 August 2005 when 80 *Oscillatoria* cells/mL were found. The filaments that broke through the filter consisted of approximately

30 cells/unit. These results show that there was as much as 5.5 log removal of total cyanobacteria and potential toxin producers by water treatment (Table 1).

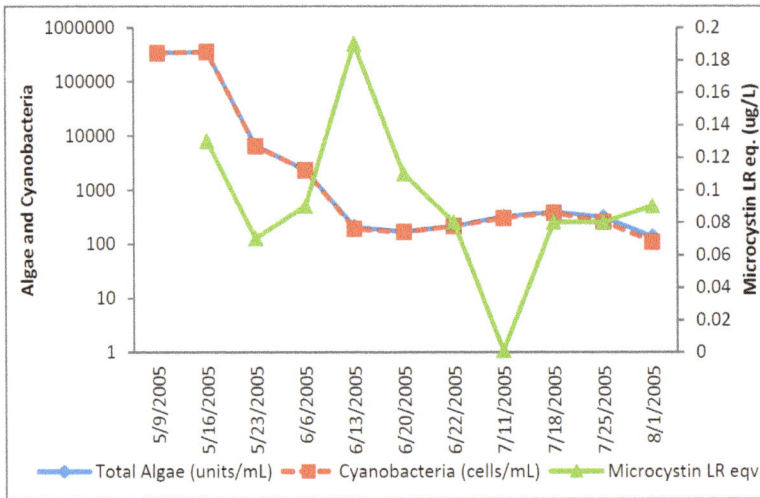

Figure 1. California algal density and ELISA microcystin concentration in raw water.

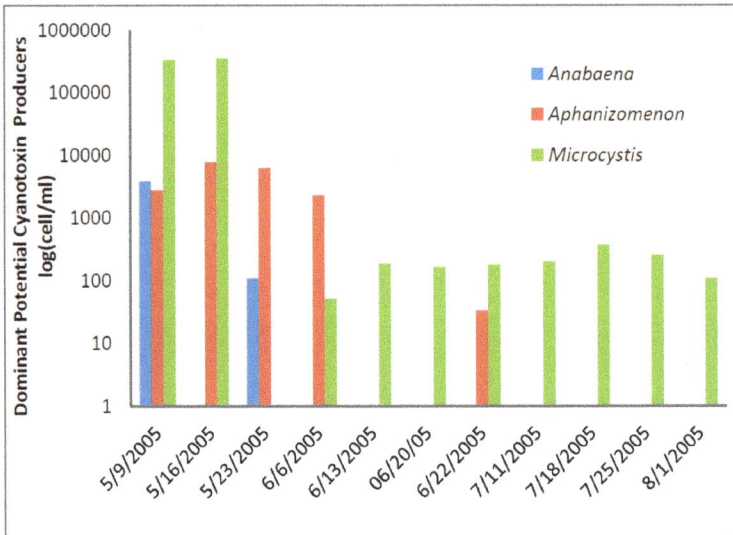

Figure 2. California site cyanobacteria potential producers of individual toxins.

Figure 1 shows that low levels of microcystin, determined by ELISA, were detected in all but the 11 July 2005 sample. The highest amount of microcystin detected by ELISA was 0.19 ug/L in the 6 June 2005 sample, which did not coincide and lagged the highest densities of *Microcystis* cells (Figure 1). This same sample, from 6 June 2005, was found to contain microcystin-LR at 0.79 ug/L when determined by HPLC/PDA. This was the only discrepancy between the ELISA (Envirologix

Inc., Portland, OR, USA) and HPLC/PDA (Waters Corporation, Milford, CT, USA) analyses at the California site. HPLC/PDA analysis did not detect microcystin in any other sample, or cylindrospermopsin or anatoxin-a in any sample of raw water. No toxins were detected by ELISA or HPLC in any finished drinking water sample.

2.1.2. Texas Plant

At the Texas site, potential toxin-producing cyanobacteria exceeded the AL 1 of 2000 cells/mL toward the end of sampling period five times (Figure 3) and AL 2 once. Total potential toxin-producers were well below 2000 cells/mL at the beginning of sampling period and generally represented less than half of the total cyanobacteria at that time. Both total cyanobacteria and total potential toxin-producing cyanobacteria increased over time so that toward the end of sampling potential toxin-producers accounted for nearly all of the cyanobacteria present. *Cylindrospermopsis* exceeded 2000 cells/mL on 18 July and 25 July and accounted for more than half of the total cyanobacteria on those dates. By 1 August 2005 the bloom became dominated by *Aphanizomenon*, which may produce cylindrospermopsin and anatoxin-a. It was present at 4700 cells/mL. The abundance of *Cylindrospermopsis* and *Aphanizomenon* near the end of sampling was responsible for the large numbers of potential cylindrospermopsin and anatoxin-a-producers at these times (Figure 4). *Anabaena* increased during the initial sampling period and exceeded 2000 cells three times, and declined after 18 July 2005 (Figure 4). It is a potential microcystin and anatoxin-a-producer.

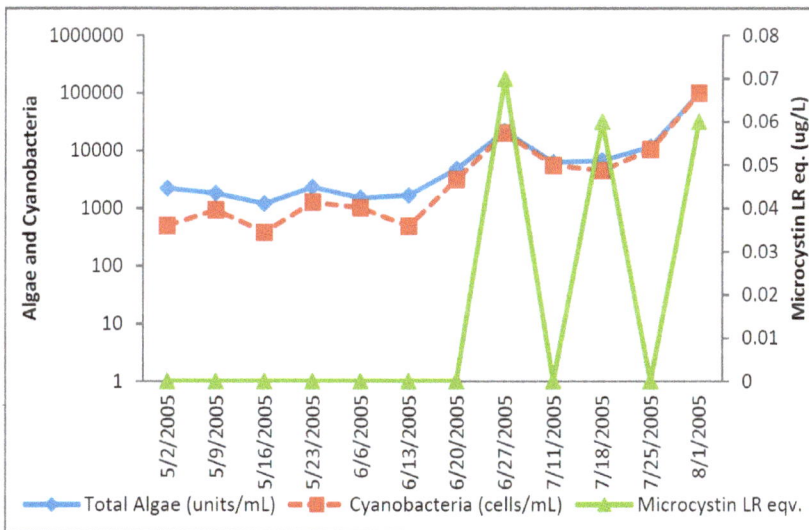

Figure 3. Texas algal density and ELISA microcystin concentration in raw water.

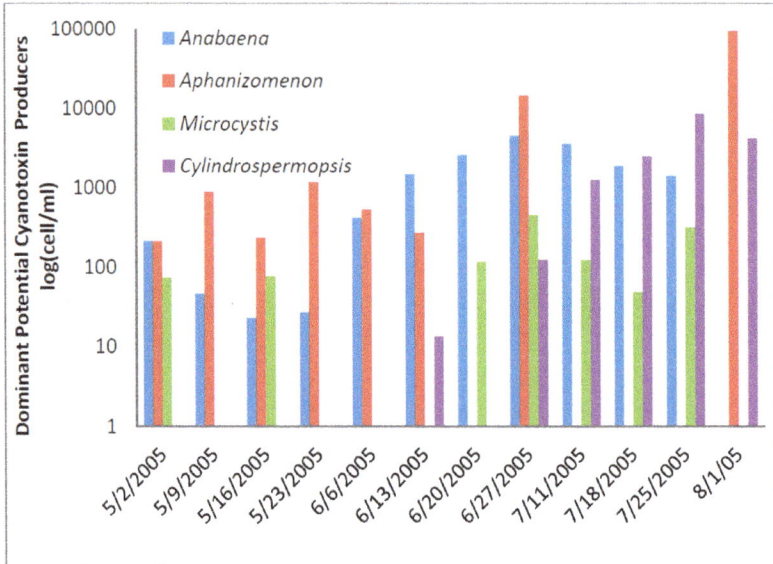

Figure 4. Texas toxin-producing cyanobacteria.

Microcystin detected by ELISA was observed in three samples at levels slightly above the detection limit during the latter part of the sampling period (Figure 4). HPLC/PDA did not detect microcystin, cylindrospermopsin, or anatoxin-a in any sample despite high densities of potential cylindrospermopsin and anatoxin-a-producers.

In the Texas DWTP finished water, 1 total algal unit/mL was detected in the 2 May, 9 May, 23 May, and 18 July 2005 samples. Additionally, less than 80 cells /mL of *Cylindrospermopsis*, *Aphanizomenon* and *Anabaena* were observed in the 11 July 2005 sample. No microcystin, cylindrospermopsin or anatoxin-a were observed in any distribution system sample. The log removal of total cyanobacteria by treatment was up to 4.0 log and about the same for the toxin-producers (Table 1).

Table 1. Range of cell removal by water treatment for total cyanobacteria and toxin-producers.

Location	Total Cyanobacteria (Range of cell removal (log_{10}))	Toxin Producers (Range of cell removal (log_{10}))
California	1.5 to >5.5	1.5 to >5.5
Oklahoma	1.6 to >3.4	0.2 to >3.2
Vermont	>2.5 to 3.1	* to >2.2
Texas	>2.8 to >4.0	>1.6 to >4.0
Florida (both sources)	1.6 to 3.8	1.6 to 3.3

* log removal cannot be determined. Toxin producer numbers were very low in the raw water, and not detected in the finished water.

2.1.3. Florida DWTP

The Florida Plant removed water from the river and pumped into a reservoir. Since the reservoir had longer than one day retention time, the reservoir was included as a second source to the utility. The Florida River exceeded the WHO Alert Level 1 monitoring level for eight of the raw water samples analyzed for cyanobacterial cells (Figure 5). Total potential toxin-producing cyanobacteria exceeded WHO Alert Level 1 for cell densities on 16 May, 23 May, and 23 July 2005, with the greatest number of 43,000/mL occurring on 16 May 2005 (Figure 6). *Aphanizomenon* was dominant. Potential toxin-producers were somewhat lower than total algal numbers during sampling but followed the same density trends in most samples. Potential cylindrospermopsin and anatoxin-a-producers increased to their highest numbers on 16 May 2005, declined through 27 June 2005 and increased thereafter. Potential microcystin-producers varied between 15,000 and 16,000 cells/mL. The potential microcystin-producers on this date consisted of *Microcystis* and *Oscillatoria*.

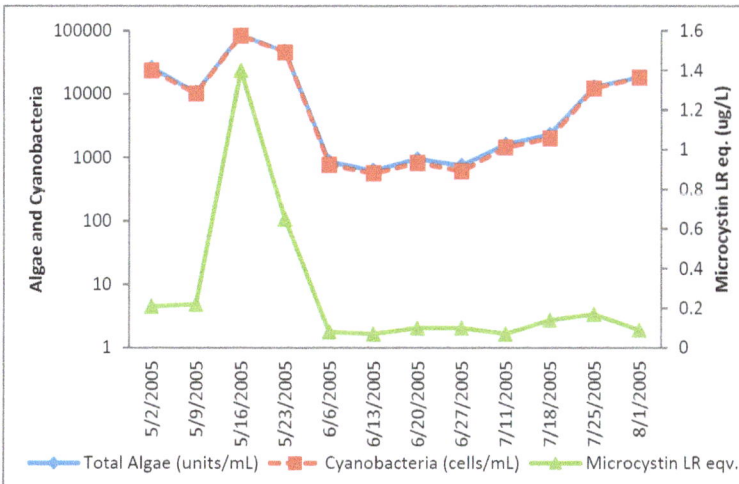

Figure 5. Florida River algal density and ELISA microcystin concentration in raw water.

The ELISA microcystin-LR equivalent analyses increased up to 1.41 ug/L microcystin-LR equivalents on 16 May 2005 before declining in later samples to levels below 0.2 ug/L. The 16 May 2005 raw water sample was the only sample in the entire study that exceeded the WHO guideline level of 1 ug/L for microcystin-LR in drinking water. Microcystin, cylindrospermopsin, and anatoxin-a were not detected by HPLC/PDA in any raw water sample. Microcystins, cylindrospermopsin, and anatoxin-a were not detected by HPLC/PDA or ELISA in any finished water sample.

The first eight finished water samples contained between 2 and 11 total and potential toxin-producer cyanobacteria per mL in the finished water, except for 23 May 2005 when 340 cells/mL of *Anaebena* and 1260 cells/mL of *Aphanizomenon* were present. After the eighth sample, finished water samples contained 0 to 20 cells of total cyanobacteria/mL. Water treatment reduced total cyanobacteria by as much as log 3.7 and toxin-producers by as much as log 3.3 (Table 1).

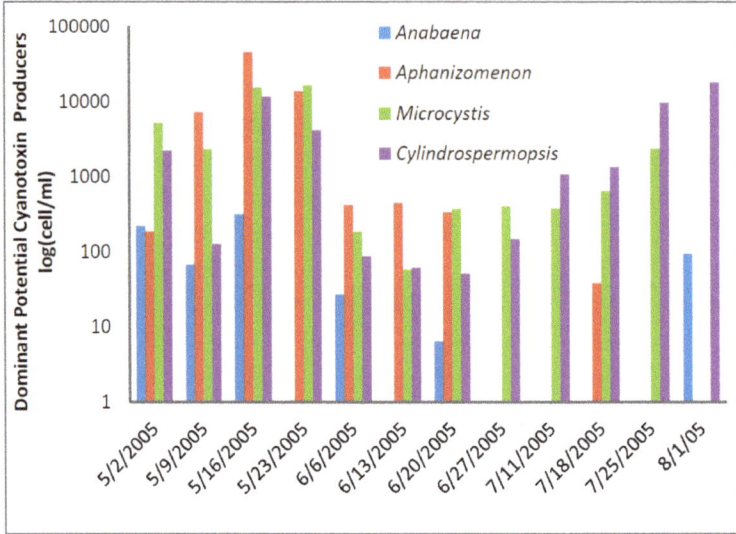

Figure 6. Florida River toxin-producers.

The total cyanobacteria exceeded AL 1 11 times in the reservoir. The potential toxin-producer cyanobacterial units were always lower than the total cyanobacteria in the Florida reservoir samples (Figures 7 and 8). The dominant genus was *Aphanizomenon*. *Microcystis* genera were uncommon and almost disappeared late in the sample period.

Microcystin as determined by ELISA was found in low concentrations in all samples except one. Microcystin, cylindrospermopsin, and anatoxin-a were not detected in the Florida reservoir samples by HPLC.

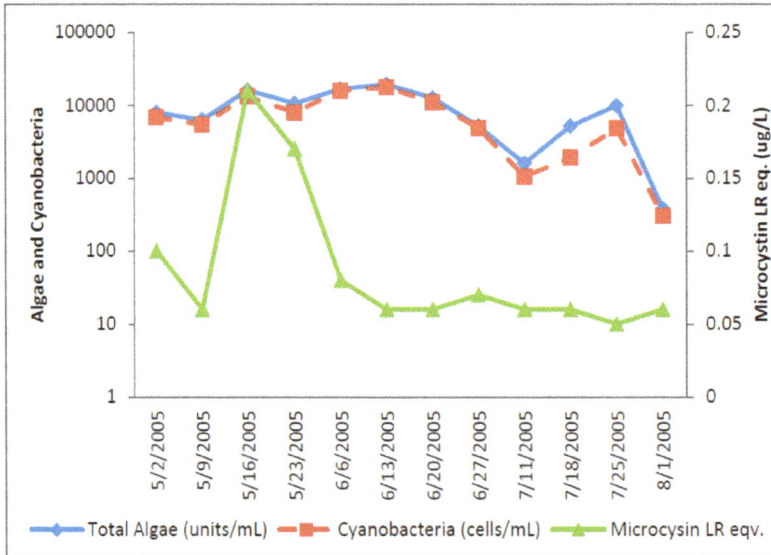

Figure 7. Florida Reservoir Cyanobacteria and Microcystin.

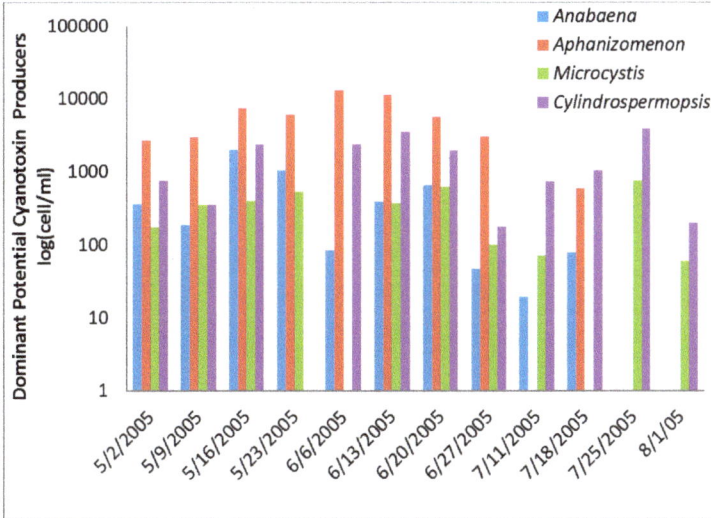

Figure 8. Florida Reservoir individual toxin producers.

2.1.4. Oklahoma

Total cyanobacteria exceeded the AL 1 10 out of 11 samples (Figure 9). *Aphanizomenon*, a potential producer of anatoxin-a and cylindrospermopsin, reached 14,600 cells/mL on 16 May 2005. *Microcystis* reached its peak of 500 cells on 20 June 2005 and accounted for 50% of the potential microcystin-producers on that day, with the remainder being *Anabaena*. *Cylindrospermopsis* reached its peak on 18 July 2005 of 17,000 cells/mL and then declined. It was the sole potential cylindrospermopsin-producer in those samples. These results shown in Figure 10 indicate that all three groups of potential toxin-producers were well represented at the Oklahoma site at some time during the study, but that cylindrospermopsin-producers reached numbers that were higher than the other types.

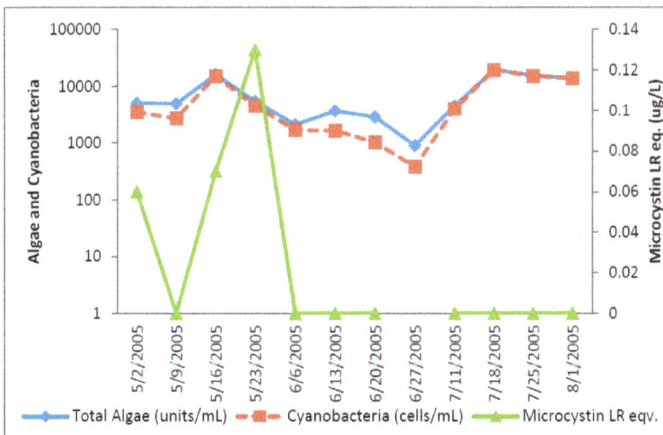

Figure 9. Oklahoma Total and toxic cyanobacteria and ELISA microcystin.

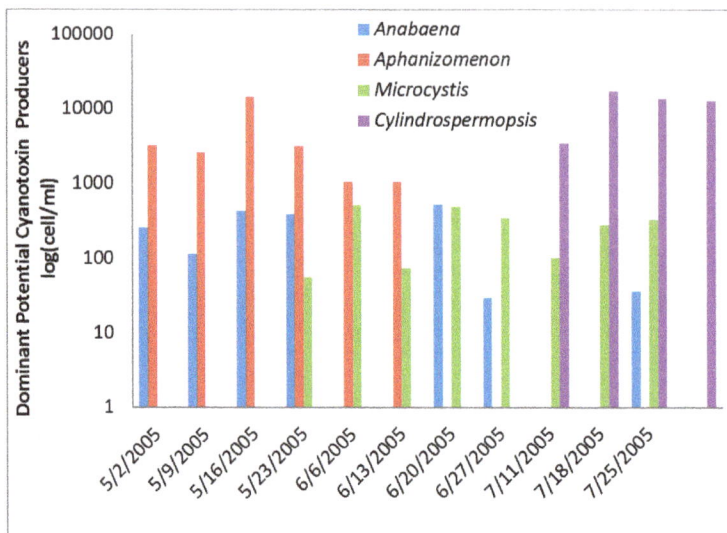

Figure 10. Individual toxin-producers at the Oklahoma site.

Microcystin as determined by ELISA was detected at very low concentrations between 0.06 and 0.13 ug/L in three samples near the start of sampling in the raw water. Microcystin-LW was detected by HPLC at a concentration of 0.9 ug/L on 13 June 2005, although it was not detected by ELISA in this sample. Cylindrospermopsin was detected by HPLC/PDA at a concentration of 0.41 ug/L on 2 May 2005. Relatively high levels of *Aphanizomenon*, 3,200 cells/mL, were found in this sample. Anatoxin-a was not detected by HPLC/PDA in any raw water sample.

The Oklahoma utility had low numbers of toxin-producing cyanobacteria in the finished water. Finished water had 46 cells/mL of *Microcystis* and 60 cells/mL of *Aphanizomenon* in the 13 June 2005 sample, 8 cells/mL of *Microcystis* in the 27 June 2005 sample, and 6 cells/mL of *Microcystis*/mL in the 1 August 2005 sample. Treatment removed between 0.2 and > 3.2 logs of toxin producing cyanobacteria for the Oklahoma distribution water (Table 1). No microcystin, cylindrospermopsin or anatoxin-a was detected in the Oklahoma distribution water by ELISA or HPLC.

2.1.5. Vermont

The total cyanobacteria never exceeded the AL 1. The total algal counts at the Vermont site reached 2600 units/mL once 16 May 2005 (Figure 11). Very low numbers of total toxin-producers were found in some samples and never approached the WHO AL 1 (Figure 12). When toxin-producers became most numerous on 22 August 2005, they only approached 500 total cyanobacteria in the sample. On this date, microcystin producers became the most numerous toxin-producer detected during sampling. No algal or cyanobacterial cells were detected in any finished water sample during sampling. Water treatment removed total cyanobacteria by as much as log 3.1 and toxin-producers by as much as log 2.2 (Table 1). Microcystin, cylindrospermopsin, and anatoxin-a were not detected in any raw water or distribution system water samples by ELISA or HPLC/PDA.

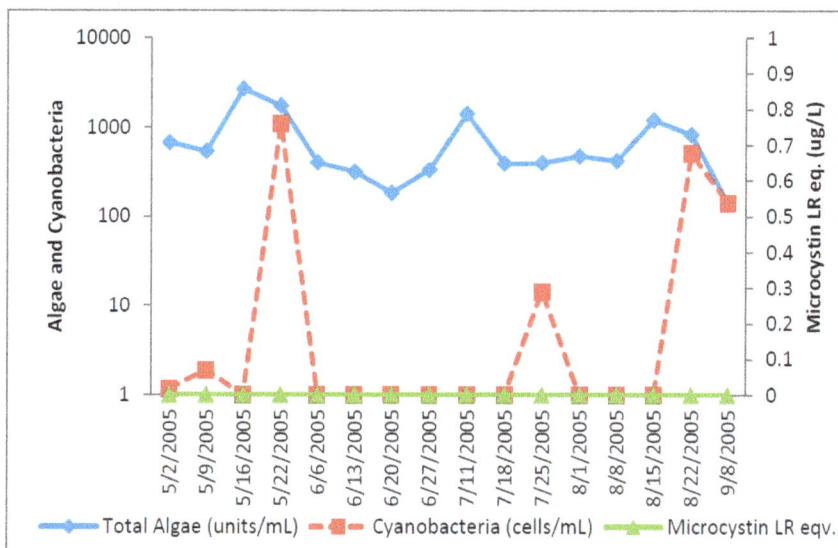

Figure 11. Vermont total cyanobacteria and total toxin-producers. Microcystin was not detected in any sample.

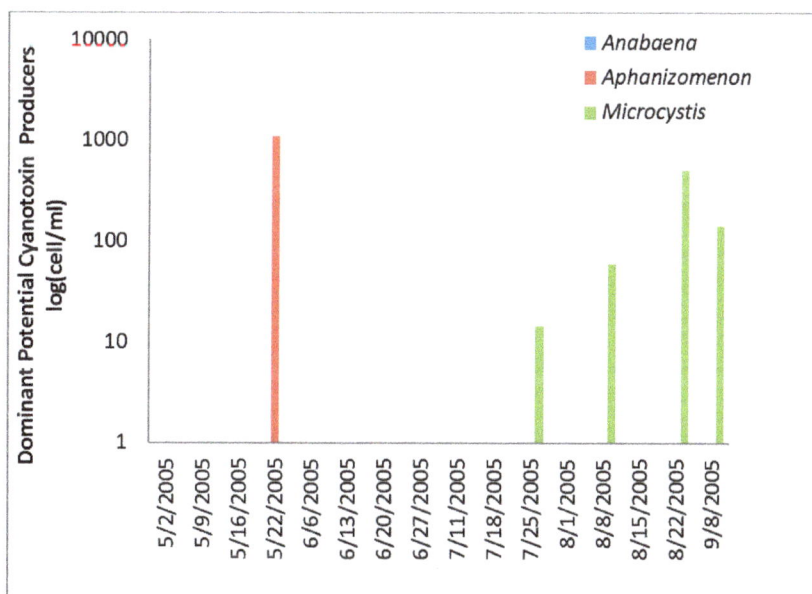

Figure 12. Individual toxin-producers at the Vermont site.

2.2. Fate of Cyanobacteria in Conventional DWTP

General observations for cyanobacteria included:

- The potential toxin-producing genera varied temporally and spatially between sites.

- *Microcystis* was the most geographically-distributed genera.
- High concentrations of cyanobacteria in the raw water did not lead to high concentrations of cyanotoxins in the raw or finished drinking water.
- Removal of cyanobacterial cells was very good in these five conventional DWTPS.
- It was observed that the filamentous cyanobacteria, especially *Aphanizomenon* are most likely to break through filters and be found in the finished water.

The concentration of cyanobacterial cells in raw water were not always related to concentrations of microcystins. This can be seen at the California site where the highest concentration of microcystin occurred after the highest concentration of potential microcystin-producer cells occurred. Possible factors causing this lack of relation could be that some strains of potential toxin-producing species did not have the toxin gene [29], or that microcystin genes may not be expressed at some times [30,31].

After conventional drinking water treatment, few cyanobacterial cells were found in the finished drinking water (Table 1). The log removal of total toxin producers ranged between log 1.5 and >log 5.5. When toxin-producers were found in finished drinking water, they were well below the WHO AL 1 level of concern of 2000 cells/mL in all cases.

In general these high removal efficiencies of cyanobacteria are encouraging with respect to *Microcystis* and microcystins. As long as the cells are intact and the bulk of the toxin is intracellular, conventional DWTPs should remove both cyanobacteria and cyanotoxins. Hoeger *et al.*[32] observed similar performance >1.5 log removal at a conventional DWTP in Germany. There is a further note of caution however. If a high percentage of microcystin is extracellular, there is a potential that PAC and oxidation may not provide sufficient removal of microcystins [32]. Furthermore, and somewhat in contrast to our study, Zamyadi *et al.* [33] observed *Aphanizomenon* and some *Pseudoanaebena* breaking through the filters into the finished water above the WHO AL 1 level (8800 cells/mL). Their study, which consisted of through-plant monitoring of cyanobacterial cell removal in a conventional DWTP, included intensive monitoring of the source, raw, clarifier, filter, sludge, and finished water for cyanobacterial cells. Their report and our observations of lower cell concentrations breaking through the filters, suggest that filamentous cyanobacteria, especially *Aphanizomenon* are likely to break through filters and to be found in the finished water. They observed these breakthroughs of filamentous bacteria when very high concentrations of the cyanobacterial were present in the raw water and clarifier sludge.

2.3. Fate of Cyanotoxins in Conventional DWTPs

Our study showed that microcystin was detected in 40 of 71 total raw water samples (56%) at less than 1 ug/L of microcystin-LR eq. Of these 40 detections, 36 were below <0.2 ug/L of microcystin-LR eq. These detections occurred in 4 of the 5 utilities sampled. Only one (1.4%) raw water sample exceeded the provisional WHO GV of 1 ug/L microcystin-LR eq. We observed no detectable microcystin in the finished water. Only one detection of cylindrospermopsin was observed in any raw water sample and none was observed in any finished water. We never observed anatoxin-a in the raw water or finished water at any DWTP in our study.

Microcystin data presented by Carmichael [22] indicated that for samples taken during bloom conditions 84% of samples contained detectable but less than 1 ug/L microcystin-LR in the raw water. Approximately 5% of the raw water samples had greater than 1 ug/L of microcystin. The remaining 11% had microcystin concentrations below detection. In contrast to our study, Carmichael observed that approximately 65% of the finished water samples contained detectable microcystin and 1% of those finished samples exceeded 1 ug/L microcystin-LR eq.

Haddix *et al.* [34] monitored 33 U.S. DWTPs collecting 206 raw water samples and 77 finished water samples. No cyanobacteria were monitored. Approximately 87% of the raw water samples had detectable MC-LR. The mean concentration was 0.307 ug/L MC-LR eq. Seven percent of the raw samples exceeded 1 ug/L MC-LR. WHO GV. Haddix *et al.* observed that 30% of their finished water samples contained detectable MC-LR. No finished water sample exceeded the WHO GV for MC-LR. The mean MC-LR eq. concentration in the finished water was 0.036 ug/L MC-LR eq.

The concentrations of microcystins in raw water reported in this work are consistent with previous studies, albeit somewhat lower given the moderately high levels of cyanobacteria present. The biggest discrepancy is in the finished water. Carmichael's observations of increased microcystin detections in finished water as compared to our study may have been due to the higher raw water microcystin concentrations entering the plants surveyed in his study.

There are several limitations that must be considered when comparing ELISA to HPLC methods. The two methods have different detection limits with ELISA being more sensitive but less specific. The ELISA also has cross reactivities to microcystin congeners ranging from 0.35 for MC-YR to 1.0 for MC-RR relative to MC-LR. There is no cross reactivity listed for MC-LW congener and the EnviroLogix ELISA kit. This may explain the discrepancy for the Oklahoma site where MC-LW was determined by PDA to be 0.9 ug/L versus 0.13 ug/L for ELISA. In the case of the California plant where MC-LR was detected at 0.7 ug/L by PDA and 0.19 ug/L by ELISA, the anomaly is probably due to differences in the sample preparation or matrix inhibition of the ELISA. In the case of the Florida samples, where MC-LR equivalents were 1.4 ug/L and the PDA had no detection, the discrepancy probably lies in the sample preparation. At low toxin levels, discrepancies between ELISA and PDA methods can be large and care should be taken to not over interpret any single result.

2.4. Application of the WHO Alert Level Framework

Watzin *et al.* [35] examined the relation of the WHO Alert Level Framework to microcystin concentration for Lake Champlain in Vermont. These investigators found that an Alert Level 1 of 2000 cells/mL was conservative, and microcystin concentrations in a developing bloom did not approach 1 ug/L until the density of potential microcystin producers was greater than 4000 cells/mL. They also found that cell density was not directly correlated with microcystin concentration. They observed that of 48 samples taken that had below 4000 cells/mL of potential microcystin-producers, nine of these samples had detectable levels of microcystin. The average and median microcystin levels found in the 39 samples with detectable microcystin were 0.42 ug/L and 0.04 ug/L respectively with a maximum of 2.42 ug/L found in one sample. These results are similar to those found in our study. Watzin *et al.* [35] also found that high toxin concentrations were rare with low cell concentrations except when a bloom was breaking down. Based on the results of our study, we concur with Watzin *et al.* [35] that the WHO Alert Level 1 framework of 2000 cyanobacteria cells/mL is overly conservative. Because of the variable nature of blooms in each source water and the high cost associated with toxin sampling and analysis, it seems prudent that each DWTPs should consider developing cyanobacterial cell count action levels that trigger toxin sampling and analysis for their local conditions. Furthermore, our results suggest that the composition should be determined and different levels set for each genera. For instance the WHO AL 1 would not be appropriate for cylindrospermopsin or anatoxin-a potential producers. Our results showed that even when these genera were present at levels in excess of 2000 cells/mL anatoxin-a and was never detected and cylindrospermopsin was only detected once at a level, below most proposed GV for this toxin.

The original WHO Alert Level framework (ALF) is based on total cyanobacterial cells/mL. This management scheme provides a useful starting point but should not be arbitrarily adopted in North America. The Water Safety Plan approach should be considered as a tool to modify the WHO ALF for local conditions including Alert Levels based on cell concentrations of locally present toxin producing genera [36]. Additionally, the expected ability of particular drinking water treatment systems to remove toxins should be included in individual water safety plans. Some countries such as the Czech Republic continue to use the original WHO framework. Other countries have based their alert levels on anywhere from 5000 to 50,000 cyanobacteria cells/mL. In the case of Australia, Health Alert Levels, are based on specific species present. However, all regular interval microscopic methods have a significant disadvantage in that they cannot capture the highly dynamic changes in cyanobacterial cell concentrations. New low-cost sensors based on phycocyanin fluorescence can overcome some of the problems inherent in infrequent microscopic monitoring and can be combined with microscopy to provide a comprehensive management system that should be given consideration in the development of a site specific water safety plan [37].

3. Experimental Section

3.1. Sampling Procedures

Five drinking water utilities where chosen for this study based on a history of the occurrence of potential toxin-producing cyanobacteria and their geographic distribution across the U.S. Utilities selected were located in the states of California, Oklahoma, Vermont, Texas, and Florida. All five utilities are conventional coagulation/filtration treatment plants. The Florida utility utilized two source waters, a river and a reservoir; samples were taken from both. The general physical and chemical treatment processes used by each utility are listed in Table 2.

Each utility was sampled at two locations; the raw water (prior to any chemical addition) and the finished water (first point of distribution). Samples were collected for 12 consecutive weeks from May to August 2005 at all utilities except California, where 11 weekly samples were taken and Vermont where 16 weekly samples were taken. Samples were collected for both cyanotoxin analysis and algae or cyanobacteria identification/enumeration. Cyanotoxin samples were collected in duplicate using 1 L amber glass bottles. Approximately 100 mg/L of ascorbic acid was added to the finished water samples to inactivate any residual free chlorine. Cyanotoxin samples were refrigerated until shipped on ice via an overnight delivery service. Cyanobacterial identification/enumeration samples were collected at each sample location and placed in 125 mL amber Nalgene™ bottles containing Lugol's reagent and mailed priority next day mail to the analysis laboratory.

Table 2. Utility Information.

Site Identification Number	State	Source Water	PAC	Coagulation/Flocculation	Clarification	Filtration	Disinfection
123	VT	Lake	-	x	x	Sand/Anthracite	Chlorine
485	FL	River/Reservoir	x	x	x	x	Chloramines
619	OK	Reservoir	x	x	x	Sand/Anthracite	Chlorine
762	CA	Reservoir	-	x	x	Sand/Anthracite	Ozone/Chloramines
929	TX	Reservoir	x	x	x	Sand/Anthracite	Chloramines

3.2. Sample Preparation and ELISA Analysis

An unfiltered 1 mL aliquot from both the raw and finished sample from each location was sonicated at 60 watts for 5 min. The Envirologix Quantiplate™ ELISA (enzyme-linked immunosorbant assay) Kit for total microcystins was employed as a screen for microcystin. The ELISA kit's high sensitivity option found in the manufacturer's directions, was used to quantify microcystin concentrations from 0.05 to 0.83 ug/L. Samples were analyzed in duplicate. Samples below 0.05 ug/L were reported as <0.05 ug/L and samples above 0.8 ug/L were repeated at 1:10, 1:100, and 1:1000 dilutions. The quality control program for the ELISA analysis consisted of a laboratory sample duplicate, laboratory fortified sample matrix and continuing calibration verification standard analyzed every seven samples. Analyses were acceptable if the quality control samples were within 15 percent of the expected value. If any value fell outside of the acceptance criteria the batch was reanalyzed.

3.3. Sample Preparation & HLPC-PDA Analysis

One liter of the cyanotoxin sample was filtered through a Whatman® Glass microfiber filter. The filters and 250 mL of the filtrate were frozen at −80 °C and archived until analysis. The archived glass-fiber filter was homogenized in 4 mL of 50% methanol. The homogenized sample was sonicated in an ultrasonic bath at 60 watts for 25 min and centrifuged for 5 min at 11,000 rpm. The supernatant was collected and the pellet was extracted by two sequential 2 mL 85% methanol extractions. Additional sonication and centrifugation was performed between extractions. All supernatants were pooled together and brought to dryness under nitrogen. Samples were reconstituted to a final volume 1 mL in 20% methanol. The filtrate was lyophilized then extracted by two sequential 2 mL 85% methanol extractions. All supernatants were pooled together and brought to dryness under nitrogen. Samples were reconstituted to a final volume 0.25 mL in 20% methanol.

Samples were analyzed for cylindrospermopsin, anatoxin-a, and microcystin-RR, LR, LA and LF using a High Performance Liquid Chromatograph with a Photodiode Array (HPLC/PDA) [38]. A standard for microcystin-YR, identified as a high priority congener by EPA, was not available and it was therefore not analyzed. Samples below the detection limit of 0.25 ug/L were reported as <0.25 ug/L and samples above the 2 ug/L were repeated at 1:10, 1:100, and 1:1000 dilutions.

The HPLC/PDA method used a 0.02% trifluoroacetic acid (TFA) acetonitrile and 0.02% TFA water gradient. The 55-min chromatographic run utilized a 5-min 2% acetonitrile isocratic period followed by a 35%, 70%, and 90% acetonitrile gradient (Figure 13). The toxins were separated on a C18 column (Atlantis®, Waters, Milford, MA, USA) in the following order; cylindrospermopsin, anatoxin-a, microcystin RR, LR, LA, and LF. Anatoxin-a was monitored at a wavelength of 227 nm and the microcystins were monitored at a wavelength of 238 nm, cylindrospermopsin was monitored at 261 nm. (Table 3) The results of the filter extract (intracellular cyanotoxins) and lyophilized filtrate (extracellular cyanotoxins) were combined to provide a total cyanotoxin concentration. The quality assurance and quality control consisted of running a sample blank, a duplicate, a fortified duplicate, and a positive control every 10 samples. The acceptance criteria for these analyses were relative errors less than 15% for duplicate and positive controls and relative recovery within 20% for the fortified duplicate.

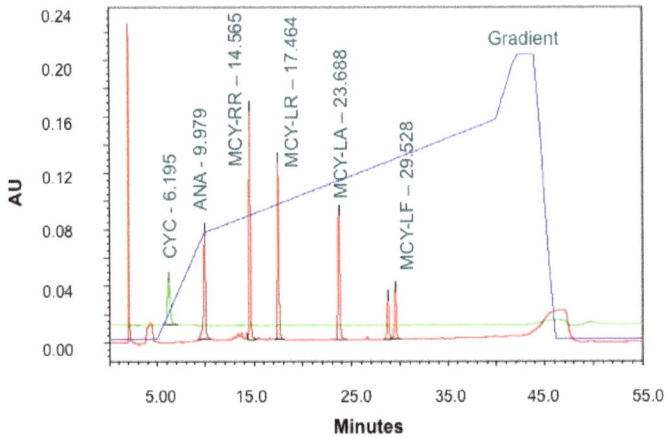

Figure 13. Chromatograph of HPLC/PDA Run.

Table 3. HPLC/PDA Analyte Parameters.

Cyanotoxin	Retention Time (min)	Wavelength (nm)	Method Detection Limit (ug/L)
Cyclindrospermopsin	6.195	261	0.25
Anatoxin-a	9.979	227	0.25
Microcystin-RR	14.565	238	0.25
Microcystin-LR	17.464	238	0.25
Microcystin-LW	29.528	238	0.25

3.4. Cell Counts by Microscopy

Twenty-five milliliter water samples were settled in Utermohl plankton sedimentation chambers for at least 24 h. A qualitative and quantitative count was performed at 200X using an inverted phase-contrast microscope. Cyanobacteria and algal identification were made using standard taxonomic references, such as Prescott [39]. A minimum of 300 cyanobacterial units or 100 microscope fields were counted per sample. This approach will yield an estimate of 10–20 percent error for the dominant genera, and 20–60 percent for the subdominant genera [5]. The cyanobacteria observed in this study grew as filaments or colonies consisting of a large numbers of cells and counted as cell-aggregations (units), rather than as individual cells. The number of cells per unit varied substantially by genera, site and sampling date. For each sample the average number of cells / unit was determined by counting individual cells/units in ten fields. Total cyanobacteria and potential toxin-producing cyanobacteria counts are reported. Because of the variable number of cells per unit for different genera and our ability to quantify 1–2 units/mL, low cell concentrations are highly variable and may not be statistically significant. The plots of specific potential toxin producers at each site were based on the following genera; microcystin- *Microcystis, Oscillatoria, Nostoc, Hapalosiphon, Anabaenopsis,* and *Anabaena*; cylindrospermopsin- *Aphanizomenon* and *Cylindrospermopsis*; anatoxin-a- *Aphanizomenon, Anabaena,* and *Oscillatoria*.

4. Conclusions

The presence of toxic cyanobacteria and microcystin in drinking water source waters is a widespread phenomenon across the U.S. Even though the concentrations of cyanobacterial cells were elevated and in many cases exceeded the WHO AL 1 cell limit of 2000 cells/mL, microcystin concentrations were low and only exceeded the WHO provisional guidance value, 1 ug/L, once. Furthermore no anatoxin-a was measured above the detection limit at any site. Cylindrospermopsin was detected once. More important, conventional treatment effectively removed most toxin producing cyanobacterial cells and toxins at levels observed in this study. When our results are combined with previous studies it emphasizes the highly variable nature of the cyanobacteria problem. The WHO AL framework is conservative with respect to the levels of cyanobacterial cells that trigger increased monitoring. It should be considered a starting point and the cyanobacterial cell levels adjusted upwards as necessary to reflect local conditions that will balance the available resources for monitoring and consumer safety.

Acknowledgments

This work was supported by USEPA contract number EP07C000149. We thank Robin Roote for performing identification and enumeration of the algae and cyanobacteria.

Author Contributions

David Szlag analyzed the data and wrote the introduction, results, and discussion sections and formatted the final paper. Ben Southwell performed the laboratory analyses, edited and contributed sections the methods sections of the manuscript. Jim Sinclair was the USEPA project manager and initiator of the study. Judy Westrick was the PI on the contract, managed the data collection and QA/QC, and was the primary contact with the DWTPs.

Conflicts of Interest

The authors declare no conflict of interest. The opinions expressed in this paper are solely those of the authors and do not reflect USEPA policy. Mention of trade names, products, or services does not convey official EPA approval, endorsement, or recommendation.

References

1. Nishiwaki-Matsushima, R.; Ohta, T.; Nishiwaki, S.; Suganuma, M.; Kohyama, K.; Ishikawa, T.; Carmichael, W.W.; Fujiki, H. Liver tumor promotion by the cyanobacterial cyclic peptide toxin microcystin-LR. *J. Cancer Res. Clin. Oncol.* **1992**, *118*, 420–424.

2. Maire, M.-A.; Bazin, E.; Fessard, V.; Rast, C.; Humpage, A.; Vasseur, P. Morphological cell transformation of Syrian hamster embryo cells by the cyanotoxin, cylindrospermopsin. *Toxicon* **2010**, *55*, 1317–1322.

3. Knappe, D.R.U.; Belk, R.C.; Briley, D.S.; Gandy, S.R.; Rastogi, N.; Rike, A.H.; Glasgow, H.; Hannon, E.; Frazier, W.D.; Kohl, P.; *et al. Algae Detection and Removal Strategies for Drinking Water Treatment Plants*; AWWA Research Foundation: Denver, CO, USA, 2004.

4. Davis, T.W.; Berry, D.L.; Boyer, G.L.; Golber, C.J. The effects of temperature and nutrients on the growth and dynamics of toxic and non-toxic strains of *Microcystis* during cyanobacteria blooms. *Harmful Algae* **2009**, *8*, 715–725.

5. Chorus, I.; Bartram, J. *Toxic Cyanobacteria in Water: A Guide to Their Public Health Consequences, Monitoring and Management*; EF&N Spon: Los Angeles, CA, USA, 1999.

6. Fristachi, A.; Sinclair, J.L.; Hall, S.; Hambrook Berkman, J.; Boyer, G.; Burkholder, J.; Burns, J.; Carmichael, W.; DuFour, A.; Frazier, W.; *et al.* Occurrence of cyanobacterial harmful algal blooms workgroup report. In *Cyanobacterial Harmful Algal Blooms: State of the Science and Research Needs*; Springer: New York, NY, USA, 2008; pp. 45–103.

7. Graham, J.L.; Loftin, K.A.; Meyer, M.T.; Ziegler, A.C. Cyanotoxin mixtures and taste-and-odor compounds in cyanobacterial blooms from the Midwestern United States. *Environ. Sci. Technol.* **2010**, *44*, 7361–7368.

8. Zhou, L.; Yu, D.; Yu, H.; Chen, K.; Shen, G.; Shen, Y.; Ruan, Y.; Ding, X. Drinking water types, microcystins and colorectal cancer. *Zhonghua Yu Fang Yi Xue Za Zhi* **2000**, *34*, 224–226.

9. Yu, S.-Z.; Zhao, N.; Zi, X. The relationship between cyanotoxin (microcystin, MC) in pond-ditch water and primary liver cancer in China. *Zhonghua Zhong Liu Za Zhi* **2001**, *23*, 96–99.

10. Falconer, I.R.; Humpage, A.R. Cyanobacterial (blue-green algal) toxins in water supplies: Cylindrospermopsins. *Environ. Toxicol.* **2006**, *21*, 299–304.

11. Fawell, J.K.; James, C.; James, H. *Toxins from Blue-green Algae: Toxicological Assessment of Microcystin-LR and a Method for its Determination in Water*; Foundation for Water Research: Denver, CO, USA, 1994.

12. Santé, O.M.D.L. *Guidelines for Drinking-water Quality*, 4th ed.; World Health Organization: Geneva, Switzerland, 2011.

13. Scotland, S.G.B.A.G. *Cyanobacteria (Blue-Green Algae) in Inland and Inshore Waters: Assessment and Minimisation of Risks to Public Health Revised Guidance 2012*; The Scottish Government: Edinburgh, UK, 2012.

14. Chorus, I. *Current Approaches to Cyanotoxin Risk Assessment, Risk Management and Regulations in Different Countries*; Federal Environmental Agency: Dessau, Germany, 2005.

15. *Announcement of the Drinking Water Contaminant Candidate List*; US EPA: Lenexa, KS, USA, 1998; Volume 63.

16. Burch, M.; Harvey, F.; Baker, P.; Jones, G. National protocol for the monitoring of cyanobacteria and their toxins in surface fresh waters. *ARMCANZ Natl. Algal Manag. Draft* **2003**, V6.0 for consideration LWBC.

17. Burch, M. The development of an alert levels and response framework for the management of blue green algae blooms. In *Blue Green Algal Blooms: New Developments in Research and Management*, Proceedings of the Australian Center for Water Quality Research and the University of Adelaide, Adelaide, SA, Australia, 17 February 1993.

18. Du Preez, H.H.; Swanepoel, A.; Van Baalen, L.; Olwage, A. Cyanobacterial Incident Management Frameworks for application by drinking water suppliers. *Water SA* **2007**, *33*, 643–652.

19. Hoeger, S.J.; Shaw, G.; Hitzfeld, B.C.; Dietrich, D.R. Occurrence and elimination of cyanobacterial toxins in two Australian drinking water treatment plants. *Toxicon* **2004**, *43*, 639–649.

20. Karner, D.A.; Standridge, J.H.; Harrington, G.W.; Barnum, R.P. Microcystin algal toxins in source and finished drinking water. *J. Am. Water Works Asoc.* **2001**, *93*, 72–81.

21. Lahti, K.; Rapala, J.; Kivimäki, A.L.; Kukkonen, J.; Niemelä, M.; Sivonen, K. Occurrence of microcystins in raw water sources and treated drinking water of Finnish waterworks. *Water Sci. Technol.* **2001**, *43*, 225–228.

22. Carmichael, W.W.; Azevedo, S.M.F.O.; An, J.S.; Molica, R.J.R.; Jochimsen, E.M.; Lau, S.; Rinehart, K.L.; Shaw, G.R.; Eaglesham, G.K. Human fatalities from cyanobacteria: chemical and biological evidence for cyanotoxins. *Environ. Health Perspect.* **2001**, *109*, 663–668.

23. Robert, C.; Tremblay, H.; DeBlois, C. *Cyanobactéries et cyanotoxines au Québec: Suivi à six stations de production d'eau potable (2001–2003)*; Service des eaux municipales, Direction générale des politiques, Développement durable, Environnement et parcs Québec: Québec, QC, Canada, 2005.

24. Boyer, G.L.; Konopko, E.; Gilbert, A.H. Rapid field-based monitoring systems for the detection of Toxic cyanobacteria blooms, ImmnuoStrips and Fluorescence-based monitoring systems. In Proceedings of the 12th International Conference Harmful Algae, Copenhagen, Denmark, 4–8 September 2006; Springer: New York, NY, USA; pp. 341–343.

25. Chiswell, R.K.; Shaw, G.R.; Eaglesham, G.; Smith, M.J.; Norris, R.L.; Seawright, A.A.; Moore, M.R. Stability of cylindrospermopsin, the toxin from the cyanobacterium, Cylindrospermopsis raciborskii: Effect of pH, temperature, and sunlight on decomposition. *Environ. Toxicol.* **1999**, *14*, 155–161.

26. Shaw, G.R.; Seawright, A.A.; Moore, M.R.; Lam, P.K.S. Cylindrospermopsin, A Cyanobacterial Alkaloid: Evaluation of Its Toxicologic Activity. *Ther. Drug Monit.* **2000**, *22*, 89–92.

27. USEPA. Creating a Cyanotoxin Target List for the Unregulated Contaminant Monitoring Rule. Available online: http://water.epa.gov/lawsregs/rulesregs/sdwa/ucmr/upload/2005_08_12_ ucmr_meeting_ucmr1_may2001.pdf (accessed on 2 February 2015).

28. Zamyadi, A.; Ho, L.; Newcombe, G.; Bustamante, H.; Prevost, M. Fate of toxic cyanobacterial cells and disinfection by-products formation after chlorination. *Water Res.* **2012**, *46*, 1524–1535.

29. Kurmayer, R.; Dittmann, E.; Fastner, J.; Chorus, I. Diversity of microcystin genes within a population of of the toxic cyanobacterium Microcystis spp. in Lake Wannsee (Berlin, Germany). *Microb. Ecol.* **2002**, *43*, 107–118.

30. Ngwa, F.F.; Chandra, C.A.; Jabaji, M.S. Comparison of cyanobacterial microcystin synthetase (mcy) E gene transcript levels, mcy E gene copies, and biomass as indicators of microcystin risk under laboratory and field conditions. *Microbiol. Open* **2014**, *3*, 411–425.

31. Gobler, C.J.; Davis, T.W.; Coyne, K.J.; Boyer, G.L. Interactive influences of nutrient loading, zooplankton grazing, and microcystin synthethase gene expression on cyanobacterial bloom dynamics in a eutrophic New York lake. *Harmful Algae* **2007**, *6*, 119–133.

32. Hoeger, S.J.; Hitzfeld, B.C.; Dietrich, D.R. Occurrence and elimination of cyanobacterial toxins in drinking water treatment plants. *Toxicol. Appl. Pharmacol.* **2005**, *203*, 231–242.

33. Zamyadi, A.; Dorner, S.; Sauvé, S.; Ellis, D.; Bolduc, A.; Bastien, C.; Prévost, M. Species-dependence of cyanobacteria removal efficiency by different drinking water treatment processes. *Water Res.* **2013**, *47*, 2689–2700.

34. Haddix, P.L.; Hughley, C.J.; LeChevallier, M.W. Source water—Occurrence of microcystins in 33 US water supplies. *JAWWA* **2007**, *99*, 118–125.

35. Watzin, M.C.; Miller, E.B.; Shambaugh, A.D.; Kreider, M.A. Application of the WHO alert level framework to cyanobacterial monitoring of Lake Champlain, Vermont. *Environ. Toxicol.* **2006**, *21*, 278–288.

36. Chorus, I. Water safety plans. In *Harmful Cyanobacteria*; Springer: New York, NY, USA, 2005; pp. 201–227.

37. Kong, Y.; Zou, P.; Miao, L.; Qi, J.; Song, L.; Zhu, L.; Xu, X. Medium optimization for the production of anti-cyanobacterial substances by Streptomyces sp. HJC-D1 using response surface methodology. *Environ. Sci. Pollut. Res.* **2014**, *21*, 5983–5990.

38. International Organization for Standardization (ISO). *WaterQuality—Determination of Microcystins—Method Using Solid Phase Extraction (SPE) and High Performance Liquid Chromotagraphy (HPLC) with Ultraviolet (UV) Detection*; ISO: Geneva, Switzerland, 2005.

39. Prescott, G.W. *Algae of the Western Great Lakes Area*; Ottokoeltz Science Publishers: Loenigstein, Germany, 1982.

Effects of Hydrogen Peroxide and Ultrasound on Biomass Reduction and Toxin Release in the Cyanobacterium, *Microcystis aeruginosa*

Miquel Lürling, Debin Meng and Elisabeth J. Faassen

Abstract: Cyanobacterial blooms are expected to increase, and the toxins they produce threaten human health and impair ecosystem services. The reduction of the nutrient load of surface waters is the preferred way to prevent these blooms; however, this is not always feasible. Quick curative measures are therefore preferred in some cases. Two of these proposed measures, peroxide and ultrasound, were tested for their efficiency in reducing cyanobacterial biomass and potential release of cyanotoxins. Hereto, laboratory assays with a microcystin (MC)-producing cyanobacterium (*Microcystis aeruginosa*) were conducted. Peroxide effectively reduced *M. aeruginosa* biomass when dosed at 4 or 8 mg L^{-1}, but not at 1 and 2 mg L^{-1}. Peroxide dosed at 4 or 8 mg L^{-1} lowered total MC concentrations by 23%, yet led to a significant release of MCs into the water. Dissolved MC concentrations were nine-times (4 mg L^{-1}) and 12-times (8 mg L^{-1} H_2O_2) higher than in the control. Cell lysis moreover increased the proportion of the dissolved hydrophobic variants, MC-LW and MC-LF (where L = Leucine, W = tryptophan, F = phenylalanine). Ultrasound treatment with commercial transducers sold for clearing ponds and lakes only caused minimal growth inhibition and some release of MCs into the water. Commercial ultrasound transducers are therefore ineffective at controlling cyanobacteria.

Reprinted from *Toxins*. Cite as: Lürling, M.; Meng, D.; Faassen, E.J. Effects of Hydrogen Peroxide and Ultrasound on Biomass Reduction and Toxin Release in the Cyanobacterium, *Microcystis aeruginosa*. *Toxins* **2014**, *6*, 3260-3280.

1. Introduction

Cyanobacterial proliferations and the formation of surface scums are among the most noticeable and malignant consequences of eutrophication [1]. Cyanobacterial blooms are a serious water quality threat, as blooms may produce nasty odors, cause high turbidity, anoxia, fish kills and food web alterations [2,3]. Furthermore, because cyanobacteria can produce a variety of potent toxins [4], cyanobacterial blooms exert strong pressure on important ecosystems services, such as recreation, aquaculture, irrigation and drinking water preparation. As a consequence, cyanobacterial blooms have severe economic impacts [5].

Because cyanobacterial blooms can deteriorate the water quality below the level that is needed for drinking water production, irrigation, industry, recreation and fishing, water managers try to control the massive development of cyanobacterial biomass. Nutrient reduction in the water body and its catchment area is clearly the most prominent effective approach to prevent cyanobacterial dominance [6]. However, reduction to sufficiently low nutrients loads may take fairly long to realize, and sometimes, it may not be feasible at all. Hence, in systems where the reduction of external nutrient loading is not economically feasible, effect-oriented (curative) measures may provide the most suitable nuisance control [7]. Such applications should be fast-acting and strongly reduce cyanobacteria biomass, so that safe water quality levels are rapidly reached [7]. In decision making for mitigating measures besides biomass also the production of cyanobacterial toxins are increasingly being taken into account [8], as these cyanotoxins make cyanobacterial blooms and surface scums a threat to environmental health and public safety [9,10]. While reducing biomass, care should be taken that the cyanobacterial toxins are not released into the water. Most cyanobacterial toxins are largely contained within the cyanobacterial cells, until lysis or damage of the cells liberates them [11,12]. Curative measures that result in the release of toxins from the cells, like the application of copper [13], endanger rather than improve water quality [4].

There are several promising curative measures to control cyanobacterial biomass. Copper is among the most applied algaecides [7], but toxicity issues using copper [4] have led to the promotion of hydrogen peroxide (H_2O_2) as an effective non-toxic alternative [14,15]. Hydrogen peroxide is a powerful oxidizing agent that acts via the formation of hydroxyl radicals ($\cdot$OH), which oxidize thiol groups in biomolecules [16]. However, it has been stated that the use of algaecides should be avoided, since it may lead to significant toxin release [4]. This finds some support in a whole lake experiment, in which both cyanobacteria biomass and the cyanotoxin microcystin (MC) strongly declined after application with H_2O_2, albeit with a two-days' time delay for MC [15], which might point towards a shift from particulate to dissolved MC and, thus, cyanotoxin release. A different technique that has been labelled as an "environmental friendly" or "green solution" to kill cyanobacteria is the use of ultrasound [17,18]. Nevertheless, a vast majority of studies on this subject have been performed with high power devices designed for cleaning and sterilizing that differ significantly from those sold on the market for controlling phytoplankton in lakes and ponds [19]. High power devices could lead to a strong increase in extracellular MC concentrations [20], but could also cause MC degradation [21,22] through peroxide formation and hydroxyl radicals [22]. The effect of commercially available ultrasound transducers on cyanobacterial toxin release is unknown. Thus, while both peroxide and ultrasound have been reported as promising measures in reducing cyanobacterial biomass, they consequently might cause a release of cyanotoxins.

Microcystins (MCs) are the most frequently occurring cyanotoxins. MCs are produced by a diverse range of cyanobacteria, of which *Microcystis* is one of the most common bloom formers [23–25]. MCs are non-ribosomal processed cyclic heptapeptides with a size between 909 Da and 1115 Da [26]. The general structure is cyclo(-D-ala-L-*X*-erythro-β-D-methylaspartic acid-L-*Z*-Adda-D-isoglutamic acid-*N*-methyldehydroalanine), where Adda is (2S,3S,8S,9S)-3-amino-9-methoxy-2,6,8-trimethyl-10-phenyldeca-4,6-dienoic acid [27] (Figure 1). *X* and *Z* are variable L-amino acids contributing mostly to the dozens of variants of MCs that have been detected [27]. MCs are potent inhibitors of protein phosphatases, but the toxicity of different variants to mice varies substantially, where replacement of the hydrophobic leucine (L) in the first variable position with a hydrophilic amino acid (e.g., arginine, R) dramatically reduces toxicity [28] (Figure 1).

Figure 1. General structure of microcystins and examples of substitutions at position X (L = leucine, R = arginine) and Y (R = arginine, W= tryptophan, F = phenylalanine) resulting in the variants microcystin MC-RR, MC-LR, MC-LW and MC-LF, if positions R1 and R2 are methylated.

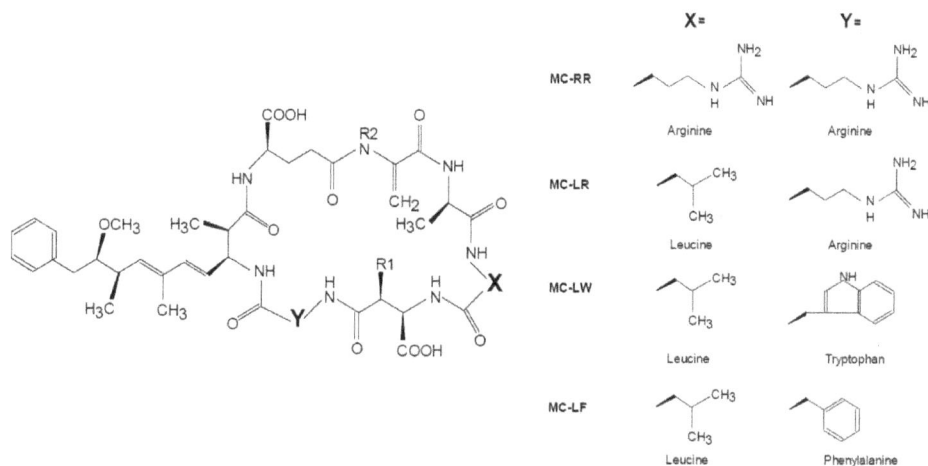

Little is known about how these different MC variants react to curative measures to control cyanobacterial biomass. The degradation rate of two MC variants (MC-LR and MC-RR, with L = Leucine and R = Arginine) upon irradiation with high power ultrasound (500 W, applied to a 22-mL reaction vessel) differed with an estimated EC_{50} of 30 min for MC-RR and 70 min for MC-LR [21]. However, the effect of commercially available ultrasound transducers on different MC variants has not been examined yet. Likewise, the few studies on H_2O_2 control of cyanobacteria that included MC analysis [15,29,30] did not specify the effects on different MC variants. Therefore, in this study, we tested the hypothesis that both H_2O_2 treatment and ultrasound from commercial transducers sold for clearing lakes are effective at strongly reducing cyanobacteria biomass, without increasing the MC concentration in the water. Furthermore, we hypothesized that all measured MC variants reacted in a similar manner to these two treatments. Hereto, we ran laboratory experiments with a *M. aeruginosa* strain that, amongst others, produces the five MC variants: dm-7-MC-LR, MC-LR, MC-LY, MC-LF and MC-LW (dm = demethylated at position R2 in Figure 1: R2 = H).

2. Results

2.1. Hydrogen Peroxide

H_2O_2 application of 4 and 8 mg L^{-1} significantly lowered the cyanobacterial chlorophyll-*a* and particle concentration after 24 h (Figure 2; Table 1). The chlorophyll-*a* concentration was reduced to approximately 200 µg L^{-1} in the highest H_2O_2 treatments (Figure 2a), but the particle concentration was reduced to ~9 × 10^4 particles mL^{-1} after 24 h in the 8-mg L^{-1} H_2O_2 treatment (Figure 2c). The photosynthetic efficiency of the cyanobacteria, expressed as photosystem II efficiency (Φ_{PSII}), was more sensitive to H_2O_2 application; it was slightly reduced at 1 and 2 mg L^{-1}, but became (virtually) zero at 4 and 8 mg L^{-1} (Figure 2b; Table 1). The H_2O_2 concentration at which 50% of the cyanobacteria were affected (EC_{50}) ranged from 2.5 mg L^{-1} for the photosynthetic efficiency, to 3.8 mg L^{-1} for cyanobacterial chlorophyll-a (Table 1).

Table 1. Statistical information on the H_2O_2 experiment for three different endpoints: chlorophyll-a concentration (Chl-a), photosystem II efficiency (Φ_{PSII}) and particle concentration (# mL^{-1}) of *Microcystis aeruginosa* PCC 7820. Homogeneous subgroups were defined by a Tukey *post hoc* comparison at $p < 0.05$ and are indicated by similar symbols (a,b,c) per column.

H_2O_2 treatment	Chl-a ($\mu g\ L^{-1}$)		Φ_{PSII} (-)		Particles (No. mL^{-1})	
			Tukey *post hoc* comparison			
Control	a		a		a	
1 mg L^{-1}	a		a,b		a	
2 mg L^{-1}	a		b		a	
4 mg L^{-1}	b		c		b	
8 mg L^{-1}	c		c		b	
repeated measures ANOVA	F	p	F	p	F	p
treatment effect ($F_{4,10}$)	367.5	<0.001	284.1	<0.001	102.4	<0.001
time effect ($F_{3,30}$)	695.3	<0.001	145.5	<0.001	80.0	<0.001
time × treatment interaction ($F_{12,30}$)	215.0	<0.001	46.5	<0.001	41.1	<0.001
nonlinear regression		r^2 adj		r^2 adj		r^2 adj
EC_{50} (mg $H_2O_2\ L^{-1}$)	3.8	0.992	2.5	0.947	2.6	0.929

MCs were determined at the start and after 24 h in the controls and the 1-, 4- and 8-mg $H_2O_2\ L^{-1}$ treatments (Figure 3). Total MC concentrations (sum of dissolved and particulate MCs) were similar at the start of the experiment (one-way ANOVA, $F_{3,11} = 3.23$; $p = 0.082$), but after 24 h, the total MC concentrations were lower in the H_2O_2-treated jars than in the controls ($F_{3,11} = 13.5$; $p = 0.002$). The total MC concentrations in the highest H_2O_2 treatments had dropped 23 to 24% compared to their initial values (Figure 3).

At the start of the experiment, on average, 6.0% (SD 1.6%) of the total MC pool consisted of dissolved MCs. After 24 h, a similar percentage (6.5%, SD 1.9%) was found for the controls and the 1-mg $H_2O_2\ L^{-1}$ treatment, whereas in the 4- and 8-mg L^{-1} treatments, the proportion of dissolved MCs had increased to 77% (4 mg L^{-1}) and 85% (8 mg L^{-1}; Figure 3). H_2O_2 application significantly increased the dissolved MC concentrations (one-way ANOVA; $F_{3,11} = 408.9$; $p < 0.001$): dissolved MC concentrations in the controls and the 1-mg $H_2O_2\ L^{-1}$ treatment were significantly lower than those in the 4- and 8-mg $H_2O_2\ L^{-1}$ treatments (Holm–Sidak comparison, $p < 0.05$).

Figure 2. (**a**) Chlorophyll-*a* concentrations (CHL-*a*, µg L^{-1}); (**b**) photosystem II efficiency (PSII); and (**c**) particle concentration (No. mL^{-1}) of *Microcystis aeruginosa* PCC 7820 exposed to different H$_2$O$_2$ concentrations for 24 h. Error bars indicate 1 SD (*n* = 3).

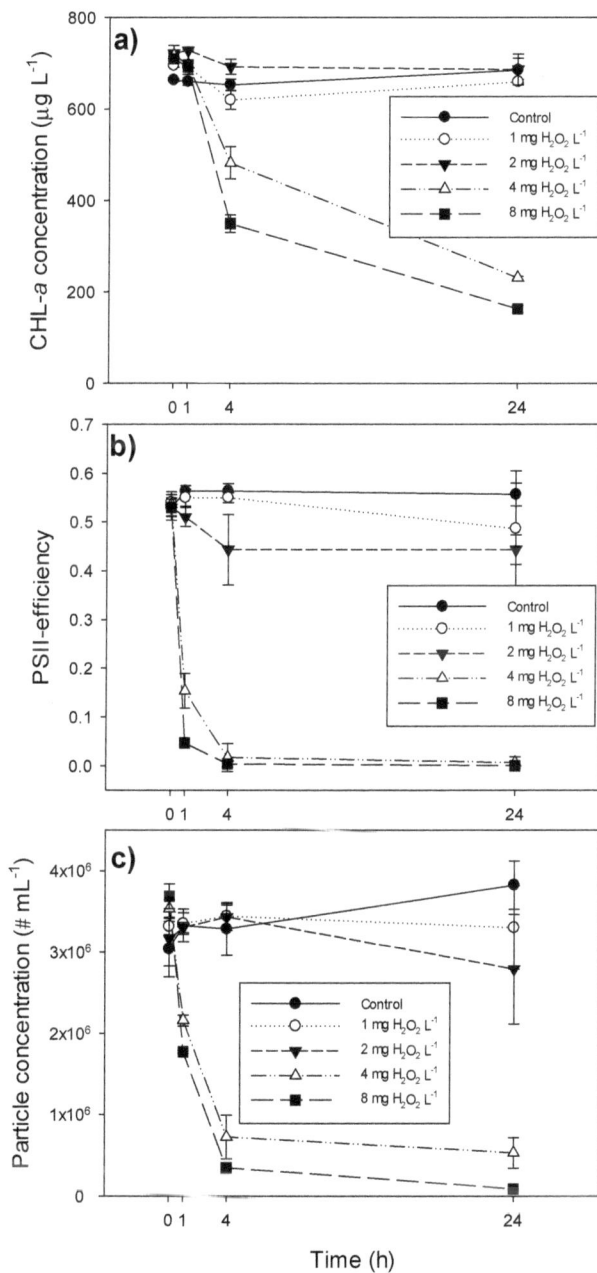

Figure 3. Total particulate and dissolved microcystin (MC) concentrations (µg L^{-1}) in *Microcystis aeruginosa* PCC 7820 at the start of the experiment (open bars) and after 24 h of exposure to different concentrations of hydrogen-peroxide (H$_2$O$_2$, in mg L^{-1}; hatched bars). Error bars indicate 1 SD ($n = 3$). Similar symbols above the bars (a,α,β) indicate homogeneous groups of total MC concentrations that are not different at the $p = 0.05$ level (Holm–Sidak comparison).

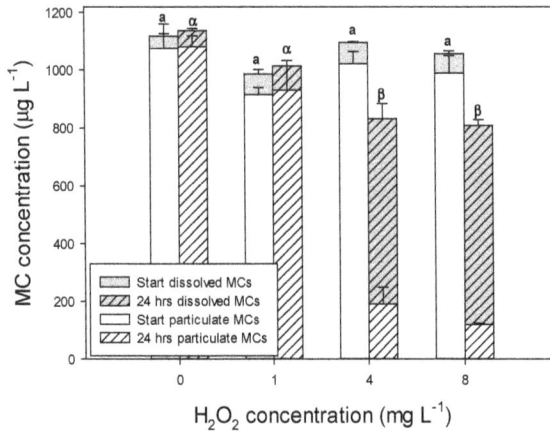

The composition of particulate MCs did not differ much during the experiment and between treatments (Figure 4a,b). MC-LR was the most abundant MC variant, making up on average 81% of the particulate MCs; MC-LF was present at 9%, MC-LW at 5% and dm-7-MC-LR at 3%, and MC-LY was the least abundant variant with 2% abundance (Figure 4a,b). The composition of the dissolved MCs at the start of the experiment deviated from the composition of particulate MCs (Figure 4a,c). This effect was strongest for the hydrophobic variant, MC-LW, which formed more than 5% of the particulate MCs, but only made up 0.6% of the dissolved MC pool at the start of the experiment (two-way ANOVA; $F_{1,23} = 969.3$; $p < 0.001$). Furthermore, the contribution of MC-LF, another hydrophobic variant, to the overall dissolved MC pool was reduced by half (to 4%) compared to the particulate pool (Figure 4a,c). Here, two-way ANOVA not only indicated a significant difference between the contribution of dissolved MC-LF and particulate MC-LF to the overall MC pool ($F_{1,23} = 969.3$; $p < 0.001$), but also revealed that in the dissolved pool, differences already appeared at the start of the experiment ($F_{3,23} = 11.0$; $p < 0.001$) with dissolved MC-LF contributions of 3% in the control and the 1-mg L^{-1} treatment and 5% in the 4- and 8-mg L^{-1} treatments (Figure 4c). At the end of the experiment, the proportion of dissolved MC-LW increased, particularly in the 4- and 8-mg L^{-1} H$_2$O$_2$ treatments. Furthermore, the proportion of dissolved MC-LF increased slightly in these treatments, at the expense of the proportion of the more hydrophilic MC-LR (Figure 4d). As a consequence, the dissolved MC profiles in the highest H$_2$O$_2$ treatments resembled the particulate MC profiles more than did the dissolved MC profiles of the control and the 1-mg L^{-1} treatment (Figure 4). Because MC-LW and MC-LF likely contribute more to the total MC toxicity than MC-LR, the dissolved MC pool of lysed cells was relatively more toxic than the dissolved pool of healthy cells.

Figure 4. Proportions of five microcystin (MC) variants in the particulate (**a,b**); and dissolved MC pools (**c,d**) of *Microcystis aeruginosa* PCC 7820 at the start of the experiment (start) and after 24 h of exposure to different concentrations of hydrogen-peroxide (H$_2$O$_2$, in mg L^{-1}; end).

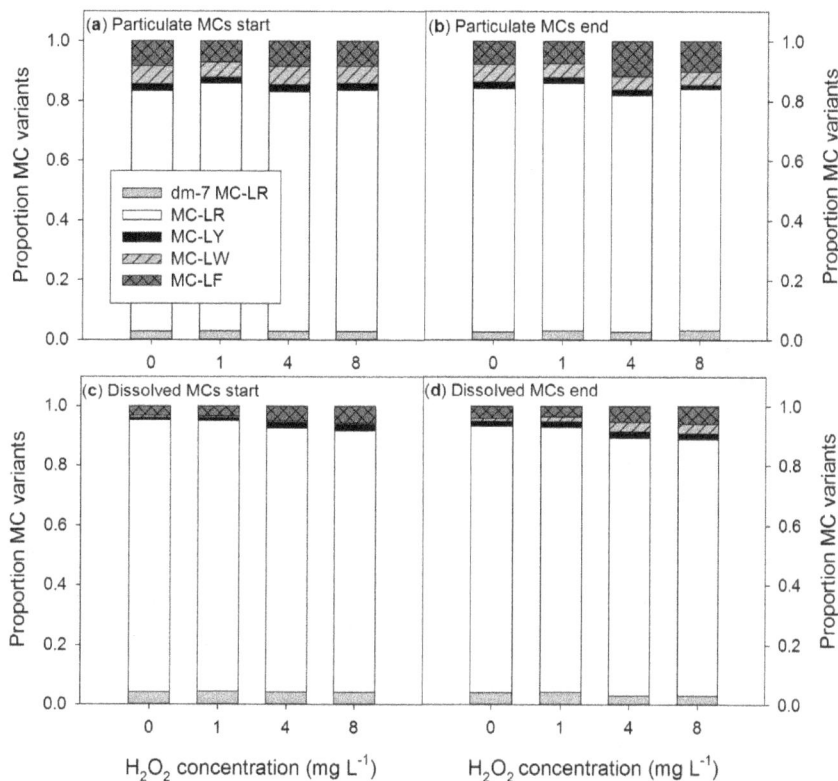

2.2. Ultrasound

Despite the application of ultrasound, chlorophyll-*a* concentrations in both ultrasound treatments increased as strongly as the control treatment during the five-day course of the experiment (Figure 5; Table 2). The particle concentration, however, increased more in the control (2.3-times) than in the two ultrasound treatments (1.2-times; Figure 5c; Table 2). The Φ_{PSII} was slightly, but significantly, reduced by the ultrasound treatments, from an average of 0.56 (SD 0.01) in the controls during the five-day exposure period, to 0.53 (SD 0.01) in the AL-05 treatments and 0.52 (SD 0.02) in the AL-10 treatments (Figure 5b; Table 2). This effect was significant, because the within group variability was very low (Figure 5b).

Figure 5. (**a**) Chlorophyll-*a* concentrations (CHL-*a*, µg L⁻¹); (**b**) photosystem II efficiency (PSII); and (**c**) particle concentration (No. mL⁻¹) in *Microcystis aeruginosa* PCC 7820 exposed to different ultrasound transducers (Flexidal AL-05 and AL-10) and in non-exposed control populations (control). Error bars indicate 1 SD ($n = 3$).

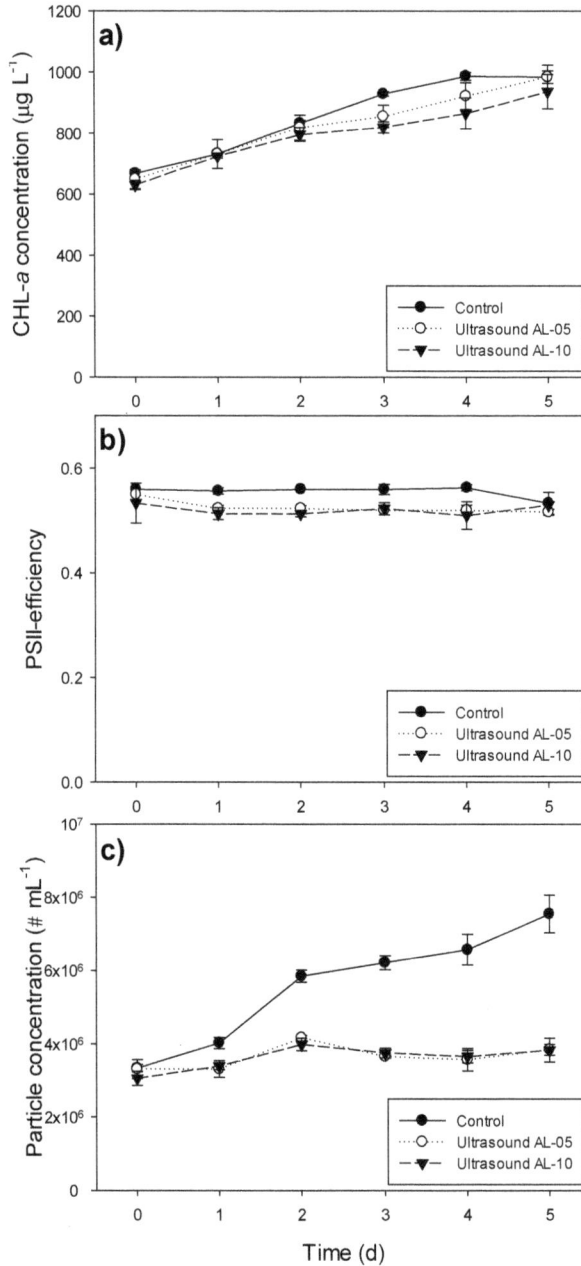

Table 2. Statistical information on the ultrasound experiment for three different endpoints: chlorophyll-*a* concentration (Chl-*a*), photosystem II efficiency (Φ_{PSII}) and particle concentration (# mL^{-1}) of *Microcystis aeruginosa* PCC 7820. Homogeneous subgroups were defined by a Tukey *post hoc* comparison at $p < 0.05$.

Treatments	Chl-*a*(μg L^{-1})		Φ_{PSII} (-)		Particles (# mL^{-1})	
	Tukey post hoc comparison					
Control	a		a		a	
AL-05	a		b		b	
AL-10	a		b		b	
repeated measures ANOVA	F	p	F	p	F	p
treatment effect ($F_{2,6}$)	3.84	0.084	64.5	<0.001	200.9	<0.001
time effect ($F_{5,30}$)	423.3	<0.001	2.35	0.065	103.8	<0.001
time × treatment interaction ($F_{10,30}$)	5.61	<0.001	1.56	0.169	42.9	<0.001

The effects of both transducers were similar; hence, only samples from the AL-05 treatments were analyzed for MCs. Total MCs significantly increased in the controls, from 1054 (SD 71) μg MC L^{-1} at the start to 1558 (SD 110) μg MC L^{-1} at the end of the experiment (*t*-test; $t = 6.67$; $p = 0.003$; Figure 6). The ultrasound treatment caused no decline in total MCs as total concentrations at the start (1023 SD 11 μg MC L^{-1}) and after five days (1079 SD 34 μg MC L^{-1}) were similar ($t = 2.68$; $p = 0.055$). The proportion of dissolved MCs after five days was significantly higher in the ultrasound treatments (19%) than in the controls (5%, $t = 6.17$; $p = 0.004$, Figure 6).

Figure 6. Particulate and dissolved microcystin (MC) concentrations (μg L^{-1}) in non-exposed (open bars) and ultrasound (Flexidal AL-05)-exposed *Microcystis aeruginosa* PCC 7820 (hatched bars). Error bars indicate 1 SD ($n = 3$).

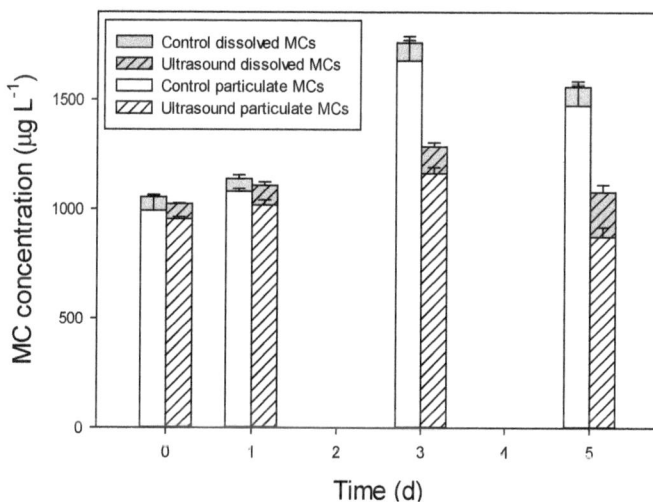

The composition of particulate MCs was similar during the course of the experiment in both controls and ultrasound treatments (Figure 7a,b) and resembled the particulate MC composition of the H_2O_2 experiment. Furthermore, the composition of dissolved MCs was similar in controls and the ultrasound treatments and remained stable during the experiment (Figure 7c,d). However, the composition of the dissolved MCs deviated slightly from the composition of particulate MCs (Figure 7). Two-way repeated-measures ANOVA revealed a significantly higher contribution of dm-7-MC-LR in the dissolved MCs (4%) than in the particulate MC pool (3%). Likewise, MC-LR was significantly more abundant in the dissolved pool (85%) than in the particulate MC pool (81%; $F_{1,8} = 124.9$; $p < 0.001$). MC-LY was present in similar proportions in both the dissolved and particulate MCs (2%; $F_{1,8} = 4.0$; $p = 0.080$), while MC-LW ($F_{1,8} = 2311$; $p < 0.001$) and MC-LF ($F_{1,8} = 65.6$; $p < 0.001$) were significantly less abundant in the dissolved MC pool (4% MC-LW and 5% MC-LF) than in the particulate MC pool, where they made up 6% (MC-LW) and 8% (MC-LF).

Figure 7. Course of the proportions of five microcystin (MC) variants in the particulate (**a,b**) and dissolved MC pools (**c,d**) of non-exposed *Microcystis aeruginosa* PCC 7820 populations (control) and populations exposed to ultrasound from Flexidal AL-05 transducers (ultrasound).

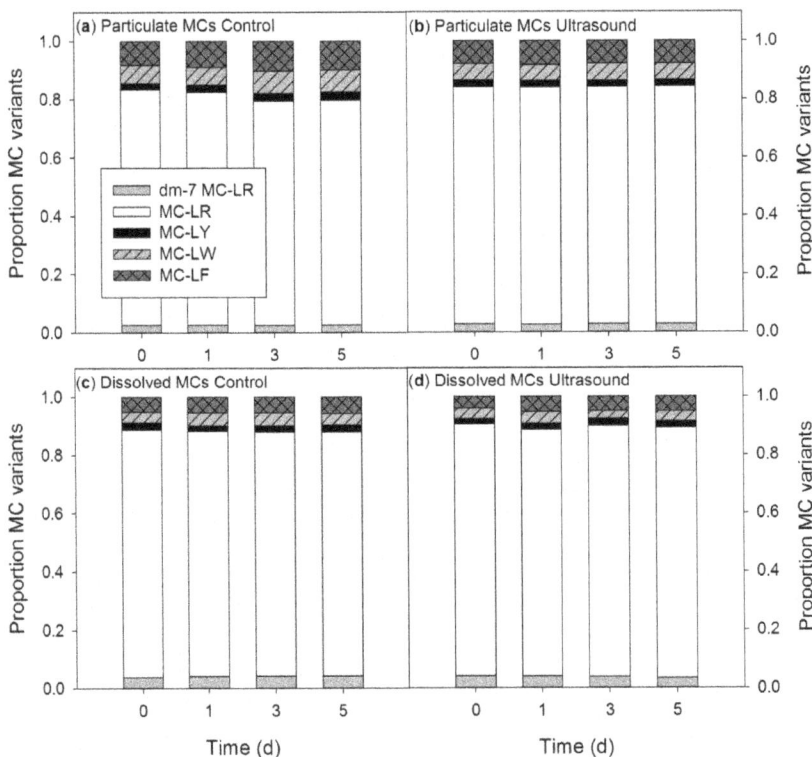

3. Discussion

3.1. Hydrogen Peroxide

H_2O_2 effectively reduced *M. aeruginosa* biomass when dosed at 4 or 8 mg L^{-1}, but not at 1 and 2 mg L^{-1}. Hence, the EC_{50}, depending on the endpoint, was between 2.5 and 3.8 mg H_2O_2 L^{-1} under our experimental conditions, which is a little higher than an EC_{50} of 0.3–0.5 mg L^{-1} reported for another strain of *M. aeruginosa* [31,32] and the dose of 2 mg H_2O_2 L^{-1} that was applied to a *Planktothrix agardhii*-dominated lake in The Netherlands, and removed 99% of the cyanobacteria [15]. However, in other field trials, 30%–40% of the cyanobacteria remained after an H_2O_2 treatment, despite the fact that dosages of 40 to 95 mg H_2O_2 L^{-1} were used [29,33]. For field collected colonial *M. aeruginosa*, a relatively high EC_{50} of about 30 mg H_2O_2 L^{-1} was found [34]. This high EC_{50} could have resulted from the use of extremely high cyanobacteria concentrations [34]. Alternatively, the mucilaginous colonies, often with quite a few bacteria attached [35], might provide *M. aeruginosa* cells protection against H_2O_2. Our strain of *M. aeruginosa* was uni- and bi-cellular; a normal growth form under laboratory conditions, but contrasting to its typical colonial appearance in the field [36]. Where an H_2O_2 concentration of 4 mg L^{-1} was sufficient to strongly reduce our strain, when blooms of colonial *Microcystis* are the target, higher concentrations may be needed. This might be a drawback in nature protection sites, as those H_2O_2 concentrations also may have an effect on non-target organisms, such as zooplankton [15,29,37].

The *M. aeruginosa* biomass reduction was probably a result of the loss of membrane integrity, followed by cell lysis [38,39]. Consequently, cell contents and cyanotoxins could be released upon treatment with H_2O_2. For instance, leakage of phycobiliproteins into the water after H_2O_2 exposure is reflected in Wang *et al.* [34], where a blue color at higher H_2O_2 dose(s) is clearly visible in their Figure 3. In our experiment, relatively high chlorophyll-*a* concentrations were present in the 8-mg L^{-1} H_2O_2 treatment after 24 h, while the particle concentration at that time had dropped to only 2.4% of the number of particles at the start of the experiment. Furthermore, after 24 h, dissolved MC concentrations in the 1-, 4- and 8-mg L^{-1} treatments had increased respectively 1.4-, 8.9- and 12-times compared to the control, which confirms compromised membrane integrity and leakage of cell contents. Similarly, lysis of cyanobacterial cells led to the appearance of dissolved MCs in the first few days after an H_2O_2 application in a waste water stabilization pond [29]. Some evidence for the release of MCs is also found in the field application of Matthijs *et al.* [15], where the MC decline was similar to the cyanobacterial biomass decline, but with a two-day delay. In contrast, a laboratory study using relatively high H_2O_2 concentrations (10.2–102 mg L^{-1}) found no increase in dissolved MCs after the H_2O_2 treatments, which was attributed to the degradation of MCs [30]. In our experiment, we found indications that part of the MCs was also lost, as after 24 h, the sum of dissolved and particulate MCs in the 4- and 8-mg L^{-1} treatments were 23% lower than at the start of the experiment. As proposed by Song *et al.* [22], the degradation pathway is probably by hydroxyl radical attack on the Adda benzene ring, causing ring hydroxylation and subsequent oxidative cleavage of the Adda structure.

At the start, and after 24 h in the control and 1-mg L^{-1} treatments, the dissolved MCs contributed 6%–6.5% to the overall MC pool. This is in agreement with literature reports that most of the total detectable toxin pool is intracellular in healthy growing cells [40–42]. The intracellular MC composition in our study is in line with findings of others; MC-LR is the most abundant MC variant in *M. aeruginosa* PCC 7820, but its relative contribution might vary (Table 3). Variation in MC variant expression might be caused by different growth conditions (e.g., [43]). However, the difference between the intracellular and extracellular MC profiles in healthy cells observed in both of our experiments (Figures 4 and 7) might point towards differences in terms of membrane crossing [44] or to different adsorption characteristics. We observed lower proportions of the more hydrophobic variants, MC-LW and MC-LF, in the dissolved fraction than in the particulate fraction of healthy cells. This difference can probably be attributed to a higher adsorption of the more hydrophilic variants on living cells. Although MCs do not easily adsorb on sediments or on suspended particulate matter [41], the more hydrophobic variants, MC-LW and MC-LF, were more associated with lipids in monolayer experiments than was the more hydrophilic MC-LR [45]. Adsorption of more hydrophobic MCs on remaining cells seems a more likely explanation than a passive diffusion mechanism [44], as that would result in a relatively higher proportion of hydrophobic MCs, as these diffuse more easily across the membrane. When most cells were lysed in the 4- and 8-mg H_2O_2 L^{-1} treatments, the proportions of the dissolved hydrophobic MCs increased (Figure 4d).

Table 3. The relative proportion (%) of different intracellular microcystin (MC) variants in *Microcystis aeruginosa* PCC 7820.

MC-variant	Our study	Ríos *et al.* [46]	Robillot *et al.* [44]
MC-LR	81.2	79.5	51.0
MC-LY	2.2	1.6	8.6
MC-LF	8.0	0.6	19.4
MC-LW	5.8	1.0	21.0
others	2.8	17.3	-

In the high H_2O_2 doses, total MC concentrations were about 23% reduced, but an H_2O_2 dose needed to oxidize all released MCs to levels below the WHO guideline of 1 μg L^{-1} would imply negative effects on non-target organisms, such as large bodied cladocerans. For example, LC_{50} values of 5–6 mg H_2O_2 L^{-1} for *Daphnia* and 2 mg L^{-1} for *Moina* have been reported [37]. Increased mortality for *Daphnia* was observed at H_2O_2 concentrations exceeding 3 mg L^{-1}; for *Moina*, this occurred already at concentrations exceeding 1 mg H_2O_2 L^{-1} [29,37], while in enclosures, cladocerans were affected by H_2O_2 concentrations exceeding 2.5 mg L^{-1} [15]. In our study, more than 75% of the MCs remained present, even when a H_2O_2 dose of 8 mg L^{-1} was applied. This implies that algicides should be avoided as much as possible, because a sudden increase in dissolved MC concentrations might present a health hazard to livestock and humans using the water for consumption [11] and could potentially affect aquatic organisms that would not readily ingest cyanobacteria (e.g., [47]).

3.2. Ultrasound

Ultrasound can have detrimental effects on cyanobacteria; it can cause gas vesicle collapse, cell wall disruption and disturbance of photosynthetic activity [17,18]. Several commercial suppliers state that their "environmental-friendly" ultrasound transducers will kill cyanobacteria rapidly [48]. However, the low power used by these commercially available transducers, in contrast to the high power cavitation-producing transducers in some laboratory settings, puts strong constraints on their efficacy [19]. Indeed, our study confirmed the findings of Lürling and Tolman [19,49] that commercial ultrasound transducers do not remove cyanobacteria. In our experiment with *M. aeruginosa*, ultrasound somewhat impaired cyanobacterial growth, but the transducer was only placed in a small volume (800 mL). When applied in larger volumes, significantly less power will be transmitted, and consequently, the impact on cyanobacteria will be far lower when such transducers are employed in ponds and lakes [18], as recommended by the manufacturer [11]. Likewise, the marginal damage to the cyanobacterial cells, reflected by the small increase in dissolved MCs, will be less in larger volumes. In addition, possible direct effects of ultrasound on MC degradation will be less in large volumes, as MC degradation is proportional to the power and duration of ultrasound [21]. Intensities used to degrade MCs are much higher than the ones employed in our study. For instance, Song *et al.* [22] used 22.7 W mL^{-1} to degrade MCs, while the intensity used in our experiment was 7.9×10^{-4} W mL^{-1}. High intensity ultrasound devices cause acoustic cavitation: a process in which compression and rarefaction create gas bubbles that may collapse [50]. On collapse of the bubbles, formation of radicals and hydrogen peroxide production may lead to degradation of MCs [22]. However, the power of the transducers applied in our study is probably insufficient to cause cavitation [19], and hence, strong ultrasound induced degradation of MCs was not observed; ultrasound caused no decline in total MCs, as total concentrations at the start of the experiment and after five days were similar.

Using high power devices to clear surface waters from cyanobacteria is not recommended, because the energy needed to treat lakes and ponds is very high, and non-target organisms will be damaged. For instance, ultrasound is used to disinfect ballast water or raw water for drinking water preparation, where it may inactivate motile plankton [51] or kill zooplankton, especially larger cladocerans [52]. Ultrasound caused cell damage in the macrophyte, *Elodea*, and in fruit flies [53]. Moreover, the commercial ultrasound transducers, as the ones we have used in our study, resulted in rapid death of the zooplankton grazer, *Daphnia* [49]. Therefore, ultrasound should not be considered "environmental friendly" [18] or a "green solution" [17] to control cyanobacteria blooms.

Some studies have reported ultrasound-induced cyanobacterial filament shortening by breakage and cell lysis at the break points [19,54]. This could lead to the release of toxins in the water. Our strain of *M. aeruginosa* was completely uni- and bi-cellular. However, in the field, *M. aeruginosa* grows mostly as large colonies, embedded in mucous. There is a possibility that application of commercial ultrasound devices could break natural colonies into smaller fragments, but no major impact, such as on toxin release, is expected.

The composition of the MC pools was not influenced by the ultrasound and the MC profiles remained similar during the experiment. The only difference was between the composition of the dissolved MC pool and the particulate MC pool that showed less hydrophobic MC-LW and MC-LF in the dissolved pool than in the particulate one, as had also been observed in the H_2O_2 experiment.

3.3. Overall

In this study, we simulated heavy bloom concentrations of *M. aeruginosa* ($\approx$700 µg chlorophyll-*a* L^{-1}) and treated them with H_2O_2 and ultrasound from commercial transducers. Where doses of 4 to 8 mg H_2O_2 L^{-1} were sufficient to kill *M. aeruginosa*, MC concentrations in the water remained high, and the majority of the particulate MCs became dissolved. The high cyanobacteria concentrations we used are not uncommon in urban ponds in The Netherlands [55], or elsewhere (e.g., [56–59]), and even higher concentrations are common in surface scums in ponds and lakes. Treating such blooms (and scums) with H_2O_2 may only be feasible if *P. agardhii* is the dominant species [60], but with *M. aeruginosa* dominating, it is not recommended, as the relatively high H_2O_2 concentrations needed for an effective treatment might harm non-target organisms and might cause a release of cell contents, including toxins and nutrients, which may fuel a subsequent bloom. Moreover, as previously reported [29,34], H_2O_2 treatment may result in surface accumulation of affected cyanobacterial cells. Such accumulation of decaying material will in itself cause nuisance and reduce water quality.

Ultrasound from the commercial available transducers was not effective at clearing a small volume of 800 mL of a cyanobacterial suspension. Hence, these devices will not be effective in larger volumes, which is in line with additional laboratory experiments [19], a tank experiment [49] and a few lake-scale experiments where ultrasound appeared ineffective at mitigating cyanobacteria nuisance [61,62]. Consequently, the application of ultrasound is not a suitable way to reduce cyanobacterial biomass.

Water authorities should perform a system analysis to determine the flow of water and sources of nutrients in systems suffering from blooms, after which the most promising set of mitigating measures can be selected. Here, source-oriented measures principally targeting the phosphorus inflow and internal loading remain essential for reducing eutrophication. However, in situations where source-oriented measures are not easily achievable, cost-effective end-of-pipe solutions might be an alternative, but these should have been proven to be effective *in situ*. For instance, coagulants in combination with a ballast can effectively precipitate positively buoyant cyanobacteria out of the water column as intact cells [63,64] without releasing cell contents and, thereby, nutrients and toxins [65,66].

4. Experimental Section

4.1. Organisms

The cyanobacterium, *Microcystis aeruginosa* (Kützing) Kützing strain PCC 7820, was obtained from the Pasteur Culture Collection (Paris, France). The culture was maintained in 250-mL Erlenmeyer flasks that contained 100 mL sterile modified WC (Woods Hole modified CHU10) medium [67] and were closed with a cellulose stopper. The flasks were placed at 25 °C in 40 µmol quanta m^{-2} s^{-1} provided in a 14:10 h light-dark cycle. Stock cultures were transferred to fresh medium every two to three weeks. These stocks were used to inoculate twenty 2-L Erlenmeyer flasks with 1.7 L sterile WC-medium to produce sufficient biomass for the experiments. The 2-L flasks were placed in a conditioned climate room at 23 °C in a 12:12 h light dark cycle at a light intensity of 100 μmol quanta m^{-2} s^{-1}. The flasks were shaken manually once a day. Regularly, a 2-mL subsample was taken for chlorophyll-*a* determination by a PHYTO-PAM phytoplankton analyzer (Heinz Walz GmbH, Effeltrich, Germany). Experiments were started with the cultured material once the chlorophyll-*a* concentration was 600–800 μg L^{-1} (equivalent to cell concentrations of on average 3.8 × 10^6 cells mL^{-1} SD 0.3 × 10^6 cells mL^{-1}). Hereto, aliquots of 800 mL cultured *M. aeruginosa* were transferred from the 2-L flasks to experimental glass jars (1 L volume). The remaining cultures in the 2-L Erlenmeyer's were replenished with fresh, sterile WC-medium and placed back for further culturing. The experiments were conducted at 23 °C in 100 μmol quanta m^{-2} s^{-1} light intensity with 12:12 h light-dark cycle in a conditioned climate room.

4.2. Hydrogen Peroxide

At the start of the experiment, suspensions of *M. aeruginosa* in WC-medium were evenly distributed over 15 replicate 1-L jars such that each contained 800 mL suspension with a chlorophyll-*a* concentration of 702 (SD 23) μg L^{-1}. Hydrogen peroxide (H$_2$O$_2$ 30%, 1.07209.0500, Merck KGaA, Darmstadt, Germany) was added in triplicate to the jars in concentrations of 0, 1, 2, 4 and 8 mg L^{-1}. H$_2$O$_2$ was gently added under continuous stirring. The jars were sealed with Parafilm with a small opening for ventilation and sampling. At 0, 1, 4 and 24 h, MC samples (8 mL, stored in glass bottles) and samples for chlorophyll-*a* and cell density measurements (10 mL) were taken from the middle of the jar after mixing with a glass stick. Cyanobacterial chlorophyll-*a* concentrations and photosystem II efficiency were measured directly after sampling by a PHYTO-PAM phytoplankton analyzer; particle concentrations were measured by an electronic particle counter (CASY cell counter, Schärfe System GmBh, Reutlingen, Germany) with a range from 1 to 120 μm equivalent spherical diameter. MCs were determined as outlined below (Section 4.4).

4.3. Ultrasound

Seven ultrasound devices (three of type AL-05 and four of type AL-10, Flexidal BVBA, Aalter, Belgium) were purchased commercially. All ultrasound transducers produced block waves at frequencies of ~20 kHz, ~28 kHz and ~44 kHz. The acoustic power of the transducers was 0.63 W (SD 0.05, *n* = 3) for AL-05 transducers [49] and 0.68 W (SD 0.23, *n* = 4) for the AL-10 transducers [19].

At the start of the experiment, suspensions of *M. aeruginosa* in WC-medium were evenly distributed over 9 replicate 1-L jars, such that each contained an 800-mL suspension with a chlorophyll-*a* concentration of 649 (SD 24) μg L^{-1}. In three jars, AL-05 transducers were placed 2 cm below the water surface; in three other jars, AL-10 transducers were placed at a similar depth; while three jars remained untreated (controls). The ultrasound transducers operated incessantly during the experiment for 5 days. Sub-samples of 10 mL for chlorophyll-*a*, photosystem II efficiency and cell density analysis (electronic particle counter) were taken daily during the experiment (Days 0 to 5) after mixing with a glass stick. MC samples (8 mL stored in glass bottles) were taken from the water column after mixing at 0, 1, 3 and 5 days. MCs were determined as outlined below (Section 4.4).

4.4. MC Analysis

The 8-mL MC samples were filtered through glass-fiber filters (Whatman GF/C, Whatman International Ltd., Maidstone, UK). Of each sample, the filtrate was collected in clean 8-mL glass tubes, while the filters were rolled gently and placed in another 8-mL glass tube. Both the filtrate and the filter samples were dried in a Speedvac (Thermo Scientific Savant SPD121P, Waltham, MA, USA), after which the filters were extracted three times at 60 °C in 2.5 mL 75% methanol-25% Millipore water (*v/v*). The extracts were dried in the Speedvac and subsequently reconstituted in 800 μL methanol, as were the dried filtrates. The reconstituted samples were transferred to 2-mL Eppendorf vials with a cellulose-acetate filter (0.2 μm, Grace Davison Discovery Sciences, Deerfield, IL, USA) and centrifuged for 5 min at $16,000 \times g$ (VWR Galaxy 16DH, VWR International, Buffalo Grove, IL, USA). Filtrates were transferred to amber glass vials for LC-MS/MS analysis.

Samples were analyzed for eight MC variants (dm-7-MC-RR, MC-RR, MC-YR, dm-7-MC-LR, MC-LR, MC-LY, MC-LW and MC-LF) and nodularin (NOD) by LC-MS/MS, as described in [68]. LC-MS/MS analysis was performed on an Agilent 1200 LC and an Agilent 6410A QQQ. The compounds were separated on an Agilent Eclipse XDB-C18 4.6×150 mm, 5-μm column by Millipore water with 0.1% formic acid (*v/v*, Eluent A) and acetonitrile with 0.1% formic acid (*v/v*, Eluent B). The elution program was 0–2 min 30% B, 6–12 min 90% B, with a linear increase of B between 2 and 6 min and a 5-min post run at 30% B. The injection volume was 10 μL; flow was 0.5 mL/min; column temperature was 40 °C. The LC-MS/MS was operated in positive mode with an electrospray ionization source, and nitrogen was used as the drying and collision gas. For each compound, two transitions were monitored in Multiple Reaction Monitoring (MRM) mode. The first quadrupole was operated in unit mode; the second quadrupole was operated in the widest mode. The dwell time was 50 ms. MS/MS settings for each compound were as in Faassen and Lurling [68]. Calibration standards were obtained from DHI LAB Products (Hørsholm, Denmark) and prepared in methanol. Samples were quantified against a calibration curve, and filter extracts were subsequently corrected for recovery. Each sample was injected once. Information on recovery, repeatability, limit of detection and limit of quantification of the analysis is given in [68].

4.5. Statistical Analysis

The chlorophyll-*a* concentrations, photosystem II efficiencies and particle concentrations were statistically evaluated by repeated measure ANOVAs in the tool pack SPSS (version 19.0, IBM statistics, Armonk, NY, USA). Homogeneous subgroups were defined by a Tukey *post hoc* comparison at $p < 0.05$. The data were checked for normality using quantile-quantile (Q-Q) plots. In case Mauchly's test indicated that the assumption of sphericity had been violated, the degrees of freedom were corrected using Greenhouse-Geisser estimates of sphericity if epsilon <0.75 or applying the Huynh-Feldt correction if epsilon >0.75.

Total MC concentrations were evaluated statistically running one-way ANOVAs in the peroxide experiment and by t-ests in the ultrasound experiment using the toolpack, SigmaPlot version 12.3 (Systat Software, Inc., San Jose, CA, USA). The composition of both the dissolved and the particulate MC pools at the start and at the end of the peroxide experiment was evaluated by two-way ANOVAs in SigmaPlot with dissolved/particulate and peroxide concentration as fixed factors. Data were checked for normality and heteroscedasticity by the normality test (Shapiro–Wilk) and the equal variance test in SigmaPlot prior to executing ANOVA. The ANOVAs were followed by pairwise multiple comparison procedures (Holm–Sidak method) to distinguish means that were significantly different ($p < 0.05$). In the ultrasound experiment, the relative contribution of each MC variant in the dissolved and particulate MC pools in controls and ultrasound exposures was evaluated over time running two-way repeated measures ANOVAs in SPSS (version 19.0, IBM statistics, Armonk, NY, USA).

5. Conclusions

Hydrogen peroxide at concentrations of 4 and 8 mg L^{-1} effectively killed *M. aeruginosa*, but caused substantial release of MCs into the water. About 23% of the total MCs was removed by these hydrogen peroxide doses. To eliminate most MCs from the water, much higher H_2O_2 concentrations will be needed, which might strongly impair non-targeted organisms, such as the grazer, *Daphnia magna*.

The application of ultrasound had no water clearing effect; it caused a minimal growth inhibition and some release of MCs into the water. Ultrasound from commercial transducers is ineffective at controlling cyanobacteria in surface waters.

The MC composition of the particulate and the dissolved fraction differed. The more hydrophobic variants, MC-LW and MC-LF, were underrepresented in the dissolved fraction of healthy cells. When cells were lysed, more hydrophobic variants appeared in the dissolved pool, but their abundance was still lower than in the particulate pool.

Acknowledgments

We thank Wendy Beekman for assistance during the experiment. E.J.F. was supported by Grant 817.02.019 from the Netherlands Organization for Scientific Research.

Author Contributions

M.L. designed the experiment, analyzed the data and wrote the manuscript. D.M. performed the experiment. E.J.F. analyzed the data and wrote the manuscript.

Conflicts of Interest

The authors declare no conflict of interest.

292

References

1. Smith, V.H.; Tilman, G.D.; Nekola, J.C. Eutrophication: Impacts of excess nutrient inputs on freshwater, marine, and terrestrial ecosystems. *Environ. Pollut.* **1999**, *100*, 179–196.
2. Paerl, H. Nutrient and other environmental controls of harmful cyanobacterial blooms along the freshwater–marine continuum. In *Cyanobacterial Harmful Algal Blooms: State of the Science and Research Needs*; Springer: New York, NY, USA, 2008; Volume 619, pp. 217–237.
3. Paerl, H.W.; Huisman, J. Blooms like it hot. *Science* **2008**, *320*, 57–58.
4. Merel, S.; Walker, D.; Chicana, R.; Snyder, S.; Baurès, E.; Thomas, O. State of knowledge and concerns on cyanobacterial blooms and cyanotoxins. *Environ. Int.* **2013**, *59*, 303–327.
5. Steffensen, D.A. Economic cost of cyanobacterial blooms. In *Cyanobacterial Harmful Algal Blooms: State of the Science and Research Needs*; Springer: New York, NY, USA, 2008; Volume 619, pp. 855–865.
6. Mackay, E.B.; Maberly, S.C.; Pan, G.; Reitzel, K.; Bruere, A.; Corker, N.; Douglas, G.; Egemose, S.; Hamilton, D.; Hatton-Ellis, T.; *et al.* Geoengineering in lakes: Welcome attraction or fatal distraction? *Inland Waters* **2014**, *4*, 349–356.
7. Jančula, D.; Maršálek, B. Critical review of actually available chemical compounds for prevention and management of cyanobacterial blooms. *Chemosphere* **2011**, *85*, 1415–1422.
8. Codd, G.A. Cyanobacterial toxins, the perception of water quality, and the prioritisation of eutrophication control. *Ecol. Eng.* **2000**, *16*, 51–60.
9. Codd, G.A.; Morrison, L.F.; Metcalf, J.S. Cyanobacterial toxins: Risk management for health protection. *Toxicol. Appl. Pharmacol.* **2005**, *203*, 264–272.
10. Funari, E.; Testai, E. Human health risk assessment related to cyanotoxins exposure. *Crit. Rev. Toxicol.* **2008**, *38*, 97–125.
11. Lam, A.K.Y.; Prepas, E.E.; Spink, D.; Hrudey, S.E. Chemical control of hepatotoxic phytoplankton blooms: Implications for human health. *Water Res.* **1995**, *29*, 1845–1854.
12. Steffensen, D.; Burch, M.; Nicholson, B.; Drikas, B. Management of toxic blue-green algae (cyanobacteria) in Australia. *Environ. Toxicol.* **1999**, *14*, 183–195.
13. Kenefick, S.L.; Hrudey, S.E.; Peterson, H.G.; Prepas, E.E. Toxin release from *Microcystis aeruginosa* after chemical treatment. *Water Sci. Technol.* **1993**, *27*, 433–440.
14. Drábková, M.; Maršálek, B.; Admiraal, W. Photodynamic therapy against cyanobacteria. *Environ. Toxicol.* **2007**, *22*, 112–115.
15. Matthijs, H.C.P.; Visser, P.M.; Reeze, B.; Meeuse, J.; Slot, P.C.; Wijn, G.; Talens, R.; Huisman, J. Selective suppression of harmful cyanobacteria in an entire lake with hydrogen peroxide. *Water Res.* **2012**, *46*, 1460–1472.
16. Russell, A.D. Similarities and differences in the responses of microorganisms to biocides. *J. Antimicrob. Chemother.* **2003**, *52*, 750–763.
17. Wu, X.; Joyce, E.M.; Mason, T.J. The effects of ultrasound on cyanobacteria. *Harmful Algae* **2011**, *10*, 738–743.
18. Rajasekhar, P.; Fan, L.; Nguyen, T.; Roddick, F.A. A review of the use of sonication to control cyanobacterial blooms. *Water Res.* **2012**, *46*, 4319–4329.

19. Lürling, M.; Tolman, Y. Beating the blues: Is there any music in fighting cyanobacteria with ultrasound? *Water Res.* **2014**, *66*, 361–373.

20. Rajasekhar, P.; Fan, L.; Nguyen, T.; Roddick, F.A. Impact of sonication at 20 kHz on *Microcystis aeruginosa, Anabaena circinalis* and *Chlorella* sp. *Water Res.* **2012**, *46*, 1473–1481.

21. Ma, B.; Chen, Y.; Hao, H.; Wu, M.; Wang, B.; Lv, H.; Zhang, G. Influence of ultrasonic field on microcystins produced by bloom-forming algae. *Colloids Surf. B* **2005**, *41*, 197–201.

22. Song, W.; De La Cruz, A.; Rein, K.; O'Shea, K. Ultrasonically induced degradation of microcystin-LR and -RR: Identification of products, effect of pH, formation and destruction ofperoxides. *Environ. Sci. Technol.* **2006**, *40*, 3941–3946.

23. Chorus, I.; Bartram, J. *Toxic Cyanobacteria in Water: A Guide to Their Public Health Consequences, Monitoring and Management*; EandFN Spon: London, UK, 1999.

24. De Figueirdo, D.R.; Azeiteiro, U.M.; Esteves, S.M.; Gonçalves, F.J.M.; Pereira, M.J. Microcystin-producing blooms—A serious global public health issue. *Ecotoxicol. Environ. Saf.* **2004**, *59*, 151–163.

25. O'Neil, J.M.; Davis, T.W.; Burford, M.A.; Gobler, C.J. The rise of harmful cyanobacteria blooms: The potential roles of eutrophication and climate change. *Harmful Algae* **2012**, *14*, 313–334.

26. Doekel, S.; Marahiel, M.A. Biosynthesis of natural products on modular peptide synthetases. *Metab. Eng.* **2001**, *3*, 64–77.

27. Dittmann, E.; Fewer, D.P.; Neilan, B.A. Cyanobacterial toxins: Biosynthetic routes and evolutionary roots. *FEMS Microbiol. Rev.* **2013**, *37*, 23–43.

28. Zurawell, R.W.; Chen, H.; Burke, J.M.; Prepas, E.E. Hepatotoxic cyanobacteria: A review of the biological importance of microcystins in freshwater environments. *J. Toxicol. Environ. Health* **2005**, *8*, 1–37.

29. Barrington, D.J.; Reichwaldt, E.S.; Ghadouani, A. The use of hydrogen peroxide to remove cyanobacteria and microcystins from waste stabilization ponds and hypereutrophic systems. *Ecol. Eng.* **2013**, *50*, 86–94.

30. Fan, J.; Peter Hobson, P.; Ho, L.; Daly, R.; Brookes, J. The effects of various control and water treatment processes on the membrane integrity and toxin fate of cyanobacteria. *J. Hazard. Mater.* **2014**, *264*, 313–322.

31. Drábková, M.; Admiraal, W.; Maršálek, B. Combined exposure to hydrogen peroxide and light: Selective effects on cyanobacteria, green algae, and diatoms. *Environ. Sci. Technol.* **2007**, *41*, 309–314.

32. Drábková, M.; Matthijs, H.C.P.; Admiraal, W.; Maršálek, B. Selective effects of H_2O_2 on cyanobacterial photosynthesis. *Photosynthetica* **2007**, *45*, 363–369.

33. Barrington, D.J.; Ghadouani, A.; Ivey, G.H. Cyanobacterial and microcystins dynamics following the application of hydrogen peroxide to waste stabilisation ponds. *Hydrol. Earth Syst. Sci.* **2013**, *17*, 2097–2105.

34. Wang, Z.; Li, D.; Qin, H.; Li, Y. An integrated method for removal of harmful cyanobacterial blooms in eutrophic lakes. *Environ. Pollut.* **2012**, *160*, 34–41.

35. Worm, J.; Søndergaard, M. Dynamics of heterotrophic bacteria attached to *Microcystis* spp. (Cyanobacteria). *Aquat. Microb. Ecol.* **1998**, *14*, 19–28.

36. Geng, L.; Qin, B.; Yang, Z. Unicellular *Microcystis aeruginosa* cannot revert back to colonial form after short-term exposure to natural conditions. *Biochem. Syst. Ecol.* **2013**, *51*, 104–108.

37. Reichwaldt, E.S.; Zheng, L.; Barrington, D.J.; Ghadouani, A. Acute toxicological response of *Daphnia* and *Moina* to hydrogen peroxide. *J. Environ. Eng.* **2012**, *138*, 607–611.

38. Mikula, P.; Zezulka, S.; Jančula, D.; Maršálek, B. Metabolic activity and membrane integrity changes in *Microcystis aeruginosa*—New findings on hydrogen peroxide toxicity in cyanobacteria. *Eur. J. Phycol.* **2012**, *47*, 195–206.

39. Fan, J.; Ho, L.; Hobson, P.; Brookes, J. Evaluating the effectiveness of copper sulphate, chlorine, potassium permanganate, hydrogen peroxide and ozone on cyanobacterial cell integrity. *Water Res.* **2013**, *47*, 5153–5164.

40. Berg, K.; Skulberg, O.M.; Skulberg, R. Effects of decaying toxic blue-green algae on water quality—A laboratory study. *Arch. Hydrobiol.* **1987**, *108*, 549–563.

41. Rivasseu, C.; Martins, S.; Hennion, M.-C. Determination of some physicochemical parameters of microcystins (cyanobacterial toxins) and trace level analysis in environmental samples using liquid chromatography. *J. Chromatogr. A* **1998**, *799*, 155–169.

42. Codd, G.; Bell, S.; Kaya, K.; Ward, C.; Beattie, K.; Metcalf, J. Cyanobacterial toxins, exposure routes and human health. *Eur. J. Phycol.* **1999**, *34*, 405–415.

43. Tonk, L.; Visser, P.M.; Christiansen, G.; Dittmann, E.; Snelder, E.O.F.M.; Wiedner, C.; Mur, L.R.; Huisman, J. The microcystin composition of the cyanobacterium *Planktothrix agardhii* changes toward a more toxic variant with increasing light intensity. *Appl. Environ. Microbiol.* **2005**, *71*, 5177–5181.

44. Robillot, C.; Vinh, J.; Puiseux-Dao, S.; Hennion, M.-C. Hepatotoxin production kinetics of the cyanobacterium *Microcystis aeruginosa* PCC 7820, as determined by HPLC-mass spectrometry and protein phosphatase bioassay. *Environ. Sci. Technol.* **2000**, *34*, 3372–3378.

45. Vesterkvist, P.S.M.; Meriluoto, J.A.O. Interaction between microcystins of different hydrophobicities and lipid monolayers. *Toxicon* **2003**, *41*, 349–355.

46. Ríos, V.; Moreno, I.; Prieto, A.I.; Soria-Díaz, M.E.; Frías, J.E.; Cameán, A.M. Comparison of *Microcystis aeruginosa* (PCC 7820 and PCC 7806) growth and intracellular microcystins contentdetermined by liquid chromatography–mass spectrometry, enzyme-linked immunosorbent assay anti-Adda and phosphatase bioassay. *J. Water Health* **2014**, *12*, 69–80.

47. Pavagadhi, S.; Gong, Z.; Hande, M.P.; Dionysiou, D.D.; de la Cruz, A.A.; Balasubramanian, R. Biochemical response of diverse organs in adult *Danio rerio* (zebrafish) exposed to sub-lethal concentrations of microcystin-LR and microcystin-RR: A balneation study. *Aquat. Toxicol.* **2012**, *109*, 1–10.

48. Flexidal Technics. Avaliable online: http://flexidal.be/nl/produktenvanflexidal_algen.asp?rubriek=algenandfotoid=8 (accessed on 26 September 2014).

49. Lürling, M.; Tolman, Y. Effects of commercially available ultrasound on the zooplankton grazer *Daphnia* and consequent water greening. *Water* **2014**, *6*, 3247–3263.

50. Neppiras, E.A. Acoustic cavitation. *Phys. Rep.* **1980**, *61*, 159–251.

51. Hoyer, O.; Clasen, J. The application of new technologies in the water treatment process of a modern waterworks. *Water Sci. Technol.* **2002**, *2*, 63–69.

52. Holm, E.R.; Stamper, D.M.; Brizzolara, R.A.; Barnes, L.; Deamer, N.; Burkholder, J.M. Sonication of bacteria, phytoplankton and zooplankton: Application to treatment of ballast water. *Mar. Pollut. Bull.* **2008**, *56*, 1201–1208.

53. Miller, D.L. A review of the ultrasonic bioeffects of microsonation, gas-body activation, and related cavitation-like phenomena. *Ultrasound Med. Biol.* **1987**, *13*, 443–470.

54. Purcell, D. Control of Algal Growth in Reservoirs with Ultrasound. Ph.D. Thesis, Cranfield University, Bedfordshire, UK, December 2009.

55. Waajen, G.W.A.M.; Faassen, E.J.; Lürling, M. Eutrophic urban ponds suffer from cyanobacterial blooms: Dutch examples. *Environ. Sci. Pollut. Res.* **2014**, doi:10.1007/s11356-014-2948-y.

56. Borics, G.; Grigorszky, G.; Szabó, S.; Padisák, J. Phytoplankton associations in a small hypertrophic fishpond in East Hungary during a change from bottom-up to top-down control. *Hydrobiologia* **2000**, *424*, 79–90.

57. Yokohama, A.; Park, H.-D. Mechanism and prediction for contamination of freshwater *bivalves* (*unionidae*) with the cyanobacterial toxin microcystin in hypereutrophic Lake Suwa, Japan. *Environ. Toxicol.* **2002**, *17*, 424–433.

58. Hirose, M.; Nishibe, Y.; Ueki, M.; Nakano, S. Seasonal changes in the abundance of autotrophic picoplankton and some environmental factors in hypereutrophic Furuike Pond. *Aquat. Ecol.* **2003**, *37*, 37–43.

59. Fairchild, W.; Anderson, J.M.; Velinsky, D.J. The trophic state 'chain of relationships' in ponds: Does size matter? *Hydrobiologia* **2005**, *539*, 35–46.

60. Bauzá, L.; Aguilera, A.; Echenique, R.; Andrinolo, D.; Giannuzzi, L. Application of hydrogen peroxide to the control of eutrophic lake systems in laboratory assays. *Toxins* **2014**, *6*, 2657–2675.

61. Govaert, E.; Vanderstukken, M.; Muylaert, K. *Evaluatie Van Effecten Van Ultrasone Straling Op Het Ecosysteem*; Katholieke Universiteit Leuven: Kortrijk, Belgium, 2007. (In Dutch)

62. Kardinaal, E.; De Haan, M.; Ruiter, H. Maatregelen ter voorkoming blauwalgen werken onvoldoende. *H₂O* **2008**, *7*, 4–7. (In Dutch)

63. Li, L.; Pan, G. A universal method for flocculating harmful algal blooms in marine and fresh waters using modified sand. *Environ. Sci. Technol.* **2013**, *47*, 4555–4562.

64. Lürling, M.; Van Oosterhout, F. Controlling eutrophication by combined bloom precipitation and sediment phosphorus inactivation. *Water Res.* **2013**, *47*, 6527–6537.

65. Drikas, M.; Chow, C.W.K.; House, J.; Burch, M.D. Using coagulation, and settling to remove toxic cyanobacteria. *J. Am. Water Works Ass.* **2001**, *93*, 100–111.

66. Chow, C.W.K.; Drikas, M.; House, J.; Burch, M.D.; Velzeboer, R.M.A. The impact of conventional water treatment processes on cells of the cyanobacterium *Microcystis aeruginosa. Water Res.* **1999**, *33*, 3253–3262.

67. Lürling, M.; Beekman, W. Palmelloids formation in *Chlamydomonas reinhardtii*: Defence against rotifer predators? *Ann. Limnol.* **2006**, *42*, 65–72.

68. Lürling, M.; Faassen, E.J. Dog poisonings associated with a *Microcystis aeruginosa* bloom in the Netherlands. *Toxins* **2013**, *5*, 556–567.

MDPI AG
Klybeckstrasse 64
4057 Basel, Switzerland
Tel. +41 61 683 77 34
Fax +41 61 302 89 18
http://www.mdpi.com/

Toxins Editorial Office
E-mail: toxins@mdpi.com
http://www.mdpi.com/journal/toxins